Basic Drug Therapy
and Arithmetic Review

GI 9147

edical Books/Bates/Arithmetic Review & Drug Therapy

nes/Optimas

ontmatter msp i

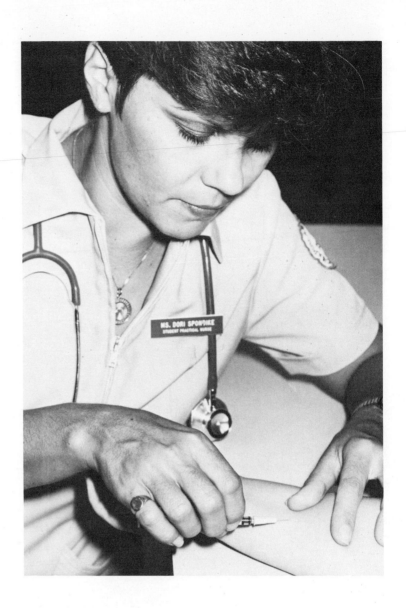

Basic Drug Therapy and Arithmetic Review

Fifth Edition

Formerly Basic Arithmetic Review and Drug Therapy

Grace Fleet Bates, R.N., M.S.

Instructor in Practical Nursing, Department of Practical Nursing, Kapiolani Community College, Honolulu, Hawaii

Grace E. Fitch, R.N., M.S.

Formerly, Associate Director of Nursing in Charge of Practical Nursing Education, Grasslands School of Practical Nursing, Valhalla, New York

Margaret A. Larson, R.N., M.S.

Formerly, Program Specialist, Health Occupations, Palm Beach County Board of Public Instruction, West Palm Beach, Florida

Marion P. Mooney, R.N., M.S.

Formerly, Practical Nursing Instructor, South Technical Education Center, Palm Beach County, Florida

MACMILLAN PUBLISHING COMPANY
New York

COLLIER MACMILLAN CANADA, INC.
Toronto

COLLIER MACMILLAN PUBLISHERS
London

Earlier edition (s), entitled *Arithmetic Review and Drug Therapy for Practical Nurses*, by Grace E. Fitch, © 1961 and copyright © 1966 by Grace E. Fitch; *Arithmetic Review and Drug Therapy for Practical/Vocational Nurses*, by Grace E. Fitch and Margaret A. Larson, copyright © 1973 by Macmillan Publishing Co., Inc.; *Basic Arithmetic Review and Drug Therapy*, by Grace E. Fitch, Margaret A. Larson, and Marion P. Mooney, copyright © 1977 by Macmillan Publishing Co., Inc.

Macmillan Publishing Company
866 Third Avenue, New York, New York 10022

Collier Macmillan Canada, Inc.
Collier Macmillan Publishers • London

Library of Congress Cataloging-in-Publication Data

Basic drug therapy and arithmetic review.

    Rev. ed. of: Basic arithmetic review and drug therapy/Grace E. Fitch, Margaret A. Larson, Marion P. Mooney. 4th ed. c1977.
        Bibliography: p.
        Includes index.
        1. Chemotherapy.   2. Pharmaceutical arithmetic.
3. Nursing.   I. Bates, Grace Fleet.   II. Fitch, Grace E. Basic arithmetic review and drug therapy. [DNLM:
1. Drug Therapy—nurses' instruction.   2. Mathematics—nurses' instruction. WB 330 B311]
RM262.B35   1987   615.5'8   86-23603
ISBN 0-02-306460-9

Printing: 1   2   3   4   5   6   7   8   Year: 7   8   9   0   1   2   3   4   5

Preface

PURPOSE

The purpose of this manual is to assist students to gather, organize, and use information needed to provide drug therapy that is safe and effective for individuals with a wide variety of medical-surgical conditions. Essential principles of pharmacology and pathophysiology are presented and correlated with specific nursing actions.

CONTENT EXPANDED AND REORGANIZED

The completely revised Fifth Edition contains eight sections. Section I contains four new chapters that introduce the student to the nurse's role in drug therapy, to concepts and nursing skills in drug therapy, and to the nursing process as it relates to drug therapy. This section concludes with an Arithmetic Pretest. Students may be referred on the basis of the pretest results to five arithmetic chapters that have been moved to Section VIII. Sections II to IV contain chapters that assist the student to use various measurement systems, calculate dose, and administer drug therapy by various routes. Chapter 12 is devoted to dose calculations for infants and children.

Sections V and VI describe drugs affecting various body systems and drugs used in various medical conditions. These greatly expanded sections contain a revised format that reflects the need for increased knowledge about drugs in order to contribute to the nursing assessment, carry out nursing orders, and select nursing actions that are based on nursing knowledge. A review of body structure and function and a description of the special condition is retained and updated at the beginning of each chapter in these sections. This is followed by an outline of actions and uses, adverse responses, and nursing implications for each major group of drugs affecting that body system or special condition. The nursing implications flow purposefully from what is known about the body and how drugs affect it. New tables provide the student with the nonproprietary name, proprietary name, adult dose range, and additional special notes for each group of drugs.

Section VIII contains the arithmetic review chapters and ends with an Arithmetic Posttest. This section has been moved at the suggestion of practical nurse educators who report that not all students require a review.

LEARNING AIDS

Each chapter in the fifth edition begins with expected behavioral outcomes to assist the student in evaluating progress in developing competencies related to drug therapy. Students are urged to also use the expected behavioral outcomes as study guides.

Each chapter concludes with a case study or other exercises that are tailored to the expected behavioral outcomes. Answers to odd-numbered case studies, exercises, and problems are provided at the end of the book so that students can assess their own progress independently. An answer key, available to instructors, contains a list of recommended audiovisual aids and the answers to even-numbered case studies, exercises, and problems.

Nursing implications have been highlighted throughout the text to reinforce learning and for quick reference. These nursing implications include specific precautions, assesment techniques, patient-teaching guidelines, and charting procedures for each drug classification.

An updated glossary and suggested readings are included in the Appendixes.

NOTE TO THE STUDENT

Basic Drug Therapy and Arithmetic Review is designed to help you learn how to administer safe and effective drug therapy to your patients. Drugs are presented in related groups according to similarities of actions and uses. To learn about a particular drug, it is important to read the information about actions and uses, adverse responses, and nursing implications for the whole group. Then, the specific drug, its nonproprietary name, adult dose range, and any additional information can be located in the Table that accompanies each group of drugs.

Acknowledgments

Now that the Fifth Edition has been completed, it is a sincere pleasure to acknowledge the essential contributions made by a comprehensive support system composed of individuals who provided professional guidance, personal support, and technical expertise. It is from these strong roots that the Fifth Edition grew.

Hundreds of patients, practical/vocational nursing students, and their teachers have played a key role. A characteristic they share is a willingness to learn and teach and a desire for excellence both in the practice of nursing and the way it is taught and learned. Sincere appreciation is extended to all those who participated in this way.

Grateful recognition and thanks is also extended to the following colleagues who reviewed portions of the manuscript and offered helpful suggestions, comments, and criticisms.

Josephine Aoki, R.N., B.S.N.
Instructor in Practical Nursing
Kapiolani Community College
Honolulu, Hawaii

Charles K. Bates, B.S.E.E., M.B.A.
Kailua, Hawaii

Roland Clements, M.S.
Program Director, Radiologic Technology
Kapiolani Community College
Honolulu, Hawaii

Sandra Barnes Fleet, B.S., R.Ph.
Staff Pharmacist
Meriden Wallingford Hospital
Meriden, Connecticut

James A. Jeffryes, M.A.
Assistant Dean of Instruction and
    Instructor in Mathematics
Kapiolani Community College
Honolulu, Hawaii

Barbara Molina Kooker, R.N., M.S., M.P.H.
Instructor, Graduate Program in Nursing
University of Hawaii
Honolulu, Hawaii

Irena M. Levy, M.A., M.Ed.
Instructor, Community College System
University of Hawaii
Honolulu, Hawaii

Joan Takao Matsukawa, R.N., M.S., M.P.H.
Chairperson, Department of Practical Nursing
Kapiolani Community College
Honolulu, Hawaii

Margot Scott Murray, R.N.C., M.S.
Instructor of Nursing
Arapahoe Community College
Littleton, Colorado

Eleuteria Yanai, R.N., M.A.
Instructor in Practical Nursing
Kapiolani Community College
Honolulu, Hawaii

The authors wish to extend thanks to family and friends who helped in numerous ways during the revision.

Special recognition is extended to Charles Kirk Bates who, in addition to providing technical assistance in completing the manuscript, provided continuing encouragement and loving support throughout the revision process.

The technical support vital to the Fifth Edition was provided by Carol Wolfe, Senior Editor—Nursing, Macmillan Publishing Company. Mrs. Wolfe's understanding, expertise, and editorial encouragement made the completion of the Fifth Edition a reality.

The Fifth Edition is dedicated to the late Mildred A. Mason, R.N., Ed.D., a pioneer in practical nurse education. Dr. Mason's gifts of caring and commitment and her unique accomplishments as a health occupations educator continue to enlighten and enrich the world she left and those who inhabit it.

G.F.B.
Kailua, Hawaii, 1987

Contents

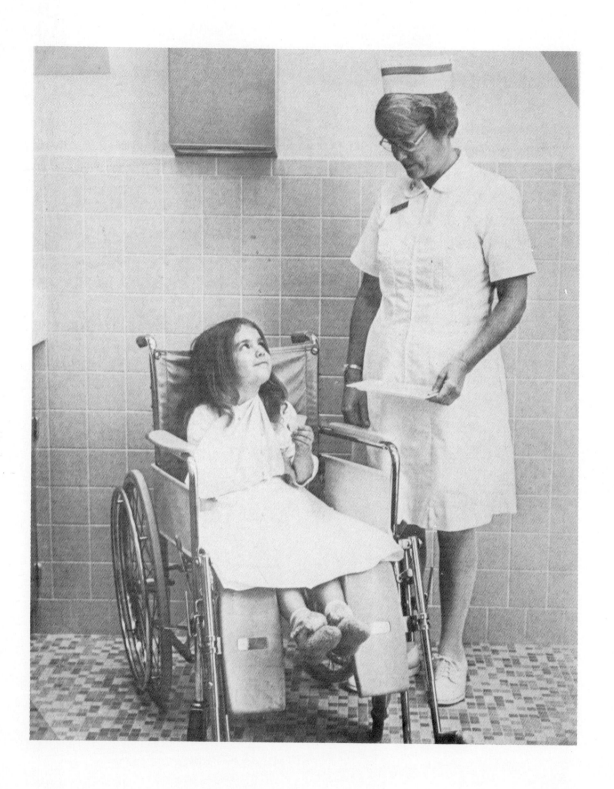

Section I

INTRODUCTION TO DRUG THERAPY

Chapter 1 | THE ROLE OF THE NURSE IN DRUG THERAPY

EXPECTED BEHAVIORAL OUTCOMES

Expected behavioral outcomes are minimum objectives that serve several purposes. First, they tell you what you are expected to know or do after reading and studying each chapter. Second, they can be used as a study guide. After completing this chapter you should return to the expected behavioral outcomes and evaluate your ability to:

1. Define *drug therapy*.
2. Describe major roles of the nurse that pertain to the patient receiving drug therapy.
3. Describe major laws that affect nursing practice related to drug therapy.
4. Identify the functions of each of the health team members that participate in drug therapy.
5. Relate how trends in drug therapy are affecting nursing practices in caring for the patient receiving drug therapy.

DEFINING DRUG THERAPY

Drug therapy is the use of substances to prevent, diagnose, treat, or cure disease or relieve its symptoms. Substances used as drugs come from animal, vegetable, mineral, and chemical sources.

A drug (from the Dutch word meaning dry) is a substance, like food, that acts upon the living protein of the body. There are hundreds of drugs available to patients today. Many of these same drugs were used by early humans, who, probably by persistent trial and error, determined which barks, herbs, roots, and spices were of medicinal value.

The use of opium dates back to 5000 B.C. when the ancient Egyptians discovered that it made patients drowsy. Cinchona bark and sassafras were first used medicinally by the people of ancient Peru. The Greeks first introduced senna and rhubarb to stimulate the activity of the intestinal tract. They advocated the need for personal cleanliness and encouraged the use of soft music and medicated wines to soothe both the body and the spirit. Hippocrates, often considered the father of modern medicine, used over three hundred drugs in his practice of medicine in ancient Greece. He believed the physician's function was to aid "nature" in allowing the body to exercise its recuperative powers. He is also credited with defining the tenets of modern medical ethics.

The Dark Ages, following the fall of Rome (approximately A.D. 400 to about A.D. 1400), brought progress in the sciences to a virtual standstill. However, in the monasteries during that time the monks were using such medicinal agents as colchicine, belladonna, henbane, and iron. They also collected and preserved many valuable manuscripts on pharmacy and medicine.

Finally, in the sixteenth century, impetus was given to the gathering and organizing of drug information. The first official pharmacopoeia was published in 1546. During the eighteenth century the first synthetic drug was produced. In 1796 smallpox vaccine was successfully introduced, leading to the development of serums, vaccines, and other substances used in the control and prevention of many communicable diseases. National pharmacopoeias were published in several countries during the nineteenth century. In 1820 the first such document was published in the United States.

The twentieth century has been a time of unprecedented progress in the drug therapy field. Some of the most notable achievements are:

1. Controls to regulate the manufacture and sale of habit-forming drugs.
2. Elimination of undesirable side effects of many drugs.
3. Advances in the field of substitution therapy. There are now many glandular products available for use, such as insulin.
4. Production of synthetic drugs. Drugs produced in this fashion frequently are less toxic and may be available in unlimited amounts.
5. Introduction of chemotherapeutic agents and antibiotics, which has revolutionized the treatment of microbial and neoplastic diseases.
6. Use of isotopes as therapeutic and diagnostic agents.
7. Advent of psychotherapeutic drugs, which include the tranquilizers and psychostimulators, has alleviated the symptoms of mental illness to such an extent that many patients are now able to leave institutions and resume the normal activities of daily living.
8. Acceptance of the use of neuroleptic analgesics, which cause general quiescence and a state of psychoindifference to environmental stimuli but do not produce sleep. The introduction of neuroleptic anesthetics.

LAWS THAT AFFECT NURSING PRACTICES RELATED TO DRUG THERAPY

In general, three kinds of laws affect the nurse administering drug therapy. The outline in Drug Legislation, below, provides a summary of major legislation during this century that relates to drugs.

I. Licensing laws. Licensing laws describe who may participate in drug therapy and how they may participate.
   A. Only licensed physicians, dentists, and veterinarians may prescribe drug therapy.
   B. The *Nurse Practice Act* in most states is the law that defines who may practice nursing or practical nursing; this law describes the legal limits of practice.
II. Food and Drug Acts. These acts are federal laws affecting the standards for purity and effectiveness of all substances classified as drugs.
III. Controlled Substance Acts. These federal laws place restrictions on the prescription, dispensing, and use of drugs known to have a potential for drug abuse.

Drug Legislation

Between 1906 and 1970 the Congress of the United States, in an effort to protect public health, passed a number of laws designed to control the use of drugs. The Comprehensive Drug Abuse Prevention and Control Act passed in 1970 supplanted a number of the earlier drug laws. Drug legislation passed during the last 64 years includes the following:

I. Federal Pure Food and Drugs Acts and amendments of 1906 (passed by Congress as a result of excessive adulteration and misbranding of foods and drugs).
   A. Named the *United States Pharmacopeia* and the *National Formulary* as official standards.
   B. Required contents of bottles or containers to conform with label statements.
   C. Established standards of safety and effectiveness for new drugs, cosmetics, and therapeutic devices.
   D. Designated the Food and Drug Administration to enforce laws related to drugs, foods, and cosmetics.
   E. Defined which drugs require a prescription and which drugs may be sold over the counter (without a prescription).
   F. Identified prescription drugs that require authorization for refills.

II. Comprehensive Drug Abuse Prevention and Control Act of 1970 (became fully effective on May 1, 1971 and repealed all other controls except the Durham–Humphrey Amendment). This act was designed to control drugs with abuse potential as designated by the Drug Enforcement Administration, Department of Justice. This act divides these drugs into five schedules.

   A. *Schedule I.* Drugs in this schedule have a high abuse potential and no currently accepted medical use in treatment in the United States. Examples include heroin, marijuana, lysergic acid diethylamide (LSD), mescaline, dihydromorphine, methylsulfonate, and nicocodeine.

   B. *Schedule II.* Drugs in this schedule have a high abuse potential and have severe psychic or physical dependence liability. These controlled substances consist of the former class A narcotics and drugs containing amphetamines or methamphetamines. Examples include opium, morphine, codeine, hydromorphone (Dilaudid), methadone (Dolophine), pantapon, meperidine (Demerol), cocaine, straight amphetamines, and methamphetamines; and phenmetrazine (Preludin), methaqualone (Sopor), amobarbital (Amytal), pentobarbital (Nembutal), and secobarbital (Seconal).

   C. *Schedule III.* The drugs in this schedule have an abuse potential less than those in Schedules I and II. Their abuse may lead to moderate or low physical dependence with a high psychological dependence. Examples include compounds or preparations containing limited quantities of codeine, hydrocodone, opium, morphine, and paregoric. Certain nonnarcotic drugs are included, such as chlorhexadol, glutethimide (Doriden), nalorphine, chlorphentermine, phendimetrazine, as well as some barbiturates.

   D. *Schedule IV.* The drugs listed in this schedule have a low abuse potential and more limited physical and psychological dependence. Examples include barbital, phenobarbital, chloral hydrate, meprobamate (Equanil, Miltown), paraldehyde, chlordiazepoxide (Librium), diazepam (Valium), flurazepam (Dalmane), and oxazepam (Serax).

   E. *Schedule V.* The drugs listed in this schedule have an abuse potential level lower than those in Schedule IV. In general, these are narcotic drugs containing nonnarcotic active medicinal ingredients as, for example, not more than 2.5 mg of diphenoxylate and not less than 2.5 mg of atropine sulfate per dosage unit. Drugs in Schedule V may be dispensed without a prescription order provided:

   1. Distribution is made only by a pharmacist.
   2. Not more than 240 ml of any Schedule V substance containing opium, or more than 120 ml of any other Schedule V substance, is distributed at retail in a 48 h period without a prescription order.
   3. Purchaser at retail is at least 18 years of age.
   4. Pharmacist obtains suitable identification.
   5. Record book is maintained that contains:
      a. Name and address of purchaser.
      b. Name and quantity of controlled substance purchased.
      c. Date of sale.
      d. Initial of pharmacist.
      e. Other federal, state, and local law does not require a prescription order.

IMPLICATIONS FOR NURSES ADMINISTERING DRUG THERAPY

1. There must be a written, dated, signed order from a licensed physician for every drug the nurse administers. Some hospitals and agencies have additional policies that guide nursing practice during an emergency or other special circumstances when a physician cannot be present to write an order. However, *no drug* may be given without a physician's order.
2. The nurse is responsible for knowing basic information about each drug he or she administers. This includes the causes and effects of a particular drug for a particular patient, the usual dose, possible adverse responses, and any special information that may affect the safety or effectiveness of a drug for a particular patient.

3. Once the physician's order is understood, the nurse must give the drug exactly as prescribed. If a drug cannot be given, the physician should be notified and a written explanation entered either on the medication administration record or the nurse's progress notes according to hospital policy.

4. Some drugs require special permission from the patient before they can be administered. Examples of such drugs include anesthesia (see Tables 16–4, 17-5), antineoplastic drugs (see Tables 25–1 to 25–5), experimental drugs, hormones, certain drugs used for the patient with mental illness, and drugs used for a placebo effect. Nurses should check the hospital or agency policy for administering these drugs.

5. Requires the pharmacist to keep a record of receipt and disposition of all controlled substances. These records must be maintained for at least 2 years and should be available for inspection.

6. Prescription orders for controlled substances in Schedule II must be typewritten, or written in ink or indelible pencil, and must be signed by the physician; such prescription orders cannot be refilled.

7. Prescription orders for drugs in Schedules III and IV may be issued either orally or in writing by a physician; they may be refilled, but not more than five times, and may not be filled or refilled more than 6 months after the date of issue. After five refills or after 6 months, the physician may write a new prescription order.

8. Drugs in Schedule V may be prescribed in the same way as drugs in Schedules III and IV; under certain conditions, they may be dispensed without a prescription.

9. The label of any controlled substance in Schedule II, III, or IV when prescribed for a patient must contain the following statement: "Caution: Federal law prohibits the transfer of this drug to any person other than the patient for whom it was prescribed."

10. In order to prescribe controlled substances, a physician must be registered with the Bureau of Narcotics and Dangerous Drugs and registration must be renewed annually. The number on the certificate of registration must be indicated on all prescription orders for controlled substances.

ROLES OF THE NURSE IN DRUG THERAPY

Most patients under nursing care receive drug therapy at some time or another. The nurse plays several essential parts in providing safe and effective drug therapy.

I. Patient's assistant.
   A. The nurse helps with those activities a person with enough knowledge, skill and energy can do alone (bathing, eating, toileting, ambulating).
   B. The nurse administers drug therapy to the hospitalized patient because there is a need for special knowledge and skill to do so safely and effectively.
II. Health team member.
   A. The nurse is a key person on the health team since he or she carries out numerous activities that are part of the patient's medical treatment plan.
   B. The nurse administers drug therapy that has been prescribed by a licensed physician.
   C. The nurse observes, records, and reports the patient's response to drug therapy.
III. Activity coordinator.
   A. The nurse helps to schedule and coordinate the many daily activities in which the patient may be involved. For example, the nurse schedules laboratory tests, x-ray examinations, mealtimes, and medication so that the patient obtains maximum benefit from each.
IV. Patient teacher
   A. The nurse teaches the patient and family how to administer prescribed medications safely and effectively outside the hospital.
   B. The nurse teaches about the drug, its purpose, how to take it, when to take it, what might go wrong, what to do if something does go wrong, where to store the drug, and similar information.

THE HEALTH TEAM AND DRUG THERAPY

A number of other members of the health team participate directly or indirectly in drug therapy. In fact, the hospitalized patient may be receiving several drugs besides those administered by the nurse. Thus, there is a special need for complete and accurate recording of drug therapy by each member of the health team. The list of health team members below illustrates which members of the health team are most likely to participate in drug therapy and how they participate.

1. Anesthesiologist. This physician specializes in prescribing and administering drug therapy to produce anesthesia, usually for a surgical procedure.
2. Licensed practical nurse (LPN)/licensed vocational nurse (LVN). The LPN/LVN is licensed to administer oral, topical, and certain parenteral drugs that have been prescribed by a licensed physician, dentist, and veterinarian. The LPN/LVN is also responsible for contributing to and participating in the nursing care plan; observing, recording, and reporting the patient's response to drug therapy; and selecting nursing actions that enhance the patient's response to drug therapy.
3. Medical assistant. The certified medical assistant may administer certain drug therapy under the direct supervision of a licensed physician employer.
4. Medical laboratory technologist/technician (MLT). The MLT participates in drug therapy indirectly by collecting and analyzing specimens of blood, urine, and other body discharges for the purpose of monitoring the patient's response to therapy. In some cases, laboratory analysis of body constituents helps the physician to determine if drug therapy is needed.
5. Nurse anesthetist. This nurse specialist administers drug therapy to produce anesthesia, usually for a surgical procedure.
6. Pharmacist. Licensed to prepare and dispense drugs. May also monitor administration of drug therapy in the hospital or long-term care facility. Acts as a resource person for other members of the health team about matters related to drug therapy.
7. Pharmacy technician. Dispenses selected drugs under the direct supervision of a licensed pharmacist.
8. Physician. Prescribes drug therapy. Monitors and evaluates the patient's response to drug therapy. Responsible for preventing, diagnosing, and treating disease. Leader of the health team.
9. Radiologist. Physician specialist in the use of x-rays to diagnose and/or treat disease. May prescribe and/or administer contrast dyes, radioactive chemicals, and similar drugs used to diagnose disease.
10. Registered nurse. Licensed to administer drugs prescribed by a licensed physician, dentist, or veterinarian. Responsible for establishing, monitoring, and evaluating the nursing care plan. Observes, records, and reports the patient's response to drug therapy. Responsible for selecting nursing actions that enhance the effectiveness of drug therapy. Supervises other nursing personnel such as the LPN/LVN.
11. Respiratory therapist. Administers drugs prescribed by the physician for inhalation. Drugs taken by inhalation may be used for diagnosis or treatment.
12. Social worker. Collects and analyzes information about the patient's social environment that influences or is influenced by drug therapy. For example, the social worker may assist the patient to obtain financial assistance to continue purchasing refills of prescribed drugs following discharge from the hospital.

TRENDS IN DRUG THERAPY

A number of trends can be seen in drug therapy, each of which has an impact on nursing practices.

1. The number of available drugs continues to expand rapidly. Thus the nurse administering drug therapy is challenged to maintain a current knowledge and skill level that is consistent with safe and effective drug therapy.

2. There is a trend, especially noticeable in the elderly, toward combination drug therapy. In other words, two or more drugs may be prescribed to treat the patient's symptoms and/or illness. This trend is especially obvious in patients with chronic illnesses such as cardiovascular diseases, chronic respiratory illnesses, kidney diseases and the like. Combination therapy enhances the likelihood of an adverse drug interaction (an unexpected effect that could not have been predicted from what is known about each of the prescribed drugs). A systematic observation method such as that described in Table 3–1 is extremely helpful to the nurse who practices early detection of complications in drug therapy.

3. There is a flow of new information available about interactions between prescribed drugs and foods or fluids consumed. Thus, the student building an information base about drugs should include whatever is known about the impact of food and fluids on the drug under study.

4. There is a trend toward a unit dose delivery system in hospitals and long-term care facilities. In this system, each dose of medication prescribed for the patient is prepackaged and labeled in the pharmacy. Then the pharmacy delivers each patient's individually packaged dosages for an 8- to 24-hr period depending upon specific hospital or agency procedure. This system is associated with greater accuracy of the dose and improved techniques for administering the drug. In practice, unit dosage cuts down on the need for dosage calculation by the nurse. However, the same careful attention to reading labels, correct pouring techniques, identification of the patient, and accurate complete recording is needed (see Chapter 13).

5. There is an increase in the number of drugs prescribed by the IV route. This trend has been made possible by improved technology both in the manufacture of drugs and in equipment available for IV therapy (see Chapter 15). In practice, nurses find that many more patients have IV lines that must be observed, protected, and otherwise cared for. In addition, calculation and observation of the flow rate have become much more frequent tasks.

6. The introduction of computers to the pharmacy, laboratory, and nursing unit provides a useful new tool for collecting, organizing, and analyzing all the patient data affecting and affected by drug therapy. In practice, this information is often kept for each patient in the form of a *drug profile* stored in the pharmacy. The clinical pharmacist studies the drug profile and alerts the physician, nurse, and other appropriate members of the health team to important changes in the profile, the potential for drug interactions, and untoward affects of drug therapy.

7. A dramatic increase in the cost of health care is associated with a trend toward shorter hospital stays and early discharge. Patients may be discharged to complete or continue drug therapy at home. Although the need for patient teaching is expanding, there is less time available for the patient and family to learn important new information and skills. Thus, the nurse should consider the need for early patient teaching, written discharge instructions, and referral for home care if necessary.

8. Currently, there is an increase in the use of drugs for recreation—"to get high." This in turn is creating new health-related issues for recreational drug users and others as well as new challenges for nurses caring for them. For example, alcohol and other drug use are major factors in automobile accidents that result in severe and often fatal injuries. A related continuing trend affecting nurses is impaired performance by physicians, nurses, and other health team members who have become addicted to prescription drugs.

Additional information about substance abuse can be located in Chapter 16. This trend enhances the likelihood of unusual drug interactions in patients. Impaired physician or nurse performance makes errors in drug therapy more likely. Therefore the nurse must remain observant at all times during drug therapy.

9. The trend toward self-medication with over-the-counter (OTC) or nonprescribed drugs continues. This multibillion-dollar industry is having major impacts on nursing practice in several areas. For example, in collecting information about drugs the patient is taking (drug history), the nurse must ask specifically about the use of nonprescribed drugs such as aspirin, acetaminophen (Tylenol), vitamins, sleeping aids, laxatives, and antacids. When teaching the patient and family about drug therapy, the nurse must also consider whether prescribed drugs will be taken along with nonprescribed drugs.

CASE STUDY 1

Mrs. Jones was admitted to the hospital for treatment of pneumonia. She was well known to the nursing staff because of several previous admissions for acute asthma. The physician's orders included:

- Chest x-ray film today.
- Sputum specimen for culture and sensitivity stat.
- After sputum collection, start ampicillin 1 g q6h IV.
- Guaifenesin (Robitussin) 15 cc orally q4h.
- Intermittent positive-pressure breathing (IPPB) therapy with normal saline stat and q4h.
- O$_2$ by nasal prongs at 2 L/min.
- Force fluids to 3,000 cc/day.
- NO SEDATIVES, OPIATES, OR TRANQUILIZERS.

QUESTIONS

1. From information provided in the case study, list the drugs prescribed for Mrs. Jones.
2. For each of the drugs identified in Question 1, tell whether it was prescribed to diagnose, prevent, or treat disease, or relieve its symptoms.
3. Using information provided in the chapter, describe each role of the nurse as it relates to drug therapy prescribed for Mrs. Jones.
4. Describe major laws affecting drug therapy for Mrs. Jones.
5. From information provided in the case study, describe how other members of the health team are likely to participate in drug therapy for Mrs. Jones.
6. Which of the trends described in the chapter are likely to affect nursing practices for Mrs. Jones? What do you think the impact will be?

Chapter 2 | CONCEPTS IN DRUG THERAPY

EXPECTED BEHAVIORAL OUTCOMES

After completing this chapter, you should return to the expected behavioral outcomes and evaluate your ability to:

1. Describe the major effects of drug therapy on body processes, thoughts and feelings, and social interaction.
2. Explain the difference between a nonproprietary name and a trade name.
3. Use a reference book to get additional information about a particular drug.
4. Give at least two examples of liquid, solid, and semisolid preparations.
5. Identify an incomplete or illegible prescription or doctor's order and seek further information.
6. List the responsibilities of the nurse for dose and dosage.
7. Describe in your own words how a drug works.
8. Define each of the adverse drug responses presented in the chapter.
9. Explain the relationship between nursing implications and nursing care.
10. List the routes of administration using a head to toe format.
11. Use the language and symbols of drug therapy.

Concepts are thoughts and ideas about what something is like and how it works. An understanding of basic concepts in drug therapy is essential to the nurse in order to provide nursing care that is safe and effective. In this chapter, most of the concepts concern the patient and the drug.

THE PATIENT

A key concept in learning about drug therapy is understanding the patient as a unique whole person. For purposes of understanding and study, human activity is often separated into several categories such as physiologic (activity related to body functions), psychological (activity related to mental and emotional function), and social (activity related to interactions with others). However, it is important to remember that individuals are not composed of separate parts but are whole entities. Thus, even when drug therapy is prescribed to alter a body function, it also affects the individual's mental and emotional processes and social interaction. Whenever drug therapy is prescribed for the patient, the nurse can anticipate the following events:

1. A change in body processes.
2. A change in thoughts and feelings.
3. A change in interactions with others.

For example, diuretic therapy was prescribed for Mr. Carson to lower his blood pressure. *Diuretics* are drugs that act in the kidney to increase the elimination of urine. As urinary elimination increases, the volume of circulating blood is reduced and the blood pressure decreases. Mr. Carson experienced the following changes while receiving diuretic therapy:

1. Increased urinary output (change in a body process).
2. Anxiety about the cost of drug therapy (change in feeling).
3. Questions about whether to take the drug in the morning or at night (change in thoughts).
4. Questions from co-workers about his frequent trips to the bathroom (change in interactions with others).

The nurse can convey understanding and respect for the patient as a whole person in many ways including:

- Active listening to the patient's concerns (Fig. 2–1).
- Careful and systematic observation of the patient's whole response to drug therapy (physical, psychological, and social responses).
- Explaining some of the changes created by drug therapy to the patient, family, physician, and others as appropriate.
- Reporting and recording unfavorable responses to the appropriate physician or nurse. Adverse drug responses are described later in the chapter in the section Adverse Responses to Drug Therapy, pp. 18–19.

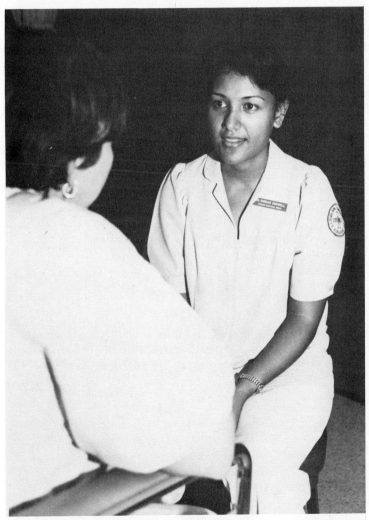

FIGURE 2-1 The nurse conveys understanding and respect for the patient by actively listening to the patient's concerns.

THE DRUG

A drug is a substance that acts on living protein of the body. The study of drug therapy encompasses several broad areas. In each of these areas, the nurse is expected to develop knowledge and skill sufficient to meet the behavioral objectives listed in the beginning of the chapter.

Pharmacology embraces the knowledge of the history, source, physical and chemical properties, compounding, biochemical and physiological effects, mechanisms of action, absorption, distribution, biotransformation and excretion, and therapeutic and other uses of drugs.* *Pharmacodynamics* refers to the study of drugs and their actions on the body. *Pharmacotherapeutics* is the study of the treatment, prevention, and diagnosis of diseases by drugs. *Toxicology* is the study of poisons or of the toxic effects produced by overdosage. *Pharmacognosy* is the study of crude drugs and their properties. *Pharmacy* is the art of preparing and compounding drugs (also the place where drugs are compounded, dispensed, and stored). *Posology* is the science of dosages, including minimum, maximum, therapeutic, toxic, and usual dose of each drug.

DRUG NOMENCLATURE

The word *nomenclature* refers to a system of naming something. In order to discuss and learn about drugs, the nurse needs to understand drug nomenclature. Every drug has several different names. One name is known as the *chemical name or designation*. Another name is called the *nonproprietary name*. A third name, given by the manufacturer, is known as the *proprietary or trade name*. A drug may have several different trade names depending upon how many companies make it. The naming of drugs often proceeds in the following way.

A newly manufactured drug is given a chemical name or designation as well as a code name by the pharmaceutical company. When the drug is placed on the market, a United States adopted name (USAN) is selected by the United States Adopted Name Council. This council is sponsored jointly by the American Medical Association (AMA), the American Pharmaceutical Association (APA), and the United States Pharmacopoeial Convention, Inc. Should the drug be admitted to the *United States Pharmacopeia* (USP), or the *National Formulary* (NF), the USAN becomes the official or nonproprietary name for the drug. Although there is a tendency to refer to the *nonproprietary* name of a drug as the generic name, actually *generic* properly denotes a pharmacologic class of drugs, such as antibiotics. Whenever possible and to avoid confusion, the nonproprietary name of a drug should be used. All the drugs included in this book are listed under their nonproprietary names. The dose mentioned in each instance is the average adult dose. It is not possible to list the average child's dose, since such doses must be determined on an individual basis (see p. 78).

DRUG PUBLICATIONS

There are a number of references that the nurse may use to identify a drug or collect important information about it. These publications include generic and proprietary names, the composition of the drug, the uses, the methods of administration, the side effects, and the precautions to be observed in administering the drug.

    I. *United States Pharmacopeia* (USP).
        A. Published first in 1820.
        B. Revised every 5 to 10 years.
        C. Contains the following information concerning drugs:
            1. Official name.
            2. Classification according to therapeutic use.
            3. Description and structural form.

*Goodman, L. S., and Gilman, A. (eds.): *The Pharmacological Basis of Therapeutics*, 7th ed. Macmillan, New York, 1985, p. 1.

    4. Source.

    5. Established purity.

    6. Biological and chemical assays.

    7. Usefulness.

    8. Usual dose and range of dose.

    9. Dosage forms, that is, tablets, capsules, and so forth.

    10. Toxicity.

    11. Methods of storage and preservation.

    12. Now published as a single volume together with the NF.

II. *National Formulary* (NF).

    A. Published first in 1888.

    B. New editions appear in the same volume as the USP.

    C. Includes drugs frequently used in prescription.

    D. Provides standards for many old remedies.

    E. All doses expressed in the metric system.

III. *AMA Drug Evaluations.*

    A. A publication issued under the supervision of the Department of Drugs of the AMA.

    B. It contains pertinent data on both old and new single-entity drugs and mixtures, arranged according to therapeutic category.

IV. *Physicians' Desk Reference.*

    A. Published annually.

    B. Supplements published as necessary.

    C. Each drug description has been prepared by the manufacturer.

    D. Frequently used by nurses as a quick reference.

V. *American Hospital Formulary Service.*

    A. Published by the American Society of Hospital Pharmacists.

    B. Annual and Supplementary Index are published.

VI. *The United States Pharmacopeia Dispensing Information* (USPDI).

    A. First published in 1980.

    B. One volume entitled *Drug Information for the Health Care Provider.*

    C. Second volume entitled *Advice for the Patient.* Contains instructions in lay language that may be given to patients.

VII. *Canadian Formulary* (CF).

    A. Published by the Canadian Pharmaceutical Association.

    B. Given official status by the Canadian Food and Drug Act.

    Note: Many drugs used in Canada are obtained from the United States.

VIII. *Pharmacopoeia International.*

    A. Published by World Health Organization.

    B. All doses are expressed in the metric system.

    C. Nomenclature is in Latin.

    D. Attempts to unify drugs in relation to:

        1. Composition.

        2. Strength.

        3. Terms used.

        4. Dosage—usual, daily, and maximum single dose.

        5. Route of administration.

SOURCES FOR OBTAINING DRUGS

Drugs are obtained from four sources.

    1. Animal kingdom. The organs of cattle, hogs, sheep, and other animals are used in the preparation of many drugs used in the treatment of disease. Some of the drugs derived from the animal kingdom include:

    a. Insulin, from the pancreas of hogs, sheep, and cattle, and used in the treatment of diabetes mellitus.

    b. Liver extract, used in the treatment of pernicious anemia.

    c. Thyroid extract, used in the treatment of hypothyroidism.

    d. Immune serums, used in the treatment of some infectious diseases.

    e. Immunizing agents, used in the prevention of some of the communicable diseases.

2. Plant kingdom. Many of the widely used drugs are prepared from barks, flowers, leaves, roots, saps, and seeds of various plants. Examples of such drugs are:

    a. Digitalis, prepared from purple foxglove and used in the treatment of diseases of the heart.

    b. *Cascara sagrada*, made from the bark of the buckthorn tree and widely used as a laxative.

    c. Caffeine, obtained from tea leaves and used as an effective heart stimulant.

    d. Morphine, derived from the white poppy, a flower of the Orient. Morphine is used for the relief of severe pain.

3. Mineral kingdom. Minerals and salts found in nature frequently are purified for use. Examples of mineral drugs are:

    a. Epsom salt or magnesium sulfate, available in a white powder or glassy crystals. This drug may be used internally as a saline cathartic or externally in solution for soaks.

    b. Sodium bicarbonate, available in tablet and powder form and used as an antacid.

4. Synthetic drugs. Drugs in this group are prepared in the chemist's laboratory from a known formula. A number of drugs prepared in this manner are duplicates of natural substances. For example, cortisone, which is found in the animal kingdom, may be prepared synthetically in the laboratory. Examples of drugs produced in this manner are:

    a. The sulfonamides, used in the treatment of many bacterial infections.

    b. Cortisone, used in the treatment of arthritis.

PREPARATION OF DRUGS

Drugs are prepared in various forms for administration. It is important for the bedside nurse to know the various ways in which drugs are prepared. Drugs are prepared in:

I. Liquid forms.

    A. Aqueous solutions—these preparations may be used internally or externally.

        1. Internal use—aromatic or volatile drugs are dissolved in water.

        2. External use—nonvolatile drugs, such as salts, are dissolved in water and used for soaks and irrigations. (Frequently these solutions are prepared by the nurse.)

    B. *Elixir*—a preparation of drugs containing sugar and alcohol.

    C. *Emulsion*—a preparation in which oils usually are dispersed in an aqueous solution.

    D. *Fluidextract*—a concentrated fluid preparation of a drug of the vegetable kingdom. *They are always 100% strength.*

    E. *Gel*—colloidal aqueous suspension of hydrated inorganic substances.

    F. *Inhalant*—drug with a vapor pressure high enough to permit it to be carried into the nasal passage with the inhaled air.

    G. *Liniment*—liquid preparation applied to the skin with friction.

    H. *Lotion*—aqueous suspension of insoluble substances used to soothe and relieve itching.

    I. *Magma*—bulky suspension of substances poorly soluble in water; tends to resemble cream or milk.

    J. *Milk*—a preparation in which an insoluble substance is suspended in water.

    K. *Mucilage*—a pharmacopeial preparation consisting of a solution in water of the gummy or starchy principles of vegetables substances; used as a soothing application to the mucous membrane.

    L. *Spirit*—an alcoholic solution of a volatile substance.

    M. *Spray*—a solution of one or more drugs in oil or water, usually sprayed into the nose and/or throat with an atomizer.

    N. *Suspension*—state of a solid when its particles are mixed, but not dissolved, in a fluid or another solid.

    O. *Syrup*—a concentrated solution of sugar in water to which a drug has been added.

    P. *Tincture*—a preparation in which a drug has been dissolved in alcohol. Tinctures vary in strengths from 10 to 20%.

II. Solid forms.

    A. *Ampule*—a small sealed glass container, the content of which is a sterile drug in either liquid or powder form.

    B. *Capsule*—a soluble shell prepared from a gelatinous substance in which drugs are encased.

        1. Hard capsule used for dispensing drugs orally.

        2. Flexible capsule used for dispensing oils and other liquids.

    C. *Pill*—a powdered drug mixed with a cohesive substance and molded into a pellet. A pill may be covered with sugar if the drug is particularly bitter. Some pills are coated with a substance that will not dissolve until they reach the small intestine. Such pills are said to be *enteric-coated*.

    D. *Powder*—a preparation of small particles of a solid.

    E. *Spansule*—a capsule containing time-released drug pellets.

    F. *Tablet*—a compressed or molded preparation of a drug. Tablets are frequently scored and usually can be dissolved or crushed easily.

    G. *Troche or lozenge*—a large flat disk that is dissolved in the mouth.

III. Semisolids.

    A. *Ointments*—drugs prepared in a fatty base. They are applied locally either to the skin or mucous membrane.

    B. *Pastes*—ointmentlike preparations containing one or more drugs and an adhesive substance that may be applied to oozing surfaces.

    C. *Suppositories*—drugs mixed with substances that melt at body temperature. Suppositories are usually cone-shaped and are inserted in such body orifices as the rectum, vagina, or urethra.

The preparation of a drug often affects its care and storage. For example, a suppository may be stored in the refrigerator. Some drugs must be stored away from strong light. Others may be affected by heat or humidity. The preparation of a drug may also affect how it is administered. For example, a spansule may not be crushed for administration through a nasogastric feeding tube without affecting its activity in the body.

ELEMENTS OF THE DRUG PRESCRIPTION

Before a drug can be administered by the licensed practical/vocational nurse, it must be prescribed in writing by a licensed physician.

  I. The prescription (Figure 2–2).

    A. Drugs are prescribed by the physician.

    B. The prescription of a drug should include:

        1. Date.

        2. Name of the patient.

        3. Drug (if it is a medication to be compounded, the names and amounts of ingredients as well as compounding directions should be included).

        4. Directions to the patient (the time, amount, and method of administration).

        5. Physician's signature.

    C. Ways of prescribing drugs:

        1. In the home or doctor's office, a prescription order is written as shown in Figure 2–2.

        2. In the hospital, the doctor usually writes the prescription order on the order sheet of the patient's chart.

```
Telephone 555-1122                                        AB1462758

                        James B. Frank, M.D.

420 N.E. 4TH AVENUE                    BOYNTON BEACH, FLA. 33435
```

Name   *Elizabeth Johns*   Age   *58*
Address *84 Third Ave., Boynton Beach*   Date *1/19/85*

R⁄   *Donnatal Extentabs 1 Tab.*
               t. i. d. as needed

Label ☒
Refill ☐1 ☐2 ☐3 ☐4 ☐5 ☐prn   *James B. Frank*   M.D.

FIGURE 2-2   Prescription order.

II. The doctor's order (Fig. 2–3).
  A. The order should be completely and legibly written.
  B. The order should include the:
   1. Patient's name.
   2. Date.
   3. Drug to be given.
   4. Amount of drug to be given (dose).
   5. Hour or hours the drug is to be given (frequency).
   6. Route of administration.
   7. Expiration date.
   8. Doctor's signature.

III. The nurse's responsibilities.
  A. Checks to see that the physician's order is complete and legible.
  B. Seeks additional information if the order is incomplete, illegible, or inconsistent with what is known about the drug and the patient.
  C. Once the prescription is known to be accurate, complete, and legible, administers the drug exactly as prescribed.
  D. Observes the patient for an adverse drug reaction; reports and records patient's response to drug therapy.
  E. Records the drug administered according to hospital agency procedures.
  F. Teaches the patient and family how to administer the drug exactly as prescribed.

11/20/85   Aspirin   0.6 g.   P.O. t.i.d.

Marian Doyle, M.D.

FIGURE 2-3   The doctor's order written on the physician's order sheet of the patient's chart.

DRUG DOSAGE

I. Common terms. The words *dose* and *dosage* mean how much. When used in connection with drug therapy, dose refers to how much of a drug has been prescribed and/or administered. Some common terms related to dose are summarized below.

A. *Average dose*—the quantity that usually produces the desired response.

B. *Lethal dose*—an amount of drug that is likely to cause death; also known as *fatal dose*.

C. *Maintenance dose*—the amount of drug necessary to produce a continuous desired effect; often smaller than the amount needed to produce the desired effect in the first place.

Dose is expressed as numbers in a system of weights and measures. For example, 25 mg is a weight that describes a specific amount of a drug. Another way that dosage is expressed is called *frequency*. Frequency is how often a drug is to be administered. Frequency is expressed in number of times per hour, day, week, or month.

II. Factors affecting dosage. In selecting a dose for a specific individual, the physician usually considers the following factors:

A. Age of the patient. Children and older people require smaller doses of medicine.

B. Sex. Women sometimes tend to be more susceptible to the effects of certain drugs than men. Body size may necessitate the administration of smaller doses. During pregnancy drugs should be kept at a minimum since some drugs may act adversely on the uterus and/or fetus.

C. Condition of the patient. The following conditions influence the amount of drug to be given:

    1. Presence of food in the stomach will delay absorption of a drug.

    2. Presence of pain and fever may increase the rate of absorption.

    3. Presence of other drugs in the body.

D. Weight and surface area of the patient. Individuals of small size require smaller doses.

E. Time the drug is given.

    1. Larger doses of sedatives are required to produce a quieting effect in the morning.

    2. Larger doses of stimulants are required to produce a wakeful state at night.

    3. Irritating drugs should be given with food, as at mealtime.

F. Method of administration. Some methods of administration require larger doses than other methods. Example: When a drug is given rectally, a larger dose is necessary than when it is given by mouth.

G. Rate of elimination. Impairment of renal and hepatic elimination may influence the use of a drug, the size of the dose, or the discontinuation of a drug. Fever may increase the rate of drug elimination.

H. Pathologic factors. Such factors as nutritional deficiencies, pulmonary disease, hyperthyroidism, and intracranial pressure may modify the effectiveness of some drugs.

I. Potential for adverse drug responses. Allergy, idiosyncrasy, drug interaction, drug tolerance are examples of adverse drug responses that may be considered. Additional information can be located in this chapter on pp. 12–13.

III. Nursing activities related to drug dosage

A. The nurse knows the average dose of every drug administered. It may be necessary to gather the information by using one or more of the references described on pp. 12–13.

B. The nurse is expected to seek additional information if the prescribed dose is different from the average dose.

C. The nurse may need to calculate the correct amount of medication to be given after the dose has been prescribed by the physician.

D. The nurse administers the dose as prescribed by the physician.

E. The nurse reports observations that indicate the patient's response to drug therapy.

F. The nurse documents on the chart all drugs given or omitted.

ROUTES OF ADMINISTERING DRUGS

Drugs are administered in several different ways to ensure their effectiveness. The routes of administration include:

1. *Oral (by mouth).* This is the most common method of administration. Tablets, pills, capsules, and liquids are given in this manner.
2. *Per rectum (by rectum).* Drugs administered in this way are given in the form of enemas or suppositories.
3. *Subcutaneous injection.* The drug is injected into the layer of tissue just under the skin. Drugs administered this way act promptly.
4. *Intramuscular injection.* The drug is injected into the muscle, and absorption takes place there.
5. *Intravenous injection.* The drug is injected into the vein either directly or by diluting it in 50 to 150 ml of intravenous solution. Drugs given in this way act very quickly. Intravenous infusion is a slow method of administering large amounts of solution.
6. *Intrathecal or intraspinal injections.* The drug is introduced into the spinal fluid. This method of administration is done by the physician.
7. *Intra-arterial injection.* The drug is introduced directly into the artery. May be done for localized effect as on a particular tissue or organ.
8. *Intraperitoneal.* The drug is introduced directly into the peritoneal cavity.
9. *Inhalation.* The drug is breathed in through a nebulizer or in steam.
10. *Inunction.* The drug is rubbed into the skin.
11. *Sublingual.* The drug is dissolved under the tongue.
12. *Topical or local methods.* Drugs may be administered by swabbing, painting, soaks, irrigations, instillations, gargles, and sprays.

HOW DRUGS WORK

Once a drug is administered, it usually enters the circulation, a process known as *absorption*. Absorption is affected by several factors including the route of administration, the characteristics of the specific drug, and the patient's fluid balance and circulatory states. The bloodstream transports the drug to receptor sites in the target tissue. The term *onset of action* describes the length of time it takes for a drug to be absorbed and reach the target tissue.

While the prescribed drug produces a certain intended effect in the target tissues, it also affects other body tissues at the same time. This is known as an unintended or *side effect*. For example, a common side effect of drug therapy is nausea, vomiting, and diarrhea. These side effects very often occur as a result of irritation of the gastrointestinal system by drugs in the oral form. Side effects may be mild or very intense. In some cases, a drug may be changed or discontinued because of side effects. A very important nursing responsibility includes observing, recording, reporting, and teaching the patient about side effects.

At the target tissues, the drug remains active until it is metabolized and finally excreted. The term *duration of action* describes how long the drug remains active.

Metabolism is the rate at which the body uses substances in maintaining vital life processes. Most drugs are metabolized in the liver. However, drugs may also be metabolized in the lungs, skin, kidneys, or intestines. In most patients, drugs are excreted by the kidneys. However, some drugs are excreted in feces, sweat by the lungs during expiration, or in breast milk.

For each of the drugs administered to the patient, the nurse is expected to have a general understanding of how it works. This understanding is translated to practice by observing, recording, and reporting the patient's response to drug therapy.

ADVERSE RESPONSES TO DRUG THERAPY

A person receiving drug therapy may experience an adverse response to the drugs prescribed. An adverse response is one that is unfavorable, unintended, and does not benefit the patient. An important responsibility of the nurse administering drug therapy is to observe the patient carefully and systematically for adverse responses and report and record them early so that the patient is not harmed. The list below describes major adverse responses.

1. *Allergic response*—a hypersensitive reaction to a drug; may take the form of a skin reaction, respiratory symptoms, gastrointestinal symptoms; symptoms may range from uncomfortable to life threatening.
2. *Drug addiction*—a pattern of drug use that involves preoccupation with getting and using drugs and a tendency to relapse after withdrawal. [Adapted from Goodman, L.S., and Gilman, A. (eds.): *The Pharmacological Basis of Therapeutics*, 7th ed. Macmillan, New York, 1985, p. 533.]
3. *Drug interaction*—an adverse effect of two or more drugs that can frequently be predicted from what is known about the effect of each drug; an adverse effect may also be produced by a drug–food interaction; some drug interactions may be beneficial to the patient.
4. *Drug tolerance*—an adverse response during which an individual does not receive the same benefit from a drug or a drug dose that has previously been helpful; more likely to occur when the drug has been taken for a long time; *cross-tolerance* is the same response to a similar drug.
5. *Idiosyncrasy*—an abnormal reaction to a drug; genetic factors have been suggested as being responsible.
6. *Physical dependence*—a condition in which a person experiences symptoms of withdrawal when a drug is discontinued.
7. *Side effects*—those responses that are unintended and unrelated to the purposes for which the drug was prescribed.
8. *Toxic effects*—those responses that result from accumulation of circulating drug; overdose.
9. *Other responses*. Unfavorable mental and emotional responses that impair benefits of drug therapy. Unfavorable social responses such as withdrawal from interaction with others, unbearable financial burden associated with drug therapy.

❏   Nursing Implications

Nursing implications is a term that describes how the nurse is expected to use information collected and organized about drug therapy to provide nursing care for the patient. For example, a nursing implication for a drug that causes gastrointestinal symptoms as a side effect could be to administer that drug either with meals or a snack. The nursing implications for a drug known to produce toxicity at a maintenance dose could be to teach the patient what, how, and when to report toxic symptoms.

Throughout this book, the student will notice that information about a drug includes examples of nursing implications. This is because the nurse is expected to have basic information about drugs and to use that information when providing nursing care. Thus, nursing implications can be thought of as a call for action and a guide to action by the nurse.

LANGUAGE AND SYMBOLS OF DRUG THERAPY

In studying drugs, drug therapy, and patient care, the student nurse needs to learn the language and symbols used by nurses, physicians, pharmacists, and other members of the health team. These language and symbols serve as a kind of shorthand way to communicate. Thus, in order to understand and use this communication, the student may study the common language and symbols listed below.

Use of Abbreviations

A number of abbreviations are used commonly in drug therapy. The nurse should become familiar with their meanings. The most commonly used abbreviations are listed in the table on page 20.

Abbreviation	Meaning	Abbreviation	Meaning
$\bar{a}$	Before	No.	Number
$\overline{aa}$	Of each	noct	Night
ac	Before meals	non rep	Do not repeat
ad lib	As desired	o	Every
agit	Shake or stir	OD	Right eye
aq	Water	OS	Left eye
bid	Twice a day	OU	Both eyes
bin	Twice a night	oz*	Ounce
BT	Bedtime	$\bar{p}$	After
$\bar{c}$	With	pc	After meals
cc	Cubic centimeter	PO	By mouth
caps	Capsule	prn	When required
comp	Compound	pt*	pint
dil	Dilute	qod	Every other day
disp	Dispense	qd	Every day
dr*	Dram	qh	Every night
elix	Elixir	q2h	Every 2 hours
et	And	q4h	Every 4 hours
fl, fld	Fluid	q6h	Every 6 hours
gal or C	Gallon	q12h	Every 12 hours
g	Gram	qid	Four times a day
gr*	Grain	qn	Every night
gtt*	Drop	qs	As much as is
h	hour		necessary
hs	hour of sleep	qt*	Quart
hypo	Hypodermic	Rx	Take
HT	Hypodermic	$\bar{s}$	Without
	tablet	SC	Subcutaneously
IM	Intramuscularly	sig	Write on label
IV	Intravenously	sol	Solution
kg	Kilogram	sos	If necessary (once only)
kl	Kiloliter	Sp	Spirit
km	Kilometer	$\overline{ss}$*	One half
m	Meter or mix	stat	Immediately
m.*	Minim	syr	Syrup
μg	Microgram	tab	Tablet
mg	Milligram	tid	Three times a day
ml	Milliliter	Tr or tinct	Tincture
mist	Mixture	ung	Ointment

*Abbreviations from the apothecaries' system.

SYMBOLS OF THE METRIC SYSTEM

The metric system is a system of weights and measurements in units of 10. The physician prescribes a dose of medication by writing how many units in the system are to be given. Although there are two systems, the metric system is preferred because it is considered more precise and it is in international use. The nurse must learn to use both systems of weights and measures because both are used in prescribing and administering drug therapy. Additional exercises to develop skill in using systems of weights and measures can be located in Section II.

Units and Symbols of the Metric System

Unit	Symbol/Abbreviation
Weights	
Gram	g
Milligram	mg
Microgram	µg
Kilogram	kg
Capacity Measurement (Wet)	
Liter	L
Cubic centimeter	cc
Milliliter	ml
Kiloliter	kl
Length	
Meter	m
Millimeter	mm
Kilometer	km

SYMBOLS OF THE APOTHECARIES' SYSTEM

The apothecaries' system is an old English system of weights and measures. The physician may prescribe a dose of medication in the apothecaries' system. In addition to abbreviations that have been starred in the list above, there are certain symbols used. These are listed in the table below.

Units and Symbols of the Apothecaries' System

Weights	
Unit	Symbol
Grain	gr
Dram	ℨ or dr
Ounce	℥ or oz
Pound	lb

Capacity Measurements (Wet)	
Unit	Symbol
Minim	m
Dram (fluidram)	ℨ or dr
Ounce (fluidounce)	℥ or oz
Pint	O
Quart	qt
Gallon	gal or C

Lengths	
Unit	Symbol
Inch	in.
Foot	ft
Yard	yd
Mile	mi

CASE STUDY 2

John Bishop is a practical nursing student who has been assigned to care for Miss Heidi Sue Mason, a 72-year-old woman with heart disease and hypertension. The physician's orders include:

- Weigh daily.
- Digoxin (Lanoxin) 0.25 mg PO qd
- Check daily for digitalis toxicity.
- Vital signs qid.
- Furosemide (Lasix) 40 mg ʒ.

QUESTIONS

1. For each of the drugs prescribed for Miss Mason, which is the nonproprietary name and which is the trade name?
2. Mr. Bishop has never heard of digoxin. What should he do?
3. What actions should Mr. Bishop take about the doctor's order for furosemide?
4. What responsibilities does Mr. Bishop have for the dosages of each drug prescribed for Miss Mason.
5. What information should Mr. Bishop have about each of the drugs before administering them? Where can this information be located.
6. What does the word *toxicity* mean?
7. List the factors in the case study that may influence the doses of drugs prescribed for Miss Mason.
8. Mr. Bishop learns that furosemide may produce depletion of potassium in the body. What are the nursing implications?
9. Define each of the symbols and abbreviations underlined in the case study.
10. After looking up each of the drugs prescribed for Miss Mason, Mr. Bishop learns that they may be administered by the oral, IM, and IV routes. What are the differences between these routes? What routes should Mr. Bishop select?
11. Describe each of the parts of a complete prescription and drug order.

Chapter 3 | NURSING SKILLS IN DRUG THERAPY

EXPECTED BEHAVIORAL OUTCOMES

After completing this chapter, you should return to the expected behavioral outcomes and evaluate your ability to:

1. Complete a systematic nursing assessment.
2. Communicate relevant oral and written information about drug therapy to the patient, family, and members of the health team.
3. Pour or prepare a drug without introducing unnecessary microorganisms.
4. Apply principles discussed in the chapter to use supplies and equipment for drug therapy in a safe, effective manner.
5. Store drugs safely and effectively.
6. Complete the arithmetic pretest with a score that demonstrates the skills sufficient to calculate dose with 100% accuracy.

NURSING ASSESSMENT

The nurse who participates in drug therapy needs to develop skill in making a nursing assessment. The word *assess* means to collect information and determine its significance. One part of assessment is observing the patient using a systematic method that includes listening, looking, touching, smelling, and asking questions. A second part of assessment is determining the significance of the information collected. In order to develop skill in making nursing assessments related to drug therapy, the nurse needs to know three things: what to look at, what to look for, and how to look for it.

In learning what to look at, the nurse assesses the whole person and considers the possible effects of drug therapy on that person. For example, the nurse may observe the patient's body to collect some information. For other kinds of information, the nurse may gather and appraise facts about the patient's *life-style* (usual way of living). For still other kinds of information, the nurse observes what the patient thinks, feels, wants, and believes. Observation of the patient's body enables the nurse to look for therapeutic and adverse effects of drug therapy. Appraisal of the patient's life-style, personal thoughts, feeling, and beliefs enables the nurse to select interventions likely to be helpful. This part of assessment is especially helpful in planning patient teaching about drug therapy.

In learning what to look for, the nurse builds on information about what is usual or expected for a particular patient. For example, a patient with infection is expected to have an elevated temperature. When administering an antibiotic, the nurse looks for changes in temperature as an indicator of the patient's response to drug therapy. If the temperature does not come down with drug therapy, the nurse knows that this is unexpected and reports the observation to the appropriate nurse or physician. A second building block in learning what to look for is information that the nurse collects about the particular drugs that have been prescribed. For example, the nurse who knows that nausea is a side effect of a particular drug specifically looks for evidence of that side effect. This may be done by observing the patient's meal tray to see how much food the patient has eaten and/or asking the patient about nausea.

In learning how to look, the nurse selects one systematic method and develops skill in using it. The method of observation of the body used most often in clinical practice is the head to toe method. The nurse looks, listens, touches, smells, and asks questions, starting with the patient's head and proceeding down the neck, trunk, and extremities. Tables 3–1 and 3–2 provide guides to the nurse in assessing the patient's body and life-style.

TABLE 3–1   A Head-to-Toe Guide for Nursing Observation

What to Observe	Observations
1. Head	
Hair	Combed or uncombed—clean or dirty
Eyes	Closed or open—puffy or sunken—reddened or yellowed sclera—wearing glasses, contact lens, or artificial eye—makes eye contact or avoids eye contact—brows knitted
Face	Shaved or unshaved
Mouth	Smiling, frowning, grimacing, breathes through mouth—lips moist or dry—color of lips—dentures present or absent—teeth clean or unclean—teeth present or absent—odor of breath—fetid, sweet, fruity—color of mucous membranes inside mouth
Nose	Breathes through nose—nostrils flaring—color reddened, pale
Speech	Talkative or silent, accent or language spoken, slurred speech, speaks very fast or very slow, initiates questions or discussion, responds only when spoken to, responses appropriate to conversation, doesn't speak
2. Neck and chest	Respirations rapid or slow, even or uneven, coughing—for a more detailed observation, see Chapter 14
3. Abdomen	Soft, taut, flat, distended
4. Extremities	Color, warmth, pulses present or absent, strong or weak, regular or irregular, body movements quick, slow, smooth, jerky, wringing hands. Fingernails and toenails clean or dirty, wears a prosthesis
5. Skin	Color, scars, warts, moles, wounds, freckles, birthmarks, operative scars, warm or cool to touch, moist or dry, perspiring, presence of body odor, clean or dirty
6. Posture	Erect or slumped, gait steady or unsteady, uses cane or walker
7. Dress	Comfortable, appropriate, color, clean, adequate for weather condition

Source: Reprinted with permission from Mason, M. A., and Bates, G. F., *Basic Medical-Surgical Nursing,* 5th ed. Macmillan, New York, 1984, p. 12.

Nursing assessment leads to a plan of action and steps to take in implementing that plan. This subject is discussed in greater detail in Chapter 4. In other words, the nurse first collects information, and then selects actions (interventions) based on an appraisal of that information. For example, Mrs. Alana, a student practical nurse, observed that a patient vomited two consecutive mornings after receiving a newly prescribed medication. Mrs. Alana's appraisal of this information was that it could represent a possible adverse drug response. She therefore took action by reporting the observation to the physician. The physician, in turn, changed the patient's medication and the vomiting stopped.

COMMUNICATION SKILLS IN DRUG THERAPY

A second skill that is important to the nurse who assists the patient receiving drug therapy is communication—the sending and receiving of messages between the patient, the nurse, the physician, the pharmacist, and other members of the health team. Successful communication about drug therapy includes spoken words, gestures, and written words and symbols. Safe and effective drug therapy requires the nurse to develop excellent communication skills. These skills include:

- The ability to read and understand basic information about the patient, the illness, and the drugs prescribed.
- The ability to send and receive accurate and complete messages that involve a wide variety of people such as the patient, family members, the physician, the pharmacist, and other nursing personnel.
- The ability to use the language of drug therapy with clarity and precision (see Chapter 2, pp. 20–21).

TABLE 3-2   Life-Style Guide

Health habits
    Eating and sleeping patterns
    Bowel and bladder habits
    Dental care
    Medical care
    Present medications
    Exercise patterns
Family relationships, role in family
    Family recreation patterns
    Type of dwelling occupied by family
Community relationships, hobbies or other interests
    Participation in community activities such as clubs, church, or po-
       litical involvement
Occupational relationships, type of work
    Work-related plans and goals

Source: Reprinted with permission from Mason, M. A., and Bates, G. F., *Basic Medical–Surgical Nursing*, 5th ed. Macmillan, New York, 1984, p. 13.

- The ability to report significant information to the appropriate health team member.
- The ability to record information related to drug therapy completely, accurately, and legibly.
- The ability to explain and translate technical information about drug therapy to the layperson.

SKILLS IN MEDICAL AND SURGICAL ASEPSIS DURING DRUG THERAPY

The nurse assisting the patient receiving drug therapy needs to be able to prepare, pour, and administer drug therapy without introducing unnecessary microorganisms. Thus the student nurse develops a practice of frequent handwashing. For drug therapy prescribed by the oral, topical, or rectal routes, the following actions help to avoid introducing unnecessary microorganisms:

1. Washing the hands before preparing the dosage.
2. Pouring the drug from its container to a cup without touching the medication with the hands.
3. Wearing gloves to administer topical or rectal medication.
4. Washing the hands between patients.

To prepare and administer drug therapy prescribed by the IM, SC, and IV routes, sterile technique and equipment are used. Additional information about these techniques can be located in Chapters 14 and 15.

USING SUPPLIES AND EQUIPMENT FOR DRUG THERAPY

The nurse uses a variety of supplies and equipment for administering drug therapy. For example, the soufflé and medicine cups shown in Figure 3-1 are used to administer oral medication. Figure 14-3 shows several kinds of syringes that may be used for parenteral injections. Chapter 15 contains several figures that demonstrate equipment that may be used for IV therapy. Since supplies and equipment are frequently updated by the manufacturer, the nurse needs to update information and skills on a regular basis. The following guidelines are suggested to help prevent errors and waste of supplies associated with accidental breakage or contamination:

1. Gather all supplies and equipment needed before preparing and/or pouring drug therapy.
2. Read *all* directions printed on packages of supplies *before* opening the package.
3. Read *all* directions *before* using a new piece of equipment.
4. Ask for a demonstration of correct use of new supplies or equipment. (Demonstrations may be provided by the manufacturer's representative, clinical instructor, charge nurse, in-service nurse, or other personnel who have been properly trained.)

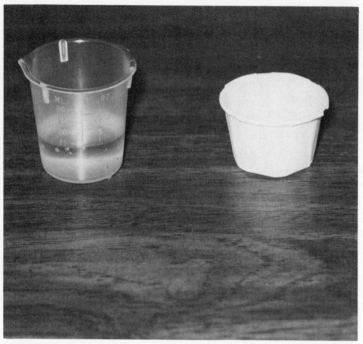

FIGURE 3-1   Supplies for administering oral medication. The medicine cup on the left is used for oral liquids; the soufflé cup on the right is used for oral solids.

5. Determine how to care for the supplies and equipment before using them (proper care should include how to troubleshoot minor problems).
6. Determine how to make the correct charge for the use of the supplies and equipment.

CARE AND STORAGE OF DRUGS IN THE HOSPITAL AND LONG-TERM CARE FACILITY

Most drugs in the hospital are stored in one of three places: a locked medicine cabinet or medicine room, a medicine cart such as the one shown in Figure 3-2, or the refrigerator. No matter where drugs are stored, the following precautions should be taken:

1. The area where drugs are stored should be locked and the key should be carried by a designated nurse.
2. Narcotics should be under double lock at all times.
3. Medicines should be arranged in an orderly manner. Medicines may be arranged in the following ways:
   a. Alphabetically—usually done when drugs are stored in a medicine cabinet.
   b. In individual patient compartments—see Figure 3-2.
   c. By storing solids in one area, liquids in another, and injectables in another.
   d. By similarity of action.
4. There should be separate storage places for external and internal drugs.
5. Every drug should have a clean label provided only by the pharmacy that contains the name of the drug, dosage strength, and route of administration.
6. The ordering of drugs should be the responsibility of a designated person such as the head nurse, medication nurse if appropriate, or pharmacist (in a unit dose delivery system).
7. The area where drugs are stored should be kept neat, clean, and free from visitors and unauthorized persons.
8. Drugs needing refrigeration such as oils, suppositories, and vaccines should be stored separately from food and drink items.

9. In general, drugs should be stored away from heat and light since these tend to speed up deterioration.
10. All poisons should be specially labeled.

CALCULATION OF DOSE

Drug manufacturers usually supply each drug in several strengths. For example, an oral tablet may be supplied by the manufacturer in tablets of 250- and 500-mg strengths. Often the strength of the medication supplied by the manufacturer is different from the dose prescribed by the physician. The nurse must then calculate how much of the drug supplied will be needed to give the exact amount prescribed by the physician. Accuracy is essential. An incorrect calculation may result in giving a patient too much or too little of the drug prescribed.

Calculation may also be needed when a prescribed drug is supplied by the manufacturer in a powder form. A solution must be added before the drug can be given. In this case, the nurse calculates the amount of solution that must be added to the powder in order to provide the dose prescribed by the physician.

A third time when calculation is needed occurs when the nurse must determine how fast (how many drops per minute) to administer IV solutions that contain electrolytes and/or drugs prescribed

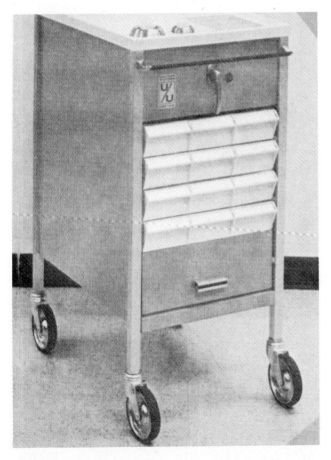

FIGURE 3-2 Example of one way in which drugs are stored in the hospital situation. Shown is the Parke, Davis Medication Cart with its individualized areas allowing each patient's drugs to be stored separately. (Courtesy of Parke, Davis and Co., Detroit, Mich.)

by the physician. Specific information about how to calculate drug dose can be located in Chapter 10. However, before this information can be used, two other skills are necessary. The first is to be able to use the language and symbols of drug therapy described in Chapter 2 on pp. 20–21. The student may wish to review those terms, symbols, and abbreviations now. The second skill is to be able to add, subtract, multiply, and divide whole numbers and fractions. An arithmetic pretest is provided at the end of Section I to help you evaluate your current skills. After completing the chapter, you should take the pretest and have it scored. If your score indicates a need for brush-up and practice, additional examples and practice are provided at the end of this book (Chapters 29–33).

CASE STUDY 3

Mr. Grant is an 82-year-old patient who was admitted to the hospital with a medical diagnosis of congestive heart failure. His color on admission was grayish, both feet were edematous, the lungs sounded congested, and the respiratory rate was 32 breaths/min and shallow. The apical rate was 110 and the skin was moist and cool. The physician's orders included:

- Digoxin 0.5 mg PO q4h × three doses then begin 0.25 mg PO qAM.
- Furosemide (Lasix) 40 mg IM now and 20 mg PO daily in AM beginning tomorrow.
- Weigh daily.
- Vital signs q3h.
- O$_2$ by nasal prongs 3 L/min.

QUESTIONS

1. Using the guide provided in the chapter and a head-to-toe method, select information from the case study that should be included in a nursing observation.
2. Using the physician's order for digoxin, prepare an oral statement that describes the purpose of this drug to a patient or family member.
3. How would you prepare a dose of digoxin without introducing unnecessary microorganisms?
4. Imagine that you are preparing an intramuscular injection of Lasix as ordered by the physician in the case study. If the equipment to be used for the injection (needle and syringe) was unfamiliar to you, what principles could you use as a guide to safe and effective practice?
5. How should digoxin and furosemide (Lasix) be stored?

Chapter 4 | THE NURSING PROCESS IN DRUG THERAPY

EXPECTED BEHAVIORAL OUTCOMES

After completing this chapter, you should return to the expected behavioral outcomes and evaluate your ability to:

1. Collect a drug history.
2. Write nursing goals and objectives related to drug therapy.
3. Describe the components of nursing orders.
4. Give an example of a nursing action related to drug therapy for each of the categories of implementation phase described in the chapter.
5. Describe what happens in the evaluation/revision phase of the nursing process.

As the roles and responsibilities of the nurse multiplied and became more complex, it was necessary to use a more systematic method of caring for the patient. That systematic method has come to be known as the *nursing* process. Nursing process is composed of several interrelated steps or phases.

I. Nursing assessment
   A. The nurse collects information from the patient, family, medical history, laboratory and x-ray studies, and nursing observations.
   B. Information is collected about past and present experiences with health and illness, and usual self-care practices related to health and illness.
   C. The *drug history* is part of this phase of the nursing history. Information is collected about past and present practices related to prescribed and nonprescribed drugs. The nurse asks about specific drugs such as laxatives, sleeping aids, cold remedies, painkillers, and alcohol (see Table 4–1). The drug history may be used by the nurse in several different ways including:
      1. To find out what the patient already knows as a basis for planning patient teaching.
      2. To correct wrong information the patient may have about drugs that are being taken.
      3. To anticipate potential problems in drug therapy.
      4. To prevent allergic reactions to drug therapy.
      5. To prevent other adverse drug reactions as described on pp. 18–19.
      6. To suggest nondrug alternatives for the patient who uses nonprescribed medication (over-the-counter medication). For example, nondrug alternatives may be suggested to promote restful sleep, healthy bowel function, weight loss, and similar activities of daily living.
      7. To identify and report previously unknown symptoms and/or illness.
   D. The nurse determines the significance of the information collected.

TABLE 4–1   Questions Included in the Drug History

1. What medicines and/or herbs are you taking at this time?
   a. What is the medicine (herb) for?
   b. How much do you take?
   c. How often do you take it?
   d. Are there special directions for taking it?
   e. Have you had any trouble as a result of taking this medicine?
2. As you think about or picture *all* the places where you keep medicines, what is on the shelf that you haven't already told me about?
3. Do you buy medicine at the drugstore for any of the following reasons? (For each nonprescribed drug taken, ask questions b through e from question 1.)
   a. Headache.
   b. Arthritis pain.
   c. To help you calm down—calm your nerves.
   d. Sleep.
   e. Help the bowels move or stop diarrhea.
   f. Acid indigestion.
   g. Vitamins.
   h. To lose weight.
   i. For a tonic.
   j. Menstrual cramps.
   k. To cure a cold.
   l. Allergy.
   m. Cough.
   n. Motion sickness.
4. Have you ever had an allergic reaction to a drug?
   a. What was the drug?
   b. What happened during the reaction?
5. About how many drinks do you have each day or week? (Include beer and wine.)
6. Do you take any other drugs that haven't come up in this discussion?

   II. Nursing diagnosis.
   A. The professional nurse makes a judgment and writes a description of a potential or actual deficit in self-care that can be helped by choosing and using specific nursing actions.
   B. The licensed practical nurse/licensed vocational nurse (LPN/LVN) contributes information for the nursing diagnosis and helps to select and implement nursing actions after the diagnosis has been made.
   C. The nursing diagnosis is made in light of information collected during the nursing assessment.
   III. Nursing goals and objectives.
   A. Nursing goals and objectives are statements about what will be achieved as a result of nursing care.
   B. Usually the nurse and the patient work together to establish the goals and objectives of nursing care.
   C. Goals are usually thought of as broader statements: By discharge, the patient will be able to take prescribed medications safely and correctly.
   D. Objectives may be viewed as smaller parts of the goal:
      1. The patient will be able to describe the name and purpose of each drug to be taken at home.
      2. For each drug to be taken, the patient will be able to describe how much is to be taken (dose), how often it is to be taken (frequency), warning signals (adverse drug responses), the proper storage precautions and foods, fluids, and activities to include and/or avoid in conjunction with taking the particular drug.
      3. The patient will be able to describe action steps to be taken if warning signals occur.
   IV. Implementation
   A. Implementation phase consists of nursing actions that will be done to help the patient reach the desired goal.
   B. Nursing actions may be called nursing orders.

C. *Nursing orders* are written statements about what is to be done to reach the goal, how often it is to be done, by whom it is to be done, and for how long it is to be done.
  1. LPN/LVN to demonstrate pouring of liquid medication at the bedside for two consecutive doses.
  2. LPN/LVN to observe patient pouring liquid medication at the bedside for three consecutive doses.
  3. The primary nurse to discuss name and action of each prescribed drug.
D. Nursing actions (nursing orders) can be placed in several broad categories for the convenience of the nurse in considering all possible actions available to reach the nursing goals and objectives. Some examples of nursing actions in each category are listed below.
  1. Developing a therapeutic relationship—actions that allow the patient to benefit from the nurse's caring.
    a. Active listening to the patient's reports about prescribed drugs.
    b. Meeting the patient's needs promptly.
    c. Calling the patient by name.
    d. Explaining tests, treatments, drug therapy in a positive or neutral way.
  2. Maintaining safety and security—actions that promote the patient's safety and prevent accidents.
    a. Raising the bedrails after administering a sedative.
    b. Placing the call bell within easy reach.
    c. Positioning the patient correctly for drug therapy.
    d. Assisting the patient to put on eyeglasses before teaching him or her how to read drug labels.
    e. Identifying the patient correctly before administering drug therapy.
  3. Assisting with foods and fluid intake—actions that relate to the influence of food and fluids on drug activity.
    a. Force fluids.
    b. Give medications after meals.
    c. Do not give antacids with water.
  4. Assisting with elimination—actions that relate to the effect of drug therapy on urinary and fecal elimination and the excretion of drugs through the urine.
    a. Measure and record intake and output q8h.
    b. Hemetest all stools for occult blood (some drugs are known to cause gastrointestinal bleeding as an adverse drug response).
    c. Report constipation or diarrhea (drug therapy often causes changes in normal bowel habits as a side effect).
  5. Assisting with ambulation, exercise, and positioning—actions that relate to the powerful impact of drug therapy on movement and position.
    a. Watch for *postural hypotension* (a sudden drop in blood pressure when the patient stands up—may cause dizziness and fainting).
    b. Instruct the patient to change position slowly.
    c. Position patient in semi-Fowler's position to swallow oral medication.
    d. Instruct the patient not to drive for 2 h after taking certain sedatives.
    e. Observe patient for extreme restlessness. High metabolic activity causes the body to use some drugs up more rapidly. An increase in dose may be indicated.
  6. Assisting with hygiene—actions that relate to the influence of drug therapy on personal hygiene needs.
    a. Oral hygiene q3h (for drugs that cause either drying of the mucous membranes or increased sputum production).
    b. Offer urinal q2h (for drugs that cause an increase in the production and/or excretion of urine).
    c. Place extra tissues at the bedside (for drugs that cause the patient to cough and expectorate more mucus).
  7. Maintaining asepsis—actions that relate to the need to prevent introduction of unnecessary microorganisms during drug therapy.

  a. Wash the hands between caring for different patients.
  b. If eyedrops are to be administered to both eyes, wash the hands again before placing drops in the second eye.
  c. Avoid resting drug therapy supplies and equipment used in caring for one patient on the bedside table of another patient.
V. Evaluation and revision.
  A. During this phase a judgment is made about whether or not the nursing goals and objectives have been achieved.
  B. If the goals and objectives have been reached, the nurse and the patient then work out a new set of goals and objectives.
  C. If the goals and objectives have not been reached, nursing personnel analyze why and make necessary adjustments.

CASE STUDY 4

Joan Guerro is a 21-year-old student nurse who was seen in the school clinic for a possible urinary tract infection. The LPN/LVN who was assigned to Ms. Guerro collected the following information during the nursing history:

1. Reason for seeking assistance. Burning on urination began about 24 h ago and has been getting worse. Last night, noticed increasing urgency, frequency, and pain (woke up to urinate at least four times during the night). This morning, noticed blood in the urine and decided to see a physician.

2. Usual self-care practices. Usually voids upon awakening. Often postpones urination after the voiding sensation is felt due to involvement with either patient care or class. Does not usually get up at night to void. No special perineal hygiene practices.

3. Drug history. ALLERGIC TO PENICILLIN. Takes birth control pills daily (does not know what brand—will ask roommate to bring in this afternoon). Occasionally takes aspirin for headache (no more than two aspirins per month). Uses nonprescribed feminine hygiene spray on weekends and daily during menstruation.

After the nursing history was obtained, the nursing diagnosis made by the primary nurse in the clinic was: Ineffective self-care practices related to urinary elimination and perineal hygiene due to knowledge deficit. The medical diagnosis was urinary tract infection. The physician's orders included:

- Collect urine for culture and sensitivities.
- Sulfisoxazole (Gantrisin) 2g PO *stat* and 1g PO q4h.
- Force fluids to 3 L/day.

Questions

1. Identify the first phase in the nursing process and list the information provided in the case study that illustrates this phase.
2. What is the difference between the nursing diagnosis and the medical diagnosis?
3. Underline the information in the case study that led to the nursing diagnosis.
4. Imagine that you are the nurse caring for Joan Guerro. Give an example of a nursing goal and objectives appropriate to her plan of care.
5. Using the guide provided in the chapter, write at least two nursing orders related to drug therapy prescribed for Joan Guerro.
6. How will the nursing staff know if the plan of care has been successful?
7. In the nursing process, what happens after evaluation?

ARITHMETIC PRETEST

Directions: In order to administer drugs safely, you must be able to solve basic arithmetic problems. This pretest is designed to assess your knowledge and skill in this area. Solve each of the following problems and circle the correct answer. After the problems have been corrected, you may need an arithmetic review. This can be located in Chapters 29 to 33.

1. 876.4×12

     a. 951.68   **b.** 10,516.8   **c.** 1,051.68   **d.** 11,615.8   **e.** 10,518

2. Change 2% to a fraction.

     a. ½   **b.** ⅕   **c.** ⅒   **d.** 1/50   **e.** 2/10

3. $0.2 \times 1,000$

     a. 2,000   **b.** 500   **c.** 20   **d.** 2   **e.** 200

4. Write the Roman numeral XXV in arabic numerals.

     a. 15   **b.** 25   **c.** 7   **d.** 3   **e.** 250

5. $5.2 \div 6.5$

     a. 0.8   **b.** 8   **c.** 0.008   **d.** 0.08   **e.** 1.25

6. Change ⅕ to percent

     a. 20%   **b.** 5%   **c.** 40%   **d.** 10%   **e.** 25%

7. How many milliliters in one L?

     a. .1   **b.** .01   **c.** 1,000   **d.** 100   **e.** 10

8. 22.5×1.105

     a. 2.4862   **b.** 24.8625   **c.** 22.505   **d.** 2.21   **e.** 25.875

9. $4\frac{1}{8} \times 6\frac{1}{2}$

     a. 24½   **b.** 32   **c.** 48¼   **d.** 26¹³/₁₆   **e.** 24¹/₁₆

10. $\frac{1}{2} \div \frac{1}{8}$

     a. 2   **b.** ¹/₁₆   **c.** 4   **d.** 8   **e.** ¼

11. 0.008×0.06

     a. 0.00048   **b.** 48   **c.** 0.0014   **d.** 4.8000   **e.** 0.0048

12. Change ¼% to a ratio

     a. 1:2   **b.** 1:20   **c.** 1:4   **d.** 1:200   **e.** 1:400

13. What do 32 oz equal?

     a. 1 qt   **b.** 1 pt   **c.** 1 gal   **d.** 1 dr   **e.** 1 lb

14. Change the fraction ¼ to a decimal.

     a. 0.4   **b.** 0.1   **c.** 0.25   **d.** 0.04   **e.** 0.20

15. Change 80% to a fraction.

     a. ⅛   **b.** ⅕   **c.** ¼   **d.** ⅘   **e.** ⅞

16. $4,684 \div 0.02$

     a. 2.342   **b.** 24.32   **c.** 234.2   **d.** 1.322   **e.** 234,200

17. Change 5% to a decimal.

     a. 0.5   **b.** 0.1   **c.** 0.2   **d.** 0.05   **e.** 5.0

18. Approximately how many milliliters in 8 fl oz?

a. 100 **b.** 240 **c.** 500 **d.** 30 **e.** 4

19. Change 0.5% to a decimal.

a. 5 **b.** 0.1 **c.** 0.05 **d.** 0.005 **e.** 2

20. $4.50 \div 0.5$

a. 90 **b.** 0.09 **c.** 0.9 **d.** 8.5 **e.** 9

21. $4\frac{1}{2} \times 1\frac{1}{2}$

a. $8\frac{1}{2}$ **b.** $5\frac{1}{2}$ **c.** $6\frac{2}{3}$ **d.** $6\frac{1}{4}$ **e.** $6\frac{3}{4}$

22. $8,407 \times 0.40$

a. 83.67 **b.** 2,562.80 **c.** 2,652.80 **d.** 25,628 **e.** 3362.8

23. $0.2 \div 0.004$

a. 50 **b.** 0.5 **c.** 0.005 **d.** 0.05 **e.** 0.02

24. $\frac{7}{8} \div \frac{1}{4}$

a. $\frac{1}{2}$ **b.** $1\frac{1}{4}$ **c.** $3\frac{1}{2}$ **d.** $3\frac{1}{8}$ **e.** $\frac{7}{32}$

25. What is the approximate equivalent of 16 oz?

a. 480 ml **b.** 1 L **c.** 1 kl **d.** 0.5 μL **e.** 2 ml

26. $640 \div 0.08$

a. 8,000 **b.** 80 **c.** 75 **d.** 7.5 **e.** 0.000125

27. Change 4% to a decimal.

a. 0.8 **b.** 0.004 **c.** 0.4 **d.** 0.2 **e.** 0.04

28. $6\frac{1}{2} \div 1\frac{1}{3}$

a. $8\frac{2}{3}$ **b.** $7\frac{1}{2}$ **c.** $4\frac{7}{8}$ **d.** $5\frac{1}{2}$ **e.** $8\frac{3}{9}$

29. $\frac{1,500,000}{3,000,000} \times 15$

a. 0.9 **b.** 2.5 **c.** 0.75 **d.** 0.5 **e.** 7.5

30. $16 \div 0.8$

a. 2 **b.** 20 **c.** 0.002 **d.** 2,000 **e.** 0.05

31. What is the equivalent of 1 m?

a. 0.039 in. **b.** 1 in. **c.** 39.370 in. **d.** 36.380 in. **e.** 3.937 in.

32. $\frac{40}{80} \times 16$

a. $\frac{5}{8}$ **b.** $\frac{1}{8}$ **c.** 4 **d.** 8 **e.** 32

33. What is the approximate equivalent of 1,000 ml?

a. 1 gal **b.** 1 qt **c.** $\frac{1}{2}$ gal **d.** 1 pt **e.** 10 qt

34. $14\frac{1}{2} \times 2\frac{1}{4}$

a. $30\frac{1}{16}$ **b.** $28\frac{1}{8}$ **c.** $29\frac{1}{8}$ **d.** $30\frac{1}{2}$ **e.** $32\frac{5}{8}$

35. $6 \div \frac{1}{3}$

a. 3 **b.** $\frac{1}{18}$ **c.** 18 **d.** 19 **e.** 2

36. At the drugstore you were sold 14 penicillin capsules for $5.60. How much did one capsule cost?

a. 30¢ **b.** 60¢ **c.** 46¢ **d.** 36¢ **e.** 40¢

37. In your first summer job you were paid $3.35 per hour and worked 5½ eight-hour days per week. How much was your first paycheck?

a. $134.00 **b.** $143.00 **c.** $26.80 **d.** $18.42 **e.** $147.40

38. What part of a 5-gr aspirin tablet would you use in order to give 2 gr?

a. $\frac{1}{5}$ **b.** $\frac{3}{5}$ **c.** $\frac{4}{5}$ **d.** $\frac{2}{5}$ **e.** 2

39. You have a cold and the doctor suggests that you increase your fluid intake to include 8 oz of fluid every 3 h. How much fluid would you drink at one time?

a. 1 glassful **b.** 1 pt **c.** 1 teacupful **d.** 0.5 L **e.** 1 qt

40. You won a $2,000 scholarship and found you had to spend $400 for textbooks. What percent of your scholarship did you spend for books?

a. 2% **b.** 20% **c.** 40% **d.** 5% **e.** 25%

41. Which fraction is the largest?

a. $\frac{1}{2}$ **b.** $\frac{1}{8}$ **c.** $\frac{1}{3}$ **d.** $\frac{1}{4}$ **e.** $\frac{1}{16}$

42. If fresh orange juice sold for 84¢ a half-gallon, how much would 1 pt cost?

a. 24¢ **b.** 42¢ **c.** 18¢ **d.** 12¢ **e.** 21¢

43. If your salary is $17,600 per year, what is your approximate weekly salary?

a. $733.33 **b.** $676.92 **c.** $338.46 **d.** $352.00 **e.** $1466.67

44. If you were asked to take 1 oz of a medication and did not have a measuring glass, which of the following measures would give you the approximate dose?

a. 1 tsp **b.** 1 tbsp **c.** 3 tsp **d.** 2 tbsp **e.** 2 tsp

45. The label on the aspirin bottle reads grains v. The doctor's prescription reads aspirin grains xv every 4 h. How many of the tablets should you take?

a. 2 **b.** 5 **c.** 4 **d.** 3 **e.** 1½

46. The patient's bill was $1,300 and the insurance company paid $780. What percent of the bill was the patient responsible for paying?

a. 60% **b.** 20% **c.** 30% **d.** 45% **e.** 40%

47. The label on the bottle reads 0.5 g of medication and the doctor ordered 0.25 g. How many of the tablets in the bottle should be given?

a. 5 **b.** 2 **c.** $\frac{1}{4}$ **d.** $\frac{1}{2}$ **e.** 4

48. If you paid 75¢ for a packet of pencils and $1.25 for a packet of lined paper, what percent of a $5.00 bill would you spend?

a. 20% **b.** 50% **c.** 15% **d.** 40% **e.** 25%

49. If you earn $800 per month and your budget includes $200 for rent, $160 for food, $60 for utilities, $80 for car payments, and $100 for insurance and incidentals, what percent of your salary would you have left for savings?

a. 25% b. 20% c. 6% d. 5% e. 75%

50. The nurses on a maternity unit recorded information on live births for 1 year. The ratio of premature to normal term births was 2:7. If there were 1,204 live births during that year, how many babies were premature?

a. 241 b. 344 c. 301 d. 349 e. 172

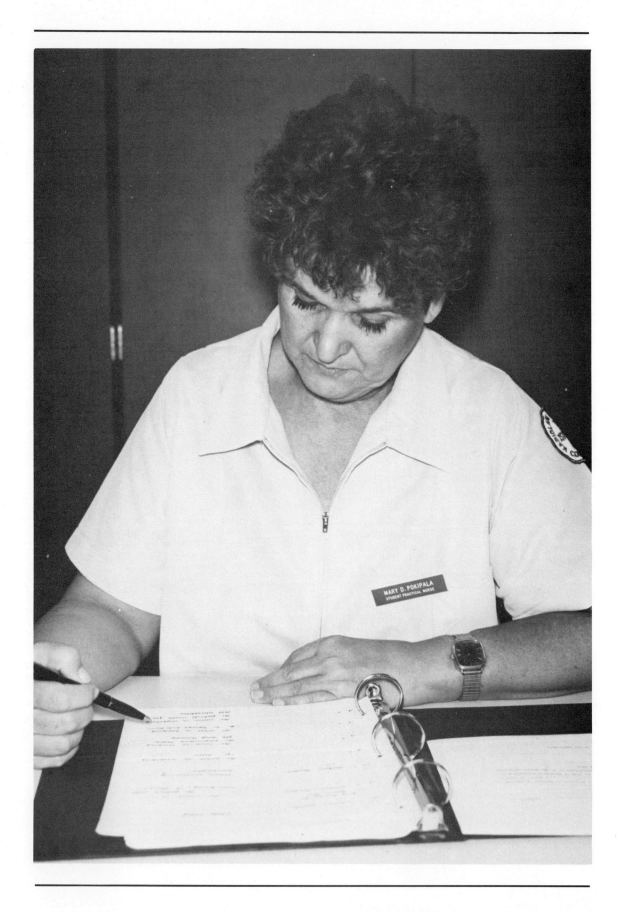

Section II

MEASUREMENTS

Chapter 5 | TEMPERATURE CONVERSION

EXPECTED BEHAVIORAL OUTCOMES

After completing this chapter, you should return to the expected behavioral outcomes and evaluate your ability to:

1. Convert a temperature reading in the Fahrenheit system to the centigrade system.
2. Convert a temperature reading in the centigrade system to the Fahrenheit system.
3. Identify the freezing and boiling points in both the centigrade and Fahrenheit systems.

Taking a patient's temperature is a common procedure performed many times a day by the nurse at the bedside. In most hospitals, the Fahrenheit (F) thermometer is used. However, an increasing number of hospitals use a thermometer calibrated with the centigrade (C) scale. This scale is also known as the Celsius scale. It is widely used in Europe.

Occasionally, the nurse may be in a situation in which it is necessary to convert a reading from one scale to another. In such situations, it is helpful to know how this is done. Figure 5-1 compares the characteristics of the Fahrenheit and centigrade scales. The differences in boiling points and freezing points in each system have been used to form an equation that allows the conversion of readings from one system to another (Table 5-1).

1. To change a centigrade reading to the Fahrenheit scale, use the following equation:

$$\frac{\text{difference between boiling and freezing F (180)}}{\text{difference between boiling and freezing C (100)}} \times \text{centigrade reading} + 32 =$$

or

$$\left(\frac{9}{5} \times \text{centigrade reading}\right) + 32 =$$

EXAMPLE: To change 60° centigrade to Fahrenheit:

$$\left(\frac{9}{5} \times 60\right) + 32 =$$

$$\frac{9}{5} \times 60 = 108 + 32 = 140°F$$

2. To change a Fahrenheit reading to the centigrade scale, use the following equation:

$$\frac{\text{difference between boiling and freezing C (100)}}{\text{difference between boiling and freezing F (180)}} \times \text{Fahrenheit reading} - 32 =$$

or

$$\frac{5}{9} \times (\text{Fahrenheit reading} - 32) =$$

EXAMPLE: To change 140° Fahrenheit to centigrade:

$$\frac{5}{9} \times (140 - 32) =$$

$$\frac{5}{9} \times 108 = 60°C$$

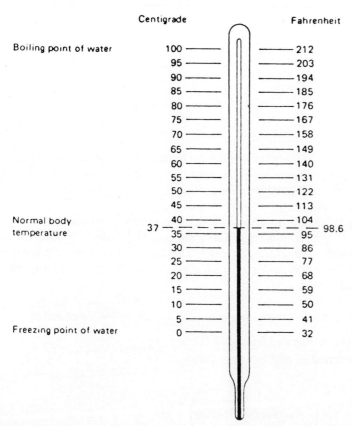

FIGURE 5-1 Thermometer showing a comparison of the Centigrade and Fahrenheit scales of heat.

TABLE 5–1 Characteristics of the Fahrenheit and Centigrade Systems

Characteristic	Fahrenheit	Centigrade
Boiling point	212°	100°
Freezing point	32°	0°
Difference between boiling and freezing points	180°	100°

3. Conversion exercises. Convert the following temperatures to the scale indicated:

1. 40°C = _____ °F.
2. 38°C = _____ °F.
3. 37°C = _____ °F.
4. 36.5°C = _____ °F.
5. 36°C = _____ °F.

6. 99°F = _____ °C.
7. 98°F = _____ °C.
8. 101°F = _____ °C.
9. 100°F = _____ °C.
10. 103°F = _____ °C.

Chapter 6 | THE METRIC SYSTEM

EXPECTED BEHAVIORAL OUTCOMES

After completing this chapter, you should return to the expected behavioral outcomes and evaluate your ability to:

1. Identify the units of length, weight, and capacity in the metric system.
2. Multiply and divide decimals to solve problems within the metric system.

UNITS IN THE METRIC SYSTEM

This system could be termed a system of decimals, since fractional and multiple parts of a unit are written as decimals. The units of measurement of the metric system are:

1. Unit of length = meter.
2. Unit of weight = gram.
3. Unit of capacity = liter.

Multiples and fractions of a unit are expressed by prefixes.

Table 6–1 illustrates prefixes used to designate multiples or fractions of a unit. Table 6–2 illustrates terms used for each unit in the metric system.

TABLE 6–1 Prefixes in the Metric System

Prefix	Decimal Equivalent	Examples
Kilo	One thousand (1,000)	Kilogram (one thousand grams)
Hecto	One hundred (100)	Hectometer (one hundred meters)
Deca	Ten (10)	Decaliter (ten liters)
Deci	One-tenth (0.1)	Decimeter (one-tenth of a meter)
Centi	One one-hundredth (0.01)	Centiliter (one one-hundredth of a liter)
Milli	One one-thousandth (0.001)	Milligram (one one-thousandth of a gram)

Review of Arithmetic for the Metric System

1. The ''decimal'' is based on the number 10.
2. The decimal point is a dot.
3. The numbers to the left of the dot or decimal point are whole numbers.
4. The numbers written to the right of the decimal point are decimals or fractional parts of a whole.

5. If the decimal point is moved to the right, the value is multiplied by 10.
  EXAMPLE: 0.1 (is one-tenth)
       1. (is one; the decimal point has been moved one place to the right, multiplying one tenth ten times)
6. If the decimal point is moved one place to the left, the value is divided by 10.
  EXAMPLE: 1. (is one—an entire unit)
       0.1 (is one-tenth; the decimal point has been moved one place to the left, thus dividing one or a whole unit into ten parts)

CONVERTING FROM ONE MEASURE TO ANOTHER IN THE METRIC SYSTEM

1. To convert from a larger measure to a smaller measure, *multiply*.
  EXAMPLE: To change 2 g to milligrams:
The multiplier must be obtained from the table. The multiplier in this case is 1,000, because there are 1,000 mg in 1 g. It is necessary to multiply because milligrams are smaller than grams.

$$2 \text{ g} \times 1,000 = 2,000 \text{ mg.*}$$

2. To convert from a smaller measure to a larger measure, *divide*.
  EXAMPLE: To change 3,000 ml to liters:
Again the divisor must be obtained from the table. Liters are larger than milliliters, so it is necessary to divide. The divisor is 1,000, because there are 1,000 ml in 1 L.

$$3,000 \text{ ml} \div 1,000 = 3 \text{ L.*}$$

Table 6–2 Metric Tables

Metric Table of Weight (Dry)*
1,000 micrograms (μg) = 1 milligram (mg)
1,000 milligrams (mg) = 1 gram (g)
1,000 grams (g) = 1 kilogram (kg)

Metric Table of Volume Capacity (Wet)†
1,000 milliliters (ml) = 1 liter (L)
1,000 cubic centimeters (cc) = 1 liter (L)
1,000 liters (L) = 1 kiloliter (kL)

Metric Table of Length‡
1,000 millimeters (mm) = 1 meter (m)
1,000 meters (m) = 1 kilometer (km)

*Note: Pills, tablets, capsules (containing powdered medicines), and powders may be measured this way.

†Note: Elixirs, emulsions, fluidextracts, milks, syrups, and solutions are measured in this way. For more complete tables, please see pp. 52–53. The tables also include the apothecaries' system equivalents.

‡Patients, such as newborn infants, may be measured in this way.

 Note: To multiply by 1,000 move the decimal point three places to the right: 2 g = 2,000 mg. To divide by 1,000 move the decimal point three places to the left: 3,000 ml = 3 L.

METRIC QUIZ

Convert the following:

1. 0.5 L   = _____ ml.
2. 30 mg   = _____ g.
3. 5,000 m   = _____ km.
4. 200 mm   = _____ m.
5. 0.25 L   = _____ ml.
6. 2 km   = _____ m.
7. 100 mg   = _____ g.
8. 700 m   = _____ km.
9. 250 mg   = _____ g.
10. 5.5 L   = _____ kL.
11. 2 mg   = _____ g.
12. 0.0003 g = _____ mg.
13. 500 mg   = _____ g.
14. 3,750 ml = _____ L.
15. 2.5 L   = _____ ml.
16. 5,500 ml = _____ L.
17. 125 ml   = _____ L.
18. 0.025 g   = _____ mg.
19. 1.5 g   = _____ mg.
20. 6,000 L   = _____ kL.
21. 1,000 mm = _____ m.
22. 0.65 g   = _____ mg.
23. 0.0025 g = _____ mg.
24. 300 ml   = _____ L.
25. 2,500 g   = _____ kg.
26. 0.75 g   = _____ mg.
27. 2,000 ml = _____ L.
28. 60 mg   = _____ g.
29. 3.5 g   = _____ kg.
30. 1,500 L   = _____ kL.

Chapter 7 | THE APOTHECARIES' SYSTEM

EXPECTED BEHAVIORAL OUTCOMES

After completing this chapter, you should return to the expected behavioral outcomes and evaluate your ability to:

1. Identify the units of length, weight, and capacity in the apothecaries' system.
2. Multiply and divide fractions to solve problems within the apothecaries' system.

THE APOTHECARIES' SYSTEM

Units in the Apothecaries' System

The apothecaries' system is very old (Table 7–1). It is a system in which abbreviations and symbols are generally used to write amounts. Roman numerals frequently are used to express whole numbers, and fractions are used to denote the parts of a whole. Included in this chapter are the English units of length. A patient's body length may be measured by the units included in Table 7–1.

Review of Special Abbreviations

1. $\overline{ss}$ is used to express the fraction ½.
2. gr is used to express grain—a small "g" is always used.
3. gtt is used to express drop. (Medications are occasionally ordered to be given in drops. This is not an equivalent term for minim. It is an approximate equivalent.)

Converting from One Measure to Another in the Apothecaries' System

1. To convert from a larger measure to a smaller measure multiply. The multiplier must be obtained from Table 7–2.

EXAMPLE: To convert ʒii (2 dr) to grains:

Grains are smaller than drams, so it is necessary to multiply. There are 60 gr in 1 dr, therefore:

$$2 \text{ dr} \times 60 = 120 \text{ gr in 2 dr}$$

TABLE 7–1　Units and Symbols of the Apothecaries' System

Weights

Unit	Symbol
Grain	gr
Dram	ʒ or dr
Ounce	℥ or oz
Pound	lb

Capacity Measurements (Wet)

Unit	Symbol
Minim	m
Dram (fluidram)	ʒ or dr
Ounce (fluidounce)	℥ or oz
Pint	O
Quart	qt
Gallon	gal or C

Lengths

Unit	Symbol
Inch	in.
Foot	ft
Yard	yd
Mile	mi

TABLE 7–2　Apothecaries' Table

Apothecaries' Table of Weight Measure (Dry)

60 grains (gr)	1 dram or ʒi
8 drams (dr)	1 ounce or ℥i
12 ounces (oz)	1 pound or lb

Apothecaries' Table of Capacity (Wet)

60 minims (m.)	1 fluidram or ʒi
8 drams (dr)	1 fluidounce or ℥i
16 ounces (oz)	1 pint or O
2 pints or 32 ounces (pt)	1 quart (qt)
4 quarts (qt)	1 gallon (gal or C)

English Units of Length*

12 inches (in.)	1 foot
36 inches (in.)	1 yard
3 feet (ft)	1 yard
5,280 feet (ft)	1 mile
1,760 yards (yd)	1 mile

*The system of length widely used in the United States. It is expected that it will be replaced shortly by the metric system (see p. 21).

2. To convert a smaller measure to a larger measure, divide. The divisor must be obtained from Table 7–2.

EXAMPLE: To convert ℥ xvi to ounces:

Ounces are larger than drams, so it is necessary to divide. There are 8 dr in 1 oz, therefore:

$$16 \text{ dr} \div 8 = 2 \text{ oz}$$

APOTHECARIES' SYSTEM QUIZ

Convert the following:

1. 4 ft   = _____in.
2. ℥ ii   = gr_____.
3. ℥ ss̄   = ʒ_____.
4. 18 in.   = _____ft.
5. ʒ vi   = ℥_____.
6. ℥ iv   = gr_____.
7. gr XLV   = ʒ_____.
8. 2,640 ft   = _____mi.
9. gr cxx   = ʒ_____.
10. ℥ xvi   = ℥_____.
11. 72 in.   = _____yd.
12. gr XC   = ʒ_____.
13. ℥ xxxii   = _____pt.
14. ℥ xvi   = _____pt.
15. 3 yd   = _____ft.
16. gr xxx   = ʒ_____.
17. ℥ iv   = ʒ_____.
18. 3.5 ft   = _____in.
19. gr CLXXX   = ʒ_____.
20. ℥ vi   = gr_____.
21. 0.25 mi   = _____ft.
22. ℥ i   = gr_____.
23. ℥ iii   = m._____.
24. 6 ft   = _____yd.
25. ℥ ss̄   = gr_____.
26. ℥ ii   = gr_____.
27. 18 in.   = _____yd.
28. ℥ viii   = _____pt.
29. ℥ viii   = ℥_____.
30. 24 in.   = _____yd.

Chapter 8 | CONVERTING UNITS OF ONE SYSTEM TO ANOTHER

EXPECTED BEHAVIORAL OUTCOMES

After completing this chapter, you should return to the expected behavioral outcomes and evaluate your ability to:

1. Remember common approximate equivalents of length, weight, and capacity in the metric and apothecaries' systems.
2. Convert units of one system to approximate equivalents in another.
3. Complete the Measurements Quiz at the end of this section (see pp. 57–60) with a passing score as determined by your instructor.

It is sometimes necessary to convert units from one system of weights and measures to another system in order to administer the dosage prescribed by the physician. When converting from one system to another, *approximate equivalents* are used. Table 8–1 contains approximate equivalents frequently used to convert units from one system to the other. Table 8–2 contains the complete list of equivalents. Exact equivalents must be used when compounding a prescription, a procedure that should be performed only by a registered pharmacist.

PROCEDURE FOR CONVERTING FROM ONE SYSTEM TO ANOTHER

1. Learn some of the approximate equivalents in length, capacity, and weight for each system (see Tables 8–1, 8–2).
2. Set up a simple proportion:

$$\frac{mg}{metric} : \frac{gr}{apothecaries'} = \frac{mg}{metric} : \frac{gr}{apothecaries'}$$

3. Place the numbers you are seeking on one side of the equation.
4. Place the approximate equivalents on the other side of the equation.
5. Change all fractions to decimals.
6. Solve the equation for the unknown quantity (usually called x), by multiplying the means and the extremes.

EXAMPLE: To convert gr ½ to milligrams:

$$60 \text{ mg}:1 \text{ gr} = x \text{ mg}:0.5 \text{ gr}$$
$$1x = 60 \times 0.5 \ (30)$$
$$x = 30 \text{ mg}$$

TABLE 8–1 Common Approximate Equivalents

Measuring Unit	Approximate Equivalent
Metric System	**Apothecaries' System**
1 m	1/60 gr
1 g	15 gr
1 ml	15 m.
Apothecaries' System	**Metric System**
1 gr	60 mg
1 oz	30 g
1 m	0.06 ml
1 fl oz	30 ml
1 pt	500 ml
1 qt	1,000 ml*
English Units	**Metric System**
1 in.	2.5 cm
2.2 lb (avoirdupois)	1 kg

*1 qt also is the approximate equivalent of 1 L.

Note: In the above equation:

1. The correct equation was used. This means that the terms of the first ratio (milligrams to grains) are in exactly the same order as the terms in the second ratio (milligrams to grams).
2. The numbers being sought were placed on one side of the equation (x mg:0.5 gr).
3. The approximate equivalents were placed on the other side of the equation (60 mg:1 gr).
4. The fraction was changed to a decimal (gr ½ to 0.5).
5. The means and the extremes were multiplied to solve for the unknown number (designated by x).

EXAMPLE: To convert 1 lb to grams:

$$1{,}000 \text{ g}{:}2.2 \text{ lb} = x \text{ g}{:}1 \text{ lb.}$$
$$2.2x = 1{,}000$$
$$x = 454 \text{ g}$$

Note: In the above equation:

1. The correct equation was used. This means that the terms of the first ratio (grams:pounds) are in exactly the same order as the terms of the second ratio (grams:pounds).
2. The numbers being sought were placed on side of the equation (x g:1 lb).
3. The approximate equivalents were placed on the other side of the equation (1,000 g:2.2 lb) – 1,000 g was obtained by changing kilograms to grams.
4. There were no fractions to change to decimals.
5. The means and extremes were multiplied to solve for the unknown number (designated by x).

EXAMPLE: To convert 20 in. to centimeters:

$$2.5 \text{ cm}{:}1 \text{ in.} = x \text{ cm}{:}20 \text{ in.}$$
$$1x = 2.5 \times 20 \ (50)$$
$$x = 50 \text{ cm}$$

Note: In the above equation:

1. The correct equation was used. This means that the terms of the first ratio (centimeters:inches) are in exactly the same order as the terms in the second ratio (centimeters:inches).

TABLE 8–2   Approximate Equivalency Tables

Weights

Apothecaries' System	Metric System
1/300 gr	0.2 mg or 0.0002 g
1/150 gr	0.4 mg or 0.0004 g
1/120 gr	0.5 mg or 0.0005 g
1/100 gr	0.6 mg or 0.0006 g
1/60 gr	1 mg or 0.001 g
1/30 gr	2 mg or 0.002 g
1/20 gr	3 mg or 0.003 g
1/12 gr	5 mg or 0.005 g
1/10 gr	6 mg or 0.006 g
1/8 gr	8 mg or 0.008 g
1/6 gr	10 mg or 0.01 g
1/4 gr	15 mg or 0.015 g
1/2 gr	30 mg or 0.03 g
3/4 gr	50 mg or 0.05 g
1 gr	60 mg or 0.06 g
1 1/2 gr	100 mg or 0.1 g
3 gr	200 mg or 0.2 g
5 gr	300 mg or 0.3 g
7 1/2 gr	500 mg or 0.5 g
10 gr	600 mg or 0.6 g
15 gr	1,000 mg or 1 g
1 dr	4 g
4 dr	15 g
1 oz	30 g

Fluid or Wet

Apothecaries' System	Metric System
1 m	0.06 ml
5 m	0.3 ml
10 m	0.6 ml
15 m	1 ml
30 m	2 ml
60 m or 1 dr	4 ml
4 dr	15 ml
1 oz	30 ml

2. The numbers being sought were placed on one side of the equation (x cm:20 in.).
3. The approximate equivalents were placed on the other side of the equation (2.5 cm:1 in.).
4. There were no fractions to change to decimals.
5. The means and extremes were multiplied to solve for the unknown number (designated by x).

OTHER PROCEDURES FOR CONVERTING

There are other procedures that can be used to convert units from one system to another. Before using these procedures, it is important to convert all fractions to decimals. This is because the metric system is a system of decimals, while the apothecaries' system contains whole numbers and fractions.

1. To convert grams to grains, multiply the number of grams by 15.

EXAMPLE: To convert 3 g to grains:

$$3 \times 15 = 45 \text{ gr in 3 g}$$

TABLE 8–2 Approximate Equivalency Tables

Metric System		English Units (Exact Equivalents)
Length		
Kilometer (km)	1,000 m	0.62 mi
Hectometer (hm)	100 m	109.36 yd
Dekameter (Dm)	10 m	32.81 ft
Meter (m)	1 m	39.37 in.
Decimeter (dm)	0.1 m	3.94 in.
Centimeter (cm)	0.01 m	0.39 in.
Millimeter (mm)	0.001 m	0.04 in.
Capacity		
Kiloliter (kl)	1,000 L	
Hectoliter (hl)	100 L	
Dekaliter (Dl)	10 L	
Liter (L)	1 L	1.057 qt
Deciliter (dl)	0.1 L	0.21 pt
Centiliter (cl)	0.01 L	0.338 fl oz
Milliliter (ml)*	0.001 L	0.27 fl dr
Weight		
Kilogram (kg)	1,000 g	2.2046 lb
Hectogram (hg)	100 g	3.527 oz
Dekagram (Dg)	10 g	0.353 oz
Gram (g)	1 g	0.035 oz
Decigram (dg)	0.1 g	1.543 gr
Centigram (cg)	0.01 g	0.154 gr
Milligram (mg)	0.001 g	0.015 gr

*cc (cubic centimeter), although a volume measurement, is often used interchangeably with milliliter, particularly on measuring devices, such as a syringe.

2. To convert milliliters to minims, multiply the number of milliliters by 15.
   EXAMPLE: To convert 5 ml to minims:

$$5 \times 15 = 75 \text{ m in 5 ml}$$

3. To convert grains to grams, divide the number of grains by 15.
   EXAMPLE: To convert 45 gr to grams:

$$45 \div 15 = 3 \text{ g in 45 gr}$$

4. To convert minims to milliliters, divide the number of minims by 15.
   EXAMPLE: To convert 60 m to milliliters:

$$60 \div 15 = 4 \text{ ml in 60 m}$$

5. To convert grams to ounces, divide the number of grams by 30.
   EXAMPLE: To convert 60 g to ounces:

$$60 \div 30 = 2 \text{ oz in 60 g}$$

6. To convert milliliters to fluidounces, divide the number of milliliters by 30.
   EXAMPLE: To convert 45 ml to fluidounces:

$$45 \div 30 = 1\frac{1}{2} \text{ fl oz in 45 ml}$$

7. To convert ounces to grams, multiply the number of ounces by 30.
   EXAMPLE: To convert 2 oz to grams:

$$2 \times 30 = 60 \text{ g in 2 oz}$$

8. To convert fluidounces to milliliters, multiply the number of fluidounces by 30.
   EXAMPLE: To convert 3 fl oz to milliliters:

$$3 \times 30 = 90 \text{ ml in 3 fl oz}$$

CONVERTING FROM ONE SYSTEM TO ANOTHER QUIZ

Convert the following:

1. gr xxx   = _____ g.
2. 15 m.   = _____ ml.
3. 80 lb   = _____ kg.
4. 1,500 ml   = _____ pt.
5. gr i   = _____ mg.
6. 28 in.   = _____ cm.
7. 2,000 mg   = gr _____.
8. 2 g   = gr _____.
9. 60 cm   = _____ in.
10. 0.5 g   = gr _____.
11. 60 m.   = _____ ml.
12. 55 cm   = _____ in.
13. gr viiss   = _____ g.
14. 4,000 ml   = _____ qt.
15. gr. i   = _____ g.
16. gr v   = _____ g.
17. 10 ml   = ℥ _____.
18. 10 lb   = _____ g.
19. 500 mg   = gr. _____.
20. 8 ml   = _____ m.
21. 150 lb   = _____ kg.
22. 15 g   = ℥ _____.
23. 15 ml   = ℥ _____.
24. 200 lb   = _____ kg.
25. gr XLV   = _____ mg.
26. ℥ vi   = _____ ml.
27. 25 in.   = _____ cm.
28. ℥ viii   = _____ ml.
29. 176 lb   = _____ kg.
30. gr x   = _____ g

Chapter 9 | HOUSEHOLD MEASUREMENTS

EXPECTED BEHAVIORAL OUTCOMES

After completing this chapter, you should return to the expected behavioral outcomes and evaluate your ability to:

1. Identify units of household measurement.
2. Multiply and divide whole numbers and fractions to solve problems within the household measurement system.
3. Convert units of household measurement to other measurement systems.

Occasionally, it may be necessary to use household measures that approximate metric and apothecaries' measurements. These measures are not accurate and should be avoided when possible. Table 9–1 lists units of household measurements. Table 9–2 contains approximate equivalencies to other measurement systems.

CONVERTING FROM ONE HOUSEHOLD MEASURE TO ANOTHER

1. To convert from a larger measure to a smaller measure, multiply. The multiplier is obtained from Table 9–1.

EXAMPLE: To convert 2 tbsp to teaspoonfuls:
Teaspoonfuls are smaller than tablespoonfuls.
There are 3 tsp in 1 tbsp.
The multiplier is 3.

$$2 \text{ tbsp} \times 3 = 6 \text{ tsp}$$

TABLE 9–1 Household Table of Measurements

60 drops (gtt)	= 1 teaspoonful (tsp)
2 tsp	= 1 dessertspoonful
2 dessertspoonfuls	= 1 tbsp
3 tsp	= 1 tbsp
6 tsp	= 1 oz
2 tbsp	= 1 oz
6 oz	= 1 teacupful
8 oz	= 1 glassful

TABLE 9–2   **Approximate Equivalents**

Household Measures	Apothecaries' Units	Metric Units
1 tsp	1 + fl dr or 60 m	5 ml
1 dessertspoonful	2 fl dr	8 ml
1 tbsp	4 fl dr	15 ml
2 tbsp	1 fl oz	30 ml
1 teacupful	6 fl oz	180 ml
1 glassful	8 fl oz	250 ml

    2. To convert from a smaller measure to a larger measure, divide. The divisor is obtained from Table 9–1.

          EXAMPLE: To convert 3 tsp to ounces:

                      Ounces are larger than teaspoonfuls.

                      There are 6 tsp in 1 oz.

                      The divisor, therefore, is 6.

$$3 \text{ tsp} \div 6 = \tfrac{1}{2} \text{ oz}$$

CONVERTING HOUSEHOLD MEASUREMENTS TO OTHER SYSTEMS

As previously mentioned, household measurements are not accurate and are avoided if at all possible when administering drug therapy. Conversions between household measurements and other systems are also not very accurate and thus, extremely rare. When a conversion of a household measurement is necessary, the following procedure is used:

    1. Set up a simple proportion:

household measurement:metric or apothecaries' = household measurement:metric or apothecaries'

    2. Select an approximate equivalent from Table 9–2.
    3. Place the numbers you are seeking on one side of the equation.
    4. Place the approximate equivalent on the other side of the equation.
    5. Multiply the means and extremes to solve for the unknown number (usually called x).

    EXAMPLE: To convert 1 tbsp to milliliters:

$$2 \text{ tbsp}: 30 \text{ ml} = 1 \text{ tbsp}: x \text{ ml}$$
$$2x = 30 \times 1$$
$$x = 15 \text{ ml}$$

Note: In the above equation:

    1. The correct equation was used. This means that the terms of the first ratio (tablespoonfuls: milliliters) are in exactly the same order as the terms in the second ratio (tablespoonfuls:milliliters).
    2. The approximate equivalent was selected from Table 9–2 (2 tbsp = 30 ml).
    3. The numbers being sought were placed on one side of the equation (1 tbsp:x ml).
    4. The approximate equivalent was placed on the other side of the equation (2 tbsp:30 ml).
    5. The equation was solved by multiplying the means and the extremes to obtain the unknown number (called x).

CONVERSION EXERCISE

Convert the following household measures:
1. 2 glassfuls   = _____oz
2. 3 teacupfuls = _____oz

3. 8 tsp = _____dessertspoonfuls
4. 3 tsp = _____oz
5. 6 tbsp = _____oz

Convert the following quantities to household equivalents:
1. 30 ml = _____tbsp
2. 2 fl dr = _____dessertspoonfuls
3. 120 ml = _____tbsp
4. 8 fl oz = _____glassfuls
5. 15 ml = _____tbsp

MEASUREMENTS QUIZ

Directions: Solve the following problems. Circle the correct answer. Circle NG if the correct answer is not given and place the correct answer next to it. Show all work.

1. Convert 1 tbsp to drams.

  a. ʒ iv **b.** ʒ viii **c.** ʒ iii **d.** ʒii **3.** NG

2. Convert gr i to milligrams.

  a. 60 mg **b.** 15 mg **c.** 30 mg **d.** 0.6 mg **e.** NG

3. Convert 20 in. to centimeters.

  a. 30 cm **b.** 10 cm **c.** 40 cm **d.** 50 cm **e.** NG

4. Convert 30 mg to grams.

  a. 0.03 g **b.** 3 g **c.** 0.3 g **d.** 0.003 g **e.** NG

5. Convert gr 1/6 to milligrams.

  a. 15 mg **b.** 10 mg **c.** 30 mg **d.** 360 mg **e.** NG

6. Convert gr viiss to milligrams.

  a. 500 mg **b.** 60 mg **c.** 0.5 mg **d.** 600 mg **3.** NG

7. Convert gr 1/300 to milligrams.

  a. 2 mg **b.** 0.0002 mg **c.** 0.1 mg **d.** 0.2 mg **e.** NG

8. Convert 2 tbsp to teaspoonfuls.

  a. 6 tsp **b.** 8 tsp **c.** 4 tsp **d.** 12 tsp **e.** NG

9. Convert gr cxx to drams.

  a. ʒ iv **b.** ʒ viii **c.** ʒ ii **d.** ʒ iii **e.** NG

10. Convert gr xv to milligrams.

  a. 500 mg **b.** 60 mg **c.** 30 mg **d.** 1,000 mg **e.** NG

11. Convert 500 mg to grams.

  a. 0.5 g **b.** 5 g **c.** 0.05 g **d.** 0.1 g **e.** NG

12. Convert 35°C to Fahrenheit.

  a. 85° F **b.** 68° F **c.** 63° F **d.** 58° F **e.** NG

13. Convert 60 m to milliliters.

        a. 1 ml **b.** 4 ml **c.** 2 ml **d.** 0.3 ml **e.** NG

14. Convert 3 ft to yards.

        a. 0.5 yd **b.** 0.3 yd **c.** 1 yd **d.** 2 yd **e.** NG

15. Convert 200 kg to pounds.

        a. 40 lb **b.** 440 lb **c.** 240 lb **d.** 400 lb **e.** NG

16. Convert 1 glassful to milliliters.

        a. 180 ml **b.** 90 ml **c.** 240 ml **d.** 150 ml **e.** NG

17. Convert 98.2°F to centigrade.

        a. 32.6°C **b.** 37.8°C **c.** 38°C **d.** 37°C **e.** NG

18. Convert 2 ml to minims.

        a. 4 m **b.** 0.5 m **c.** 60 m **d.** 30 m **e.** NG

19. Convert 100 mg to grains.

        a. gr i **b.** gr x **c.** gr ½ **d.** gr ¼ **e.** NG

20. Convert 36 in. to feet.

        a. 1½ **b.** 2 ft **c.** 3 ft **d.** 1 ft **e.** NG

21. Convert 96.8°F to centigrade.

        a. 37°C **b.** 32°C **c.** 36°C **d.** 37.6°C **e.** NG

22. Convert 0.5 g to grains:

        a. gr v **b.** gr i **c.** gr viiss̄ **d.** gr iii **e.** NG

23. Convert gr v to milligrams.

        a. 0.2 mg **b.** 500 mg **c.** 10 mg **d.** 100 mg **e.** NG

24. Convert 39°C to Fahrenheit.

        a. 70.2°F **b.** 101.8°F **c.** 102.2°F **d.** 100.2°F **e.** NG

25. Convert 29 in. to centimeters.

        a. 57 cm **b.** 80 cm **c.** 72.5 cm **d.** 75 cm **e.** NG

26. Convert 0.03 g to grains.

        a. gr v **b.** gr i **c.** gr s̄s̄ **d.** gr x **e.** NG

27. Convert 98°F to centigrade.

        a. 37°C **b.** 36°C **c.** 38°C **d.** 36.7°C **e.** NG

28. Convert 60 lb to kilograms.

        a. 27.3 kg **b.** 24.4 kg **c.** 30 kg **d.** 244 gr **e.** NG

29. Convert 8 mg to grains.

        a. gr ½ **b.** gr i **c.** gr ⅛ **d.** gr 1/50 **e.** NG

30. Convert 0.01 g to grains.

       a. gr v **b.** gr ¼ **c.** gr ⅙ **d.** gr $\overline{ss}$ **e.** NG

31. Convert 100°F to centigrade.

       a. 36°C **b.** 37.8°C **c.** 39°C **d.** 40°C **e.** NG

32. Convert 30 in. to centimeters.

       a. 72 cm **b.** 73 cm **c.** 72.5 cm **d.** 75 cm **e.** NG

33. Convert l lb to grams.

       a. 600 g **b.** 60 g **c.** 220 g **d.** 454 g **e.** NG

34. Convert 37°C to Fahrenheit.

       a. 68.2°F **b.** 98.6°F **c.** 99°F **d.** 98.8°F **e.** NG

35. Convert ʒ xvi to milliliters.

       a. 250 ml **b.** 30 ml **c.** 500 ml **d.** 1,000 ml **e.** NG

36. Convert ʒ i to milliliters.

       a. 15 ml **b.** 30 ml **c.** 8 ml **d.** 4 ml **e.** NG

37. 0.5 ml to minims.

       a. 8 m **b.** 15 m **c.** 30 m **d.** 2 m **e.** NG

38. Convert 0.6 mg to grains.

       a. gr ⅙ **b.** gr ½ **c.** gr ¼ **d.** gr ¹/₁₀₀ **e.** NG

39. Convert 40°C to Fahrenheit.

       a. 72°F **b.** 68°F **c.** 102°F **d.** 101.4°F **e.** NG

40. Convert 6.5 L to milliliters.

       a. 650 ml **b.** 65 ml **c.** 500 ml **d.** 0.65 ml **e.** NG

41. Convert 130 lb to kilograms.

       a. 59.1 kg **b.** 60 kg **c.** 2,860 kg **d.** 2,660 kg **e.** NG

42. Convert ʒ ii to drams.

       a. ʒ xvi **b.** ʒ viii **c.** ʒ xxxii **d.** ʒ xii **e.** NG

43. Convert 99°F to centigrade.

       a. 36.8°C **b.** 37.2°C **c.** 39°C **d.** 37.8°C **e.** NG

44. Convert 6,000 ml to liters.

       a. 60 L **b.** 600 L **c.** 6 L **d.** 6.5L **e.** NG

45. Convert 15 mg to grams.

       a. 0.015 g **b.** 0.l5 g **c.** 15 g **d.** 1.5 g **e.** NG

46. Convert 3 pt to liters.

       a. 1,500 L **b.** 1 L **c.** 1.5 L **d.** 3 L **e.** NG

47. Convert 1 qt to liters.

a. 0.75 L **b.** 0.5 L **c.** 1 L **d.** 1,000 L **e.** NG

48. Convert 39.2°C to Fahrenheit.

a. 106.2°F **b.** 104.4°F **c.** 100.6°F **d.** 102.6°F **e.** NG

49. Convert gr xxx to grams.

a. 2 g **b.** 0.2 g **c.** 5 g **d.** 0.5 g **e.** NG

50. Convert 200 lb to kilograms.

a. 100 kg **b.** 140 kg **c.** 90 kg **d.** 99 kg **e.** NG

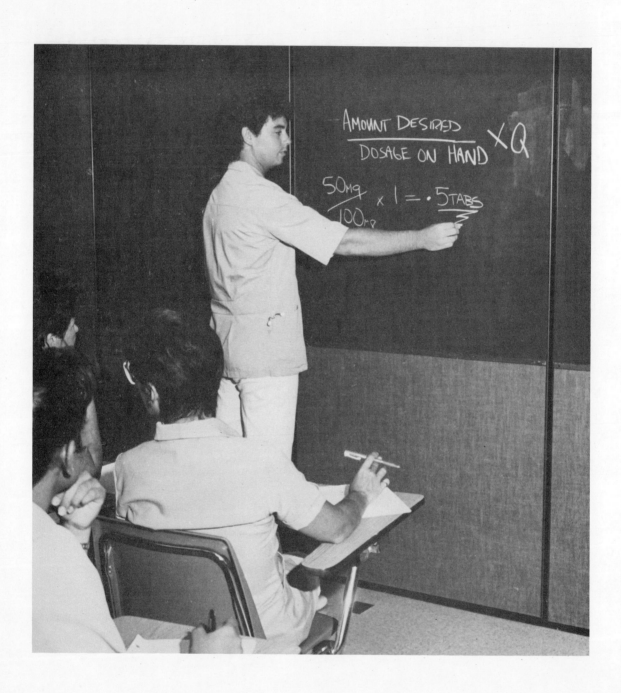

Section III

CALCULATING

DRUG DOSES

Chapter 10 | DOSES FOR ORAL ADMINISTRATION AND PARENTERAL INJECTION

EXPECTED BEHAVIORAL OUTCOMES

After completing this chapter, you should return to the expected behavioral outcomes and evaluate your ability to:

1. Identify the desired dose, the dose on hand, and the quantity in a dosage problem.
2. Use a formula to calculate the dosage of liquids and solids with 100% accuracy.
3. Add diluent (solvent) to a powder according to label directions and calculate the correct dosage from the resulting solution.

DOSAGE CALCULATION—SOLIDS

Many drugs are administered as solids in the form of tablets, capsules, or pills. Solids are usually supplied by the manufacturer in several strengths. When the strength of the drug supplied by the manufacturer is different from the dose prescribed by the physician, dosage calculation is needed. In other words, the nurse must calculate how much of the drug supplied is needed to provide the exact amount prescribed by the physician. Several terms are used to describe the various parts of dosage calculation:

1. *Dose desired*—the dose prescribed by the physician.
2. *Dose on hand*—the dose supplied by the drug manufacturer.
3. *Quantity*—the number of units or volume holding the dosage. It may be the number of tablets if the drug is a solid. It may be stated in cubic centimeters, ounces, or some other measure if the drug is in solution.

To find the proper dosage, the following equation can be used:

$$\frac{\text{dose of drug desired}}{\text{dose of drug on hand}} \times \text{quantity} = \text{amount to be given}$$

EXAMPLE: The physician's order reads: ampicillin 500 mg IM q6h. The label on the vial reads: ampicillin 250 mg/ml.

$$\frac{500\ \text{mg}}{250\ \text{mg}} \times 1 = 2\ \text{ml}$$

To solve the dosage problem the nurse needs to answer the following questions:

1. Are the units of measure in the desired dose and the dose on hand the same?
   Yes, both doses are given in milligrams. If the units of measurement are different, conversion of one measuring system is needed as described in Chapter 8.
2. Is the unit of measurement for the quantity the same as the unit of measurement for the quantity being sought? Yes, both quantities are given in capsules. If the units of measurement are different, the nurse must first convert to one measuring system. This was described in detail in Chapter 8.
3. What am I looking for? I am trying to find out how many capsules of ampicillin to give to the patient.
4. What is the desired dose and quantity? Five hundred milligrams, but I don't know the quantity yet.
5. What is the dosage on hand and quantity? Two hundred and fifty milligrams per each (1) capsule.
6. What formula shall I use? $\dfrac{\text{dose of drug desired}}{\text{dose of drug on hand}} \times \text{quantity} = \text{amount to be given}$

The above problem may also be solved by setting up the following equation (also known as a *ratio* or *proportion*):

$$\text{desired dose: quantity} = \text{dose on hand:quantity}$$

$$500 \text{ mg}:x \text{ capsules} = 250 \text{ mg}:1 \text{ capsule}$$
$$250x = 500$$
$$x = 500 \div 250$$
$$x = \text{two capsules}$$

To use this equation, the nurse answers the same questions described above. After answering the questions, the equation is solved in the following way:

1. Let x represent the quantity of drug to be given.
2. The first and fourth numbers are the extremes.
3. The second and third numbers or symbols are the means.
4. To solve the equation:
   a. Multiply the means.
   b. Multiply the extremes.
   c. The product of the means equals the product of the extremes.
5. Keep the product of the means (containing x) to the left of the equation mark.
6. Keep the product of the extremes to the right of the equation mark.
7. The coefficient (number accompanying x) becomes the divisor of the number on the right of the equation mark.
8. Divide the number on the right by the number on the left.
9. The answer is the quantity of capsules to be given.

DOSAGE CALCULATION—LIQUIDS

Some drugs are supplied by the manufacturer in liquid form. A liquid drug is also known as a *solution*. Solutions may be administered orally or injected parenterally. A solution is composed of two parts: the *solute* (the drug) and the *solvent* (liquid in which the drug is dissolved). Labels on a vial or bottle of solution usually tell the dose of drug per unit of solution. For example, a label may read 250 mg/ml. This means that each ml of solution contains 250 mg of the drug. In calculating doses of solutions, the following terms are used:

1. *Desired dose*—The dose prescribed by the physician.
2. *Dose on hand*—The dose of solute indicated on the label.*
3. *Quantity*—The specific volume of solvent holding the dose on hand.*

To find the proper dosage, the following equation can be used:

$$\frac{\text{dose of drug desired}}{\text{dose of drug on hand}} \times \text{quantity} = \text{amount to be given}$$

The reader can see that this formula is exactly the same as the one used to calculate the dosage of solid preparations. Supposing, instead of capsules, the physician prescribes the same drug and dosage to be injected as a solution.

EXAMPLE: The physician's order reads: ampicillin 500 mg IM q6h. The label on the vial reads: ampicillin 250 mg/ml.

$$\frac{500 \text{ mg}}{250 \text{ mg}} \times 1 = 2 \text{ ml}$$

To solve this dosage problem, the nurse answers exactly the same questions as in the previous example:

1. Are the units of measure in the desired dose and the dose on hand the same?
   Yes, both doses are given in milligrams.
2. Is the unit of measurement for the quantity the same as the unit of measurement for the quantity being sought? Yes, both quantities are in milliliters.
3. What am I looking for? I am trying to find out how many milliliters to inject into the patient to provide the desired dose of 500 mg.
4. What is the desired dose and quantity? Five hundred milligrams, but I don't know the quantity yet.
5. What is the dosage on hand and the quantity? Two hundred and fifty milligrams per each (1) ml.
6. What formula shall I use?

$$\frac{\text{dose of drug desired}}{\text{dose of drug on hand}} \times \text{quantity} = \text{amount to be given}$$

The above problem may also be solved by setting up the problem using a proportion as demonstrated on p. 66.

$$500 \text{ mg}: x \text{ ml} = 250 \text{ mg}: 1 \text{ ml}$$

$$250x = 500$$
$$x = 500 \div 250$$
$$x = 2 \text{ ml}$$

Caution: The label on most containers of liquid also states the total volume of liquid inside. This is *not* the same as the quantity in the calculation formula. The term *quantity*, in the calculation formula should be thought of as the strength or concentration.

PREPARING INTERNAL SOLUTIONS

Most drugs for oral and parenteral administration are prepared by the manufacturer in a stock solution. Some drugs deteriorate quickly after being dissolved, however. For these drugs, the manufacturer supplies a powder and directions on the label that instruct the pharmacist and/or the nurse

*These terms taken together also may be called the *strength* or *concentration* of the solution.

about what solvent to use and how much solvent to add to the powder in order to obtain the strength (concentration) desired. The nurse selects the strength that most nearly resembles either the exact dose desired or a multiple of that dose. The nurse follows the directions on the label exactly because unusual amounts of solvent may be added to some powders. This is because the addition of liquid to some powders causes them to expand thus affecting the amount of drug per unit of volume. After the drug has been mixed, dosage calculation may be needed to determine how much of a solution will be needed to administer the correct dose. If part of the solution remains in its container after the correct dose has been calculated, a label is prepared by the nurse and fixed to the bottle or vial containing the remaining solution. The label includes the date the solution was prepared, the strength (concentration) of the solution, and the nurse's name or initials, depending upon local custom.

EXAMPLE: The physician's order reads: penicillin G potassium 300,000 U IM q6h. The label on the bottle reads: penicillin G potassium one million U.

The label on the vial also reads:

Preparation of Solution

Add Aqueous Diluent	Concentration of Solution
19.6 ml	50,000 U/ml
9.6 ml	100,000 U/ml
3.6 ml	250,000 U/ml
1.6 ml	500,000 U/ml

To solve this dosage problem, the nurse answers the same questions presented earlier in the chapter.

1. Are the units of measure for the desired dose and the dose on hand the same? Yes, both doses are given in units.
2. Is the unit of measurement for the quantity the same as the unit of measurement for the quantity being sought? Yes, both quantities are cubic centimeters (milliliters).
3. What am I looking for? This question has two parts. First I am looking for how much diluent (solvent) to add to the powder. Next, I am looking for how many cubic centimeters (milliliters) of solution will be needed to administer the prescribed dose of 300,000 U.
4. What is the desired dose and quantity? Three hundred-thousand units but the quantity (volume) depends upon how much diluent (solvent) I add to the powder.
5. What is the dosage on hand and its quantity? The dosage on hand will be the concentration of solution. This depends upon how much diluent (solvent) I add to the powder. I will select the concentration that comes closest to providing either the exact dose or a multiple of it. Since the solution is to be injected into a muscle, I will also select a concentration that makes it possible to inject a small volume.
6. What formula shall I use? The equation to be used for this calculation is the ratio.

$$\text{desired dose:quantity} = \text{dose on hand:quantity on hand}$$
$$300,000 : x = ?$$

The concentration that comes closest to the desired dose in this example is 250,000 U/ml. To prepare this concentration, the nurse consults the label and adds 3.6 ml of diluent (solvent) to the powder in the vial. This results in a dose on hand of 250,000 U/ml. In other words, the concentration or strength of the solution prepared by the nurse becomes the dose on hand in the formula for calculation. After labeling the vial as described earlier, the nurse calculates the correct dosage using the ratio:

$$\text{desired dose:} x = 250,000 : 1 \text{ ml}$$
$$300,000 \text{ U:} x = 250,000 \text{ U:} 1 \text{ ml}$$
$$300,000 x = 250,000$$
$$x = 300,000 \div 250,000$$
$$x = 1.2 \text{ ml}$$

PREPARING EXTERNAL SOLUTIONS

Most of the solutions prepared by the nurse are for internal use via oral, intradermal, SC, IM, or IV routes. Occasionally, however, a solution must be prepared for external use. A typical situation occurs when the physician prescribes a specific concentration of a solution for a soak or for a wet to dry dressing. The solution is prepared with a solute such as crystals, powder, or tablets. The solute is dissolved with a solvent such as water, saline, alcohol, or distilled water, In some cases, a stock solution is available but it must be diluted to the concentration prescribed by the physician. In both of these instances, calculation of dose is required.

Understanding Concentration

A first step in the preparation of external solutions includes understanding the meaning of various terms that express concentration or strength. The amount of pure drug in a definite quantity of solution determines the strength of the solution. The strength of a solution may be indicated in several ways. Each of the terms below is a way of describing the relationship of parts to the whole. It may be expressed as—

1. *Percent*. Example—a 2% solution is a solution in which there are two parts of drug in 100 parts of solution (percent means in 100).
2. *Ratio*. Example—a 1:1,000 solution is a solution in which there is 1 part of drug in 1,000 parts of solution.
3. *Definite amounts*. Example—a solution label may read "units 40 in each milliliter." This means that the solution has been prepared so that each milliliter of solution contains 40 U of the drug.

It may be necessary to prepare a solution from:

1. *Full-strength drugs*. These may be solids or liquids and are 100% in strength unless otherwise stated. Examples of such drugs are sodium chloride, boric acid, and glycerin.
2. *Tablets*. These contain a definite amount of drug and are labeled accordingly. An example of such a drug is potassium permanganate.
3. *Stock solutions*. These are relatively strong solutions that are kept on hand. Many stock solutions are too strong to be used safely and must be diluted before they can be administered. An example of a stock solution is benzalkonium chloride (zephiran chloride). This drug may be available in a stock solution of 1:1,000 and be diluted to a much weaker solution when used externally.

Calculating Doses

In preparing solutions for external use, the nurse needs to answer two basic questions: How much solute should I use and how much solvent should I use to prepare the prescribed concentration? The ratio formula is used to find those amounts and slight variations of the usual six questions help the nurse to set up the formula correctly.

$$\text{desired dose:quantity} = \text{dose on hand:quantity}$$

EXAMPLE: The physician's order reads: Soak the right foot qid for 15 min in 500 ml of a 2% saline solution.

x mg:500 ml = 2:100   1. Answer questions below to set up formula correctly.

$100x = 500 \times 2$ 2. Multiply the means; multiply the extremes.

$100x = 100$ 3. Place x on the left side of the equation.

$x = 1$ mg   4. Solve the equation for the unknown amount.

The nurse would add 1 mg of sodium chloride to 500 ml tap water to make the prescribed solution.

1. Are the units of measure in the problem the same? The only measure given is in the metric system (500 ml). Therefore all units in the ratio formula must be in the metric system.
2. What am I looking for? I am trying to find out how much sodium chloride to add to 500 ml of water to prepare a 2% solution.
3. What is the desired dose and quantity? I don't yet know what the dose of sodium chloride is. The desired quantity is 500 ml.
4. What is the dose and hand and the quantity? The answer to this question is the strength of the solution which the physician has prescribed. Thus, the dose on hand is 2 parts sodium chloride to 100 parts water—a 2% solution.
5. What formula shall I use? desired dose:quantity = dose on hand:quantity

DOSAGE CALCULATION—USING A CALCULATOR

A calculator may be used to solve dosage problems. However, in order to use the calculator correctly, the six questions presented earlier in the chapter are used to identify the dose desired, dose on hand, and quantity. These numbers are placed in the correct formula first. Then, a calculator is used to multiply and divide.

EXAMPLE: The physician's order reads: prednisone 7.5 mg PO. The label on the container reads: prednisone 5 mg/tablet.

1. The nurse answers the six questions to identify each part of the formula to be used in dosage calculation and reaches the following conclusion:

$$\frac{\text{dose desired}}{\text{dose on hand}} \times \text{quantity} = \text{amount to be given}$$

$$\frac{7.5 \text{ mg}}{5 \text{ mg}} \times 1 \qquad = x$$

2. After the formula has been set up, the calculator is used by entering the numbers and symbols exactly as they appear in the formula:

$$7.5 \boxdot 5 \boxtimes 1 \boxminus 1.5 \text{ tablets}$$

If a ratio formula is used, the means and extremes must be multiplied first before the calculator is used.

EXAMPLE: The physician's order reads: ampicillin suspension 500 mg PO. The label on the bottle reads: ampicillin suspension 125 mg/5 cc.

1. The nurse answers the six questions to identify each part of the formula to be used in dosage calculation and reaches the following conclusion:

$$\text{dose desired:quantity::dose on hand:quantity}$$
$$500 \text{ mg}:x::125 \text{ mg}: 5 \text{ cc}$$
$$125x = 500 \times 5$$
$$x = 500 \times 5 \div 125$$

2. After the formula has been set up, the calculator is used by entering the numbers and symbols exactly as they appear in the formula. (Note that the x to the left of the equals (=) sign represents the amount of drug to be given; thus it is not entered on the calculator.)

$$500 \boxtimes 5 \boxdot 125 \boxminus 20 \text{ cc}$$

DOSAGE CALCULATION PROBLEMS

Directions: Use the questions provided earlier in this chapter as a guide to help you calculate the following dosages. Show all work.

1. The doctor's order reads digoxin 0.125 mg and the label on the bottle reads digoxin 0.25 mg/tablet.

2. Furosemide 80 mg is ordered by the doctor and the label on the bottle reads furosemide 20 mg/tablet.

3. The doctor's order reads prednisone 2.5 mg and the label on the bottle reads prednisone 5 mg/tablet.

4. Cimetidine hydrochloride 300 mg is ordered by the doctor and the label on the bottle reads cimetidine hydrochloride 100 mg/tablet.

5. The doctor's order reads clonidine hydrochloride 0.1 mg and the label on the bottle reads clonidine hydrochloride 0.05 mg/tablet.

6. The label on the 40-ml stock bottle reads penicillin V 125 mg per 5 ml, and the doctor's order reads penicillin V 250 mg.

CALCULATING DRUG DOSAGES QUIZ

1. Penicillin G potassium 20,000 U was ordered, and the label on the 60-ml bottle reads penicillin G potassium 100,000 U/5 ml.

2. The doctor's order reads penicillin G potassium 200,000 U and the label on the 80-ml bottle reads penicillin G potassium 200,000 U/5 ml.

3. The doctor's order reads give penicillin G benzathine 50,000 U and the label on the 10-ml vial reads penicillin G benzathine 150,000 U/ml.

4. Dicloxacillin 125 mg was ordered by the doctor, and the label on the 150-ml bottle reads dicloxacillin 62.5 mg/5 ml.

5. The label on the 5-ml stock bottle of cyanocobalamin (vitamin B_{12}) reads 30 μg/ml, and the doctor's order reads give cyanocobalamin 10 μg.

6. The label on the 30-ml stock bottle reads meperidine hydrochloride (Demerol) 100 mg/ml, and the doctor's order reads give meperidine hydrochloride 80 mg.

7. The label on the 10-ml ampule reads procainamide hydrochloride 100 mg/1 ml, and the doctor's order reads give procainamide hydrochloride 25 mg.

8. The label on the 5-ml ampule reads quinine hydrochloride 100 mg/ml, and the doctor's order reads quinine hydrochloride 125 mg.

9. The label on the 10-ml vial reads methoxamine hydrochloride 10 mg/ml, and the doctor's order reads methoxamine hydrochloride 0.015 g.

10. The doctor's order reads atropine sulfate gr $\frac{1}{150}$ and the label on the bottle reads atropine sulfate 0.4 mg/ml. *Hint*: Be sure to answer all questions on p. 67 to calculate correctly.

11. The doctor's order reads aspirin gr x and the label on the bottle reads aspirin 325 mg/tablet. *Hint*: Be sure to answer all questions on p. 67 to calculate correctly.

12. Secobarbital gr iii is ordered by the doctor and the label on the bottle reads secobarbital 0.1 g/capsule.

13. Potassium gluconate elixir 20 mEq is ordered by the doctor and the label on the bottle reads potassium gluconate elixir 5 mEq/ml.

14. The doctor's order reads nitroglycerin gr $\frac{1}{100}$ and the label on the bottle reads nitroglycerin gr $\frac{1}{200}$ per tablet.

The label of a vial reads: penicillin G potassium 1 million U.

Preparation of Solution

Amount of Aqueous Diluent	Concentration of Solution
19.6 ml	50,000 U/ml
9.6 ml	100,000 U/ml
3.6 ml	250,000 U/ml
1.6 ml	500,000 U/ml

For each of the following doctor's orders, tell how many milliliters of diluent you would add to the vial. Then, calculate the correct dosage. A table has been provided to assist you. Show all work.

Doctor's Order	Amount of Diluent to Be Added	Amount to Be Given
15. 1 million U		
16. 750,000 U		
17. 150,000 U		
18. 600,000 U		
19. 400,000 U		
20. 100,000 U		
21. 75,000 U		
22. 50,000 U		
23. 125,000 U		
24. 325,000 U		

WORK SPACE

Chapter 11 | DOSES FOR INSULIN INJECTION

EXPECTED BEHAVIORAL OUTCOMES

After completing this chapter, you should return to the expected behavioral outcomes and evaluate your ability to:

1. Draw up a prescribed dose of insulin into an appropriately calibrated syringe.
2. Calculate an insulin dose in milliliters and minims when a calibrated insulin syringe is unavailable and another syringe must be used.

Insulin is a hormone manufactured in the pancreas that is essential to life. A person who does not manufacture enough circulating insulin to meet body requirements has a condition called *diabetes mellitus*. Drug therapy is often a very important part of the medical treatment plan. Insulin may be administered by the SC route. The source for insulin administered in this way may be either animal insulin or human insulin manufactured through a special new process called *biosynthesis*. There are three basic forms of insulin, each with a different onset, peak, and duration of action (see Chapter 22 for additional information).

Insulin is supplied by the manufacturer in vials containing a total of 10 ml. Several strengths are available. U100 is the most common strength used in the United States. This means that there are 100 U of insulin in each milliliter of solution. Another strength is called U40. This means that there are 40 U of insulin in each milliliter of solution. In the past, insulin was also available in a strength called U80; however, this is no longer being used.

Special syringes are used to administer insulin. Insulin syringes are calibrated (measured and marked) in units instead of minims or milliliters as other syringes (Fig. 11–1). The units on the insulin syringe should be the same as the strength (concentration) of the insulin being used. For example, if a certain dose of U100 insulin is prescribed by the doctor, a U100 syringe is used to administer it. The nurse simply draws up the number of units prescribed to the corresponding number marked on the insulin syringe (Fig. 11–2).

Occasionally, the nurse may find that insulin syringes are not available. A typical situation occurs when the patient is at home in a rural setting and runs out of insulin syringes. Another situation may develop when the diabetic individual travels and runs out of insulin syringes. In such situations, a temporary substitution may be made with one of the following syringes until insulin syringes can be obtained:

1. One-milliliter tuberculin syringe calibrated in tenths and hundredths of a milliliter and in minims.

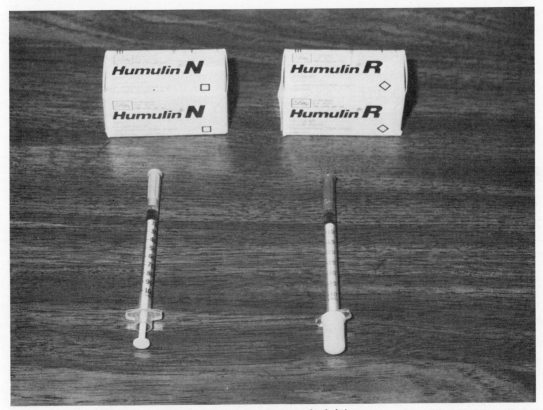

FIGURE 11-1 Insulin syringes and insulin. The syringe on the left is used when U100 insulin is ordered. The syringe on the right is used when U40 insulin is ordered.

   2. Two-, 2.5-, or 3-ml (cc) syringe calibrated in minims and milliliters (cc).

If it is necessary to use one of the substitute syringes, dosage calculation is required. The usual formula is used:

$$\frac{\text{dose desired}}{\text{dose on hand}} \times \text{quantity} = \text{amount to be given}$$

In answering the six questions presented in Chapter 10, the nurse uses the following information about insulin:

   1. The dose of insulin is always prescribed in units and supplied by the manufacturer in units per milliliter.

   2. The desired dose is the number of units prescribed by the physician.

   3. The dose on hand is always the strength (concentration) of the insulin in units as printed on the label. This is almost always U100.

   4. The quantity is usually 1 ml because the strength (concentration) is almost always supplied in units per milliliter.

   5. The answer is always the amount to be given in either milliliters or minims.

EXAMPLE: The physician's order reads: Give 32 U lente insulin U100 now SC. The label on the vial reads: Lente insulin U100. Insulin syringes are not available so the dosage must be calculated in minims or milliliters.

$$\frac{32 \text{ U}}{100 \text{ U}} \times 1 = \text{amount to be given in milliliters}$$

$$32 \div 100 \times 1 = 0.3 \text{ ml}$$

If the nurse decides that minims will provide a more accurate dosage, the formula would be set up in the following way:

$$\frac{32\ U}{100\ U} \times 15\text{--}16 = \text{amount to be given in minims*}$$

$$32 \div 100 \times 15\text{--}16* = 5\ m.$$

EXERCISES

Calculate the following doses of U100 insulin in minims and milliliters.

Doctor's Order	Minims	Milliliters
1. U-50		
2. U-40		
3. U-60		
4. U-80		
5. U-55		
6. U-100		
7. U-75		
8. U-45		
9. U-30		
10. U-25		

Take examples 2, 9, and 10 and calculate the dose of insulin U40 in minims and milliliters.

On each of the U100 insulin syringes in the left-hand column, draw a dark line at the calibration that corresponds to the prescribed dose in the right-hand column.

U100 Insulin Syringes	Prescribed Dose of U100 Insulin
	55 U
	70 U
	88 U
	12 U
	34 U

*One milliliter is equal to 15 to 16 m.

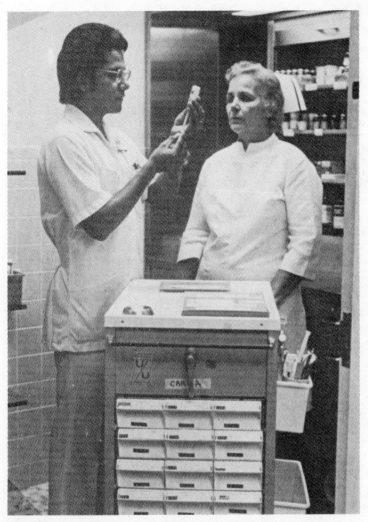

FIGURE 11-2   Insulin being measured for a diabetic patient. (Courtesy of Palm Beach County Practical Nursing Program, The School Board of Palm Beach County, Fla.)

Chapter 12 | DOSES FOR INFANTS AND CHILDREN

EXPECTED BEHAVIORAL OUTCOMES

After completing this chapter, you should return to the expected behavioral outcomes and evaluate your ability to:

1. Calculate the dose for an infant or child when the drug and/or dose prescribed is unfamiliar.
2. Provide information to other members of the health team about a calculated dose for an infant or child during an emergency.

Infants and children require smaller doses of medicine than adults. Several rules, based on either age or weight, or surface area may be used to calculate a fraction of the adult dose to be given to an infant or child. The physician uses these rules to prescribe the correct dose; however, the nurse also uses these rules in several ways:

1. To check the prescribed dose when a drug and/or usual dosage is not familiar.
2. To provide information to the physician or others when drug therapy is part of emergency care provided for an infant or child.

The rules most frequently used are:

1. Clark's rule. This rule uses the weight of the child to determine the dose.

$$Formula: \frac{\text{weight of child in pounds or kilograms}}{150 \text{ lb or } 68 \text{ kg (average adult weight)}} \times \text{adult dose} = \text{child's dose}$$

EXAMPLE: The adult dose of a drug is 100 mg. What is the dose for a child weighing 15 lb?

$$\frac{15}{150} \times 100 = \frac{1,500}{150} = 10 \text{ mg (child's dose)}$$

2. Fried's rule. This rule is used for infants.

$$Formula: \frac{\text{age in months}}{150 \text{ months (approx. 12.5 years)}} \times \text{adult dose} = \text{infant dose}$$

EXAMPLE: The adult dose of a drug is 100 mg. What is the dose for a 5-month-old infant?

$$\frac{15}{150} \times 100 = \frac{500}{150} = 150 \overline{)500.0} \quad \begin{array}{r} 3.3 \text{ mg} \\ \hline 450 \\ \hline 50\ 0 \\ 45\ 0 \\ \hline \end{array}$$

3. Young's rule. This rule is used for children from 2 to 12 years of age.

$$\textit{Formula}: \quad \frac{\text{age of child}}{\text{age of child} + 12} \times \text{adult dose} = \text{child dose}$$

EXAMPLE: The adult dose is ʒ i (60 m). What is the dose for a 3-year-old child?

$$\frac{3 \text{ (age)}}{3 \text{ (age)} + 12} \times 60 \text{ m (adult dose)} = \frac{3}{15} \times 60 = 12 \text{ m}$$

FRACTION DOSES OF LIQUID DRUGS FOR ORAL ADMINISTRATION TO CHILDREN

Liquid drugs can be prepared for administration to children in the following ways:

1. If the drug is ordered in doses of 5 ml or more, it is poured directly into a calibrated medicine glass.
2. If the dose ordered in less than 5 ml, the nurse may use a 1-, 3-, or 5-ml syringe to measure the dose. The syringe may be used to deposit the medication directly in the child's mouth with the child's head elevated.
3. If the liquid medication is a suspension, it should be shaken well first.

EXERCISES

Directions: Calculate the doses by using one of the rules described on pp. 78–79. Show all work.

1. The adult dose is 0.5 g. What is the dose for an 8-year-old child?

2. The adult dose is gr ⅙. What is the dose for a child weighing 25 lb?

3. The adult dose is 60 mg. What is the dose for a 10-month-old infant?

4. The adult dose is 250 mg. What is the dose for a 12-year-old child?

5. The adult dose is gr x. What is the dose for a child weighing 50 lb?

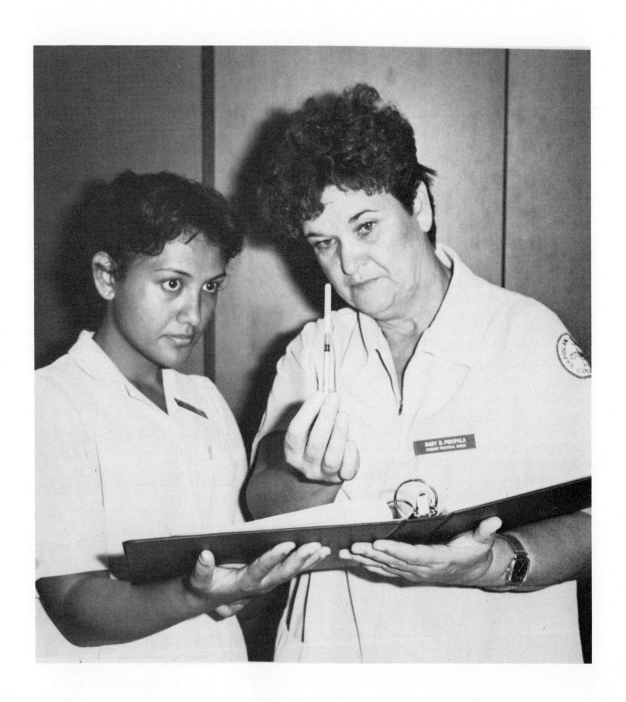

Section IV

DRUG

ADMINISTRATION

Chapter 13 | ADMINISTERING DRUG THERAPY

EXPECTED BEHAVIORAL OUTCOMES

After completing this chapter, you should return to the expected behavioral outcomes and evaluate your ability to:

1. Use the rules of drug therapy as a guide to safe and effective administration.
2. Gather information needed about patients who will receive drug therapy.
3. Use agency or hospital procedures to verify each drug order.
4. Assemble appropriate supplies and equipment for drug therapy.
5. Pour oral solids and liquids without introducing unnecessary microorganisms.
6. Record medication correctly after it has been administered.
7. Take appropriate action if a medication error is made.

I. Rules for administering drug therapy.
   A. The nurse assigned to administer drug therapy keeps all medication stored in a locked compartment. The same nurse holds the key to the locked compartment and carries it at all times.
   B. The nurse gives only drugs that have been ordered in writing by a licensed physician.
   C. The nurse carries out written orders for drug therapy only if they are complete and clearly understood. Incomplete or unclear orders are further clarified before a drug is administered.
   D. For every drug administered, the nurse knows the usual dosage range, desired effect on the particular patient, main side effects, and nursing implications.
   E. The nurse prepares medication in a quiet environment with few interruptions.
   F. Once the physician's orders are complete and understood, the nurse gives medications exactly as prescribed.
      1. The *right* patient.
      2. The *right* drug.
      3. The *right* dose.
      4. The *right* route.
      5. The *right* time.
   G. The nurse administers only those medications prepared by herself or himself.
   H. The nurse administers medications without introducing any unnecessary microorganisms.
   I. The nurse administers drugs only from properly labeled containers and packages.
      1. In a unit dose system, drugs may be labeled in single-dose packages that are supplied in strips or individual containers. (Figs. 13–1, 13–2). Every individual container or dose is labeled with the name of the drug and its dose.
      2. In traditional pharmacy systems, the pharmacy dispenses a certain supply of the prescribed drug and labels the container with the name and dose.

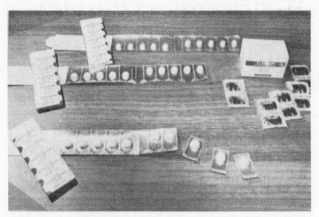

FIGURE 13-1 Examples of dry drugs in single-dose packages. These packages are usually available in strips. One unit containing a single dose is detached from the strip and administered to the patient. (Courtesy of Parke, Davis and Co., Detroit, Mich.)

3. In a unit dose system, the pharmacy may prepare parenteral injections and/or IV fluids containing additives. All syringes and IV fluids dispensed by the pharmacy in this system should be labeled with the name of the drug and its dose; the date of preparation.

J. The nurse double-checks all dosage calculations with another person.

K. The nurse does not leave medications unattended at any time.

L. The nurse selects actions that enable the patient to take prescribed drugs safely and effectively.

M. The nurse records that a drug has been administered as soon as possible after administration (Fig. 13–3).

N. The nurse reports a medication error immediately.

II. Procedures for administering drug therapy.

    A. Gather information.

        1. Attend report to gather information about patients who will be receiving drug therapy.

            a. Note the names of patients who are NPO.

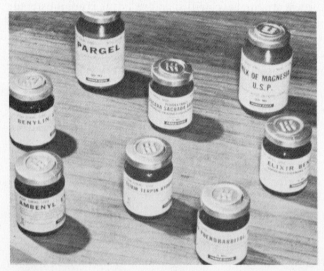

FIGURE 13-2 Examples of liquid drugs in single-dose packages. The cap is removed and the patient drinks the drug directly from the container. (Courtesy of Parke, Davis and Co., Detroit, Mich.)

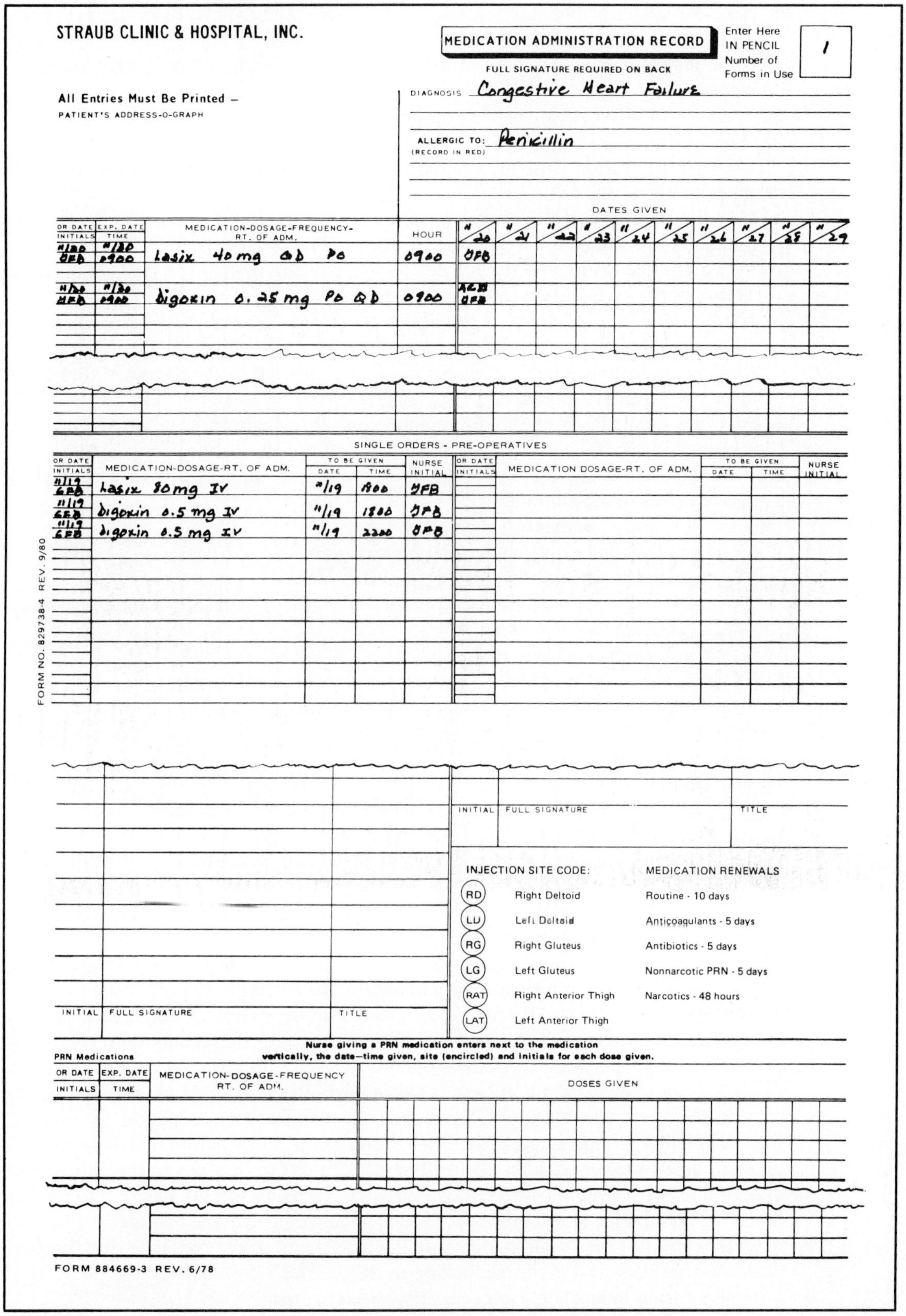

STRAUB CLINIC & HOSPITAL, INC.

MEDICATION ADMINISTRATION RECORD

FULL SIGNATURE REQUIRED ON BACK

Enter Here IN PENCIL Number of Forms in Use: 1

All Entries Must Be Printed —

PATIENT'S ADDRESS-O-GRAPH

DIAGNOSIS: Congestive Heart Failure

ALLERGIC TO: Penicillin

(RECORD IN RED)

DATES GIVEN

OR DATE INITIALS	EXP. DATE TIME	MEDICATION-DOSAGE-FREQUENCY-RT. OF ADM.	HOUR	11/20	11/21	11/22	11/23	11/24	11/25	11/26	11/27	11/28	11/29
11/20 GFB	11/30 0900	Lasix 40 mg QD PO	0900	GFB									
11/20 MFB	11/30 0900	digoxin 0.25 mg PO QD	0900	ACB GFB									

SINGLE ORDERS - PRE-OPERATIVES

OR DATE INITIALS	MEDICATION-DOSAGE-RT. OF ADM.	TO BE GIVEN DATE	TO BE GIVEN TIME	NURSE INITIAL	OR DATE INITIALS	MEDICATION DOSAGE-RT. OF ADM.	TO BE GIVEN DATE	TO BE GIVEN TIME	NURSE INITIAL
11/19 GFB	Lasix 80 mg IV	11/19	1800	GFB					
11/19 GFB	digoxin 0.5 mg IV	11/19	1800	GFB					
11/19 GFB	digoxin 0.5 mg IV	11/19	2200	GFB					

FORM NO. 829738-4 REV. 9/80

INITIAL	FULL SIGNATURE	TITLE

INITIAL	FULL SIGNATURE	TITLE

INJECTION SITE CODE:

- (RD) Right Deltoid
- (LD) Left Deltoid
- (RG) Right Gluteus
- (LG) Left Gluteus
- (RAT) Right Anterior Thigh
- (LAT) Left Anterior Thigh

MEDICATION RENEWALS

- Routine - 10 days
- Anticoagulants - 5 days
- Antibiotics - 5 days
- Nonnarcotic PRN - 5 days
- Narcotics - 48 hours

PRN Medications

Nurse giving a PRN medication enters next to the medication vertically, the date—time given, site (encircled) and initials for each dose given.

OR DATE INITIALS	EXP. DATE TIME	MEDICATION-DOSAGE-FREQUENCY RT. OF ADM.	DOSES GIVEN

FORM 884669-3 REV. 6/78

FIGURE 13-3 All medications administered by the nurse are recorded on the patient's medication administration record (MAR). (Courtesy of Straub Clinic and Hospital, Honolulu, Hawaii.)

    b. Note the names of patients scheduled for surgery, x-ray films, other special procedures.

    c. Note names of patients on fluid restrictions, force fluids, intake-output measurements.

  2. Assemble medication cards/medication profiles on all patients receiving drug therapy (see Fig. 13-3).

  3. Check each medication card/medication profile according to agency procedure. This must be done in a systematic way.

    a. If medication cards are used, they are assembled in the same sequence as the medication appears on the patient's Kardex/medication profile. A check for errors is made by reading the drug from the Kardex and comparing that to the medication card. This prevents oversights in the event of lost or missing medication cards.

    b. If a medication profile is used, it may be compared with the patient's Kardex. The check should be made in a sequence starting with the top line and moving down the Kardex line by line. The medication profile is compared to the Kardex if that is the agency or hospital procedure.

    c. All drugs should be checked in this manner including single dose and prn orders.

  4. Clarify any drug orders if necessary by calling the physician or pharmacy.

  5. Seek additional information about unfamiliar drugs from an authorized source such as a reference book or the pharmacist.

B. Assemble supplies and equipment.

  1. Water, juice, applesauce, or puddings if necessary to mix with drugs.

  2. Soufflé cups, medicine cups, drinking cups, straws, napkins, spoons.

  3. Various sizes of syringes and needles, disposal container for used supplies.

  4. Alcohol swabs, adhesive bandages.

  5. Medicine dropper, mortar and pestle, file.

  6. Medication cards/profiles for every patient; notes from morning report.

  7. Medications as supplied by the pharmacy. (These should be locked at all times.)

  8. Medication trays or cart.

C. Pour the prescribed drug.

  1. Wash the hands.

  2. Place all the medicine cards/profiles in order after they have been checked.

  3. Read the first medicine card or medication on the first line of the profile.

  4. Remove the drug from the storage container and compare the label to the medicine card/profile.

  5. Calculate the correct dose, if necessary. Cross-check all calculations with another nurse.

  6. Dispense solid medication by removing the cap of the container and pouring the correct number of pills, tablets, or capsules into the cap. Then pour the dose from the cap in a soufflé cup. If the drug is dispensed in a unit dose, the correct dose is unpackaged at the bedside and placed in a soufflé cup before giving it to the patient. Compare the label to the medication card or medication administration record for the second time.

  7. Dispense liquid medication by placing the medicine cup on a flat surface at eye level. Check the cap to be certain it is secure. Shake the bottle if directed by rolling it gently between the palms of both hands. Place the label of the container against the palm of your hand and pour the correct dose. Wipe the lip of the bottle before replacing the cap. In a unit dose system, select the correct number of units to be given to the patient and shake if directed by rotating the container between the palms of both hands. The patient drinks the liquid directly from the bottle after it is unwrapped at the bedside.

  8. After the drug has been poured, compare the label again to the medicine card/profile. Place the drug right next to the medication card.

  9. Administer drugs immediately after they have been poured.

D. Administer medication to the patient.

  1. Take the medication cart or tray to the patient's bedside.

  2. Wash the hands and introduce yourself to the patient.

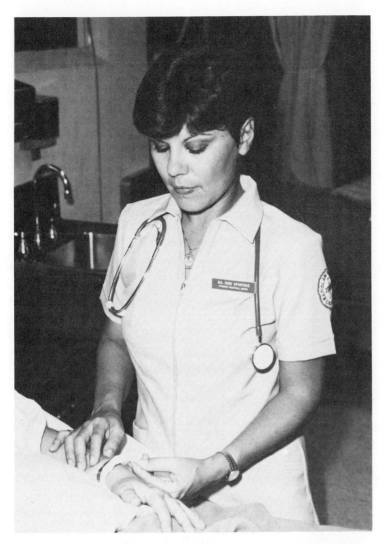

FIGURE 13-4   The student LPN/LVN is checking the patient's identification band before administering medication.

3. Read the medicine card/profile and compare the name on it to the name on the patient's identification band and bed.
4. Address the patient by name and explain that it is time for his or her medication. Position the patient if necessary.
5. Pour water or juice if the medication is a solid.
6. If the medication is in unit dose, again compare the label to the medication profile before unwrapping the package.
7. Give the medication to the patient. Solids first followed by water or juice. Liquids are given next. (Water should not be given following cough syrup.)
   a. Medication with an unpleasant taste may be given with applesauce, pudding, or fruit juice.
   b. Tablets and pills may be crushed if the patient is unable to swallow them. *Never* crush capsules without asking the pharmacy if this procedure will alter the drug action.
   c. Administer sublingual and buccal drugs last. Sublingual drugs are placed under the tongue. Buccal drugs are placed between the gum and the cheek.
8. Remain with the patient until all medication has been taken. Do not leave any medication at the bedside.

9. Raise the siderails if indicated. Place the call bell close at hand. Reposition the patient if needed.
10. Record fluid intake if ordered.
11. Note any unusual events or occurrences and report them to the nurse in charge.
12. Chart the medication immediately after administering it. Record also if the medication was withheld or refused.

III. Procedures for medication errors.
 A. Report the error as soon as it is discovered to the charge nurse.
 B. Notify the physician if it has not already been done by the nurse in charge.
 C. Observe the patient carefully for an adverse drug reaction. Seek additional information from a reference book or the pharmacy about adverse reactions if necessary.
 D. Carry out any precautionary measures ordered by the physician.
 E. Chart the error and what was done.
 F. Fill out an incident report as required by the hospital.

CHECKLIST FOR ADMINISTERING MEDICATIONS

1. Gather and record all pertinent information about the patients to whom you will be giving drugs.
2. Assemble medication cards or medication administration records (MAR) according to hospital or agency policy.
3. Verify each medication to be given using hospital or agency procedure. Start with the top line and move down in sequence line by line until every drug to be given has been verified.
4. Clarify drug orders if necessary. Look up essential information in authorized drug references or consult with the pharmacist.
5. Gather all necessary supplies.
6. Wash hands and repeat between patients and at other appropriate times while administering medications.
7. Remove drug container and check label by comparing it either to the medication card or the MAR.
8. Calculate dose if necessary and cross-check calculations with another nurse.
9. Check label for the second time.
10. Pour drug or draw it up without soiling the label or introducing unnecessary microorganisms. Turn container caps upside down before setting on a counter.
11. Complete third label check.
12. Introduce yourself to the patient and call the patient by name during the introduction.
13. Briefly describe the medication to be given using language the patient can understand. Answer the patient's questions or refer them to the registered nurse or physician as needed.
14. Identify the patient formally by comparing his or her identification bracelet to the medication card or MAR.
15. Take whatever nursing actions are appropriate before administering the drug. (For example, check for adverse responses; take blood pressure or apical pulse; measure output; check the IV administration site.)
16. Position the patient appropriately according to the route of administration.
17. Administer the medication and remain with the patient until all medication has been taken.
18. Reposition the patient and make him or her comfortable.
19. Record all medication administered; medications withheld; medications refused.
20. Record fluid intake if the patient's intake and output is measured.
21. Record the patient's response to medication on the nurses' progress notes as needed. Report appropriate information to the registered nurse.
22. Complete all necessary forms when administering narcotics and other controlled substances.
23. Clean and replenish the medication area as needed.
24. Make all necessary charges for medication and supplies.
25. Monitor the patient's response to drug therapy on a continuing basis.

Chapter 14 | ADMINISTERING PARENTERAL INJECTIONS

EXPECTED BEHAVIORAL OUTCOMES

After completing this chapter, you should return to the expected behavioral outcomes and evaluate your ability to:

1. Define common terms associated with parenteral injections.
2. List indications for drug therapy using the parenteral route.
3. List disadvantages of drug therapy using the parenteral route.
4. Identify parts of a needle and syringe.
5. Withdraw medication for injection from an ampule or a vial without introducing any microorganisms.
6. Identify appropriate injection sites for each parenteral route.
7. Use the correct procedure for injecting medication by each of the parenteral routes.

COMMON TERMS

1. *Ampule*—a small sealed glass container that holds sterile contents (Figure 14–1).
2. *Aspirate*—pull the plunger of a syringe back away from the needle to withdraw something.
3. *Hypodermic*—given or introduced beneath the skin.
4. *Hypodermoclysis*—introduction of fluid into the SC tissue to replace excessive losses or insufficient intake.
5. *Intradermal*—a parenteral route in which medication is injected between the layers of the skin.
6. *Intramuscular*—within the muscle.
7. *Parenteral*—by a route other than the gastrointestinal tract.
8. *Subcutaneous*—beneath the skin.
9. *Vial*—a small bottle (Fig. 14–1).

INDICATIONS FOR DRUG THERAPY BY THE PARENTERAL ROUTE

1. The medication is inactivated or destroyed by the gastrointestinal system.
2. A speedy action is desired.
3. The patient is unable to swallow oral medication.
4. The patient is unwilling to swallow oral medication.
5. There is a need for more predictable absorption of the drug.

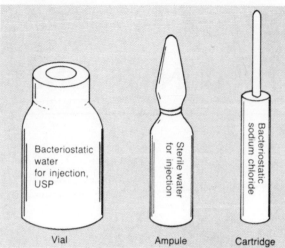

FIGURE 14-1 **Containers for parenteral medications.** (Reprinted with permission from Atkinson, L. D., and Murray, M. E., *Fundamentals of Nursing: A Nursing Process Approach.* Macmillan, New York, 1985.)

DISADVANTAGES OF DRUG THERAPY BY THE PARENTERAL ROUTE

1. The skin barrier is broken by the needle thus exposing the patient to possible infection.
2. The rapid action associated with the parenteral route may result in more rapid onsets of adverse drug actions that are difficult to prevent or control.
3. The injection procedure causes trauma and injury to the involved tissue.
4. Incorrect identification of the injection site may result in temporary or permanent injury to important nerves, blood vessels, and bones.

RULES FOR ADMINISTERING PARENTERAL INJECTIONS

The general rules listed on pp. 83–88 that guide administration of drug therapy also apply to parenteral injections. In addition, the following rules are used:

1. The nurse maintains sterility of any substance or equipment used for parenteral injections.
2. All solutions to be injected are thoroughly mixed, usually by rotating the container gently between the palms of both hands. There should be no sediment or particles in the solutions to be injected.
3. Needles and syringes are kept under lock and key.
4. Needles and syringes are destroyed before they are discarded and special containers are used to prevent accidental puncture with a used needle.
5. Injection sites are rotated when multiple injections are needed.
6. Injection sites are avoided if there is a rash or lumps in the area.

SYRINGES AND NEEDLES

Parenteral injections are given with a syringe and needle. The syringe consists of two primary parts—the barrel and the plunger (Fig. 14-2). All medications and equipment that will penetrate the skin must remain sterile. Therefore, in preparing a parenteral injection, the only parts of the syringe that may be touched by human hands are the outside of the barrel, the flange, and the end of the plunger. Several different syringes are available. Most in current use are made of plastic but some are glass (Fig. 14-3).

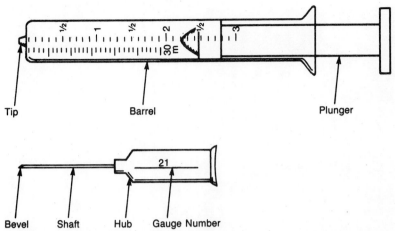

Tip   Barrel   Plunger

Bevel   Shaft   Hub   Gauge Number

FIGURE 14-2   Parts of a needle and syringe. (Reprinted with permission from Atkinson, L. D., and Murray, M. E., *Fundamentals of Nursing: A Nursing Process Approach.* Macmillan, New York, 1985.)

1. Hypodermic syringe—usual size is 2½–3 ml but other sizes also available. Calibrated in cubic centimeters and minims. May come packaged with the needle already attached.
2. Tuberculin syringe—used for intradermal injections and administering less than 1 ml of medication. Calibrated in tenths of cubic centimeters and in minims.
3. Insulin syringe—used only to administer insulin. Calibrated in units that correspond to strength of insulin. One brand comes with a very small-gauge needle that is permanently attached. Thus it cannot be changed.
4. Cartridge injection systems—a metal or plastic holder and plunger used with glass cartridges containing premeasured medication doses and a needle that is permanently attached to the cartridge (Fig. 14–4).

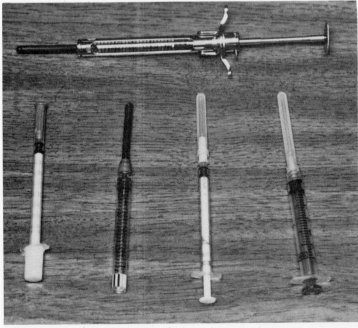

FIGURE 14-3   Examples of syringes commonly used for parenteral injections. The syringe at the top is an example of a cartridge injection system. From left to right: insulin syringe, cartridge, tuberculin syringe, and 3-ml syringe.

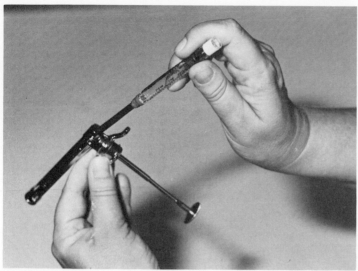

FIGURE 14-4 In this cartridge injection system, the metal holder with its plunger is being loaded with a glass cartridge that includes a permanently attached needle and a premeasured dose of medication.

Needles are made of metal and come in various lengths and gauges. The length of the needle is measured from the hub to the point. The needle selected for injection must be long enough to reach the desired site. Thus longer needles are selected for the intramuscular route or when the patient is obese. Shorter needles may be selected for the intradermal route or for patients who are thin or wasted. The *gauge* of the needle means the size of the lumen. Numbers are assigned to the gauge. The larger the number, the smaller the lumen of the needle. Gauge sizes range from 14 to 27. Thicker medications generally are administered with a larger-gauge needle such as 20 or 21 gauge. This prevents the thick medication from clogging the needle.

Most needles in current use are disposable and come covered with a needle cover and enclosed in a plastic and paper package. Some needles are already attached to syringes. In preparing medication for parenteral injection, no part of the needle should come in contact with human hands. Only the needle cover can be touched. Some experts recommend changing the needle after the medication has been prepared so that the patient's skin is broken by a needle that has never been used.

In preparing medication for parenteral injection, a common problem is a tight or sticky plunger. This can be managed easily by pulling back the end of the plunger once or twice to loosen it. Another common problem is difficulty in removing the needle cover without having the needle detach from the syringe. It sometimes helps to attach the needle firmly to the syringe first. Then rock the needle cover gently forward and backward once or twice before trying to remove it.

After a disposable needle and syringe has been used, they are discarded in a special way. The needle is broken either with a needle cutter or by rocking the cap back and forth to bend and break the needle. The syringe tip is broken with a special cutter if available (Fig. 14–5). The needle and syringe are then discarded in a special box.

PROCEDURE FOR PREPARING A NEEDLE AND SYRINGE

1. Select the appropriate needle and syringe according to the amount of medication to be given, the consistency of medication, and the route of administration.
   a. Volumes of 1 ml or less are easier to measure if a tuberculin syringe is used (Fig. 14–3).
   b. Needle size for the IM route should usually be 1 to 2½ in. and 19 to 23 gauge.
   c. Needle size for the intradermal route should usually be ½ in. and 24 to 27 gauge.
   d. Needle size for the SC route should usually be ½ to 1 in. and 24 to 27 gauge.

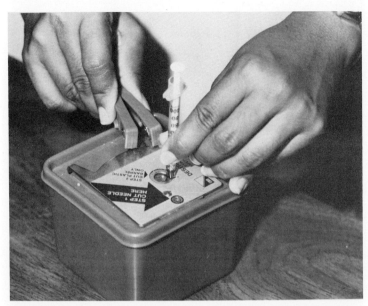

FIGURE 14-5   The nurse is destroying the syringe and needle with a needle and syringe cutter. After it is destroyed, the syringe is placed in a special receptacle for disposal.

2. Prepare the needle and syringe by removing them from the package.
3. Attach the needle to the syringe if necessary, making sure that the syringe tip and the needle hub remain sterile.
4. Loosen the needle cover by rocking it gently back and forth.
5. Remove the needle cover and inspect the needle for imperfections. During the inspection, be sure not to touch the needle or the opening of the cover. Replace the needle if necessary.
6. After replacing the needle cover, pull back on the plunger handle gently several times to make sure the plastic parts are not stuck together. Do not touch the plunger below the flange.

PROCEDURE FOR WITHDRAWING MEDICATION FROM AN AMPULE (FIG. 14–6)

1. Tap the stem of the ampule to make certain that all of the drug is contained in the ampule proper.
2. Wipe the stem with an alcohol pledget.
3. Hold the ampule in one hand and, with an alcohol pledget, break off the stem at the scored area with the other hand.
4. Place the ampule on a level surface.
5. Remove the needle cover from the needle.
6. Insert the needle into the ampule and withdraw the prescribed dose.
7. Remove air from the syringe using the following suggested steps:
    a. Position the syringe in your hand so that the needle is pointing up.
    b. Tap the side of the syringe gently until the air rises to the top toward the needle.
    c. Carefully move the plunger forward to push air out through the needle. This should be done without pushing medication out. In other words, only air should be expelled from the needle.
    d. Recheck the dosage.
    e. If medication has leaked out of the syringe and down onto the needle, change the needle.
    f. Cover the needle with the needle cover.
8. Discard the ampule in a receptacle for glass.

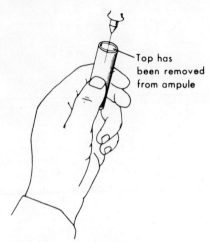

FIGURE 14-6 Removing solution from ampule.

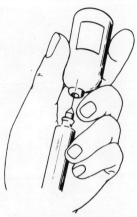

Top has been removed from ampule

FIGURE 14-7 Removing solution from vial.

PROCEDURE FOR WITHDRAWING MEDICATION FROM A VIAL

1. Remove the metal disk that seals an unopened vial if necessary.
2. Cleanse the rubber stopper of the vial with an alcohol swab using rotary motion and friction.
3. While the alcohol is drying on the rubber stopper, pull the plunger of the syringe back to the calibration that indicates the prescribed dose.
4. Inject that volume of air into the vial by inserting the needle into the rubber cap. Leave the needle in the vial.
5. Invert the vial and syringe and pull the plunger back slowly until the correct dose is measured (Fig. 14–7). To avoid air bubbles in the syringe, be sure that the tip of the needle is in the liquid before pulling back on the plunger.
6. Remove air from the syringe using the steps outlined above.
7. Cover the needle with the needle cover.
8. Discard vial if it contained a single dose—be sure to discard in a glass receptacle. Mark multiple-dose vials with the date and time opened and return to the usual storage place.

PROCEDURE FOR ADMINISTERING A PARENTERAL INJECTION

1. Take the medication cart or tray containing the syringe and an alcohol swab to the patient's bedside.
2. Wash the hands. Introduce yourself to the patient.
3. Read the medicine card/profile and compare the name on it to the name on the patient's indentification band and bed.
4. Address the patient by name and explain that it is time for his or her injection.
5. Select the injection site using the procedures outlined in separate sections in this chapter.
6. Cleanse the injection site with an alcohol swab using rotary motion and friction. Start at the center of the site and use circular motion to create ever-widening circles. An area about 2-in. in diameter should be cleansed.
7. Inject the needle into the skin according the specific route of administration described in separate sections.
8. Pull back on the plunger slightly to determine if the needle has entered a blood vessel. If blood appears in the syringe, remove the needle and replace it with a sterile one. Then repeat the injection procedure starting with step 5. If substantial blood appears, discard the needle and syringe, and begin again.

9. If blood does not appear in the syringe, inject the drug slowly by pushing the plunger forward toward the needle.
10. When the syringe is empty, quickly withdraw the needle and press the alcohol swab over the needle site.
11. Unless contraindicated, massage the injection site gently in a circular motion with the alcohol swab. This helps to distribute the medication.
12. Check the injection site for bleeding. If bleeding is present, apply gentle pressure for 1 full minute and recheck.
13. Make the patient comfortable.
14. Use hospital procedure to dispose of needle and syringe.
15. Chart the medication.

ADMINISTERING AN INTRADERMAL INJECTION

An intradermal injection is given into the dermal layer of the skin (Fig. 14–8). This route is used primarily to determine sensitivity or susceptibility to: allergens such as pollen and house dust; diseases such as tuberculosis; drugs such as antitoxins.

1. Select the injection site.
    a. Inner aspect of forearms are frequently used.
    b. Upper back may also be used.
    c. Dorsal and lateral surfaces of the upper arm are occasionally selected.
2. Select the syringe and needle.
    a. Because amounts to be administered are generally very small (0.1 to 0.3 ml), a tuberculin syringe is used.
    b. A ⅜- to ½-in. 25 to 27 gauge needle is used.
3. Cleanse the skin as previously explained.
4. After removing the needle cap, hold the syringe between the thumb and four fingers (Fig. 14–9).
5. Retract (pull back) the skin of the injection site with your free hand.
6. Holding the syringe flat against the skin (10 to 15° angle), insert the needle with the bevel up so that only the bevel of the needle actually penetrates the skin. The bevel should be visible beneath the top skin layer.
7. Remove your free hand and use it to hold the barrel of the syringe. Then aspirate (pull back) the plunger to be sure the needle has not penetrated a blood vessel.
8. Inject the medication slowly so that it forms a visible wheal (small raised bump that resembles a mosquito bite).
9. Withdraw the needle from the injection site. Apply pressure to the site with the alcohol swab but DO NOT MASSAGE THE SITE.

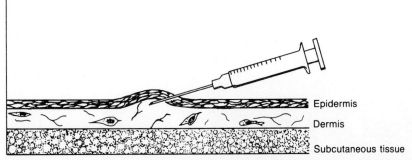

FIGURE 14-8 Medication is inserted under the epidermis in an intradermal injection. (Reprinted with permission from Atkinson, L. D., and Murray, M. E., *Fundamentals of Nursing: A Nursing Process Approach.* Macmillan, New York, 1985.)

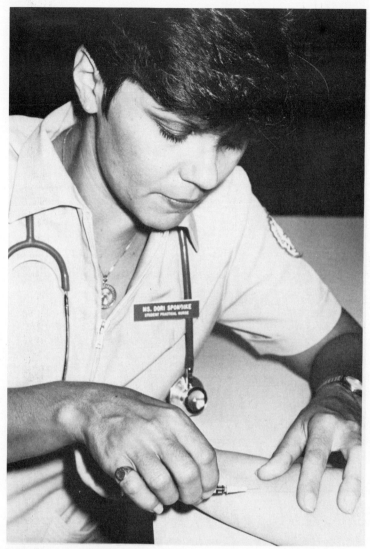

FIGURE 14-9   The nurse is administering an intradermal injection.

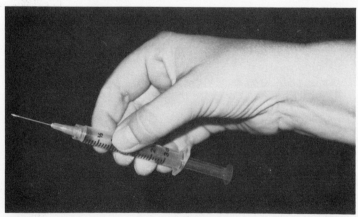

FIGURE 14-10   The syringe may be placed between the thumb and four fingers of the dominant hand for an SC injection.

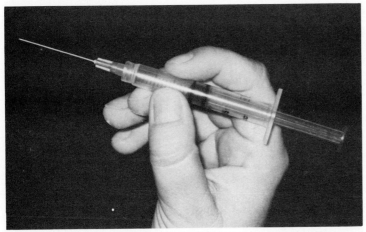

FIGURE 14-11   The syringe may be held like a pencil for either an SC or IM injection.

PROCEDURE FOR ADMINISTERING A SUBCUTANEOUS INJECTION

An SC injection is given beneath the skin.

1. Select the needle and syringe.
   a. Because the amounts to be used vary, a 1-, 2-, 2.5-, or 3-ml syringe may be used.
   b. Needles may vary from ½ to 1 in. and the needle gauge ranges from 24 to 27 gauge.
2. Select the injection site.
   a. A common site is the fleshy portion of the arm behind the deltoid muscle.
   b. Abdominal sites may also be used—select the fleshy portions of the anterior and lateral abdomen.
   c. Fleshy tissue of the anterior and lateral thighs may be used.
   d. Fleshy tissue of buttocks may be used.
3. Cleanse the skin as previously explained.
4. After removing the needle cap, the syringe may be held either between the thumb and four fingers as shown in Fig. 14–10 or as a pencil as shown in Fig. 14–11.

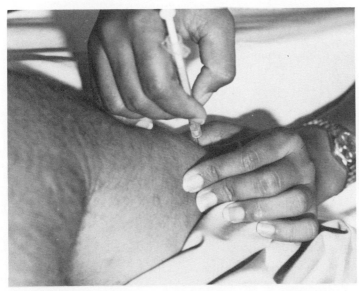

FIGURE 14-12   Administering an SC injection.

5. Using the thumb and fingers of your free hand, grasp and pull up 1 to 2 in. of that fleshy injection site that has just been cleansed.
6. Holding the needle and syringe at a 45° angle, inject the needle into the skin you are holding with your free hand (Fig. 14–12).
7. Remove your free hand and use it to hold the barrel of the syringe. Then aspirate (pull back) the plunger to make certain the needle has not entered a blood vessel. *Note*: When injecting an anticoagulant such as heparin sodium, this step is omitted.
8. After the drug has been injected slowly, withdraw the needle, apply pressure to the needle site and massage it as explained earlier. *Note*: When injecting an anticoagulant such as heparin sodium, massage is not used.

ADMINISTERING AN INTRAMUSCULAR INJECTION

An intramuscular injection is given into a muscle. The intramuscular route may be prescribed when the volume to be injected is more than 2 ml, when rapid absorption is desired, or when the prescribed drug is irritating to the injection site. No more than 3 ml should be injected into each site. The procedure for administering an IM injection is very similar to that for the SC route. A special feature of the IM route is the need for careful site selection in order to prevent injury to nerves and blood vessels.

  I. Select the appropriate needle and syringe.
    A. The needle gauge ranges from 19 to 23 and the needle length ranges from 1 to 2½ in. The needle must be long enough to penetrate skin and SC tissue and get into the muscle.
    B. The syringe capacity is usually 2 ml or more. However, a 1-ml syringe or a tuberculin syringe may be used for very small amounts.
 II. Select the injection sites.

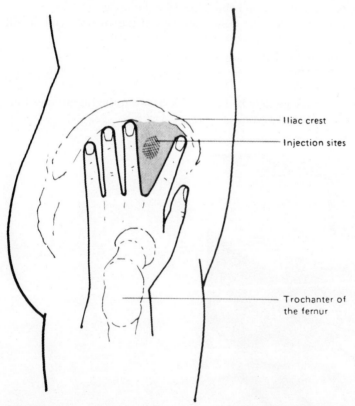

Iliac crest

Injection sites

Trochanter of the femur

FIGURE 14-13 Ventrogluteal injection site is demonstrated, showing the position of the hand over the greater trochanter of the femur and the forefinger pointing toward the anterior iliac crest.

A. The *ventrogluteal muscle* is a highly recommended site for children and adults when injections are delivered in the prone, supine, sitting, or standing position. The muscle is thick and can accept large volumes of medication. There are no major nerves or blood vessels in the area. The skin over the sites is relatively insensitive, thus, the injection may be less painful. The site is located by placing the palm of the opposite hand over the greater trochanter of the patient's opposite femur. The index finger of the hand is placed over the anterior superior iliac spine of the hip. The middle finger is placed toward the posterior iliac crest. The injection site lie in a *V* between the two fingers (Fig. 14–13).

B. The *vastus lateralis* muscle in the anterior portion of the thigh may be used for both children and adults. There is easy access when the patient is in supine, prone, or sitting position (Fig. 14–14). There are no important blood vessels or nerves in the immediate area; however, penetration of the fascia lata may be painful. The site is located by placing one hand around the thigh just above the knee. The other hand is placed around the upper thigh just below the greater trochanter of the femur. The injection sites lie in the narrow band spanning from the midlateral thigh to the midanterior thigh (Fig. 14–14).

C. The *gluteus medius* or dorsogluteal area is the most commonly used site for intramuscular injections in the adult (Fig. 14–15). The muscle mass is large and can accept greater amounts of drugs and repeated injections. This site is not recommended for children under 3 years of age or for patients who are malnourished. There are two major blood vessels (the gluteal arteries) and the sciatic nerve in this area. Therefore, the nurse uses extreme caution in selecting the site in order to prevent damage to those structures. The site is located by placing the patient in the prone position with the toes pointed inward and the entire buttock fully exposed. An imaginary line is drawn horizontally across the buttock at the top of the gluteal

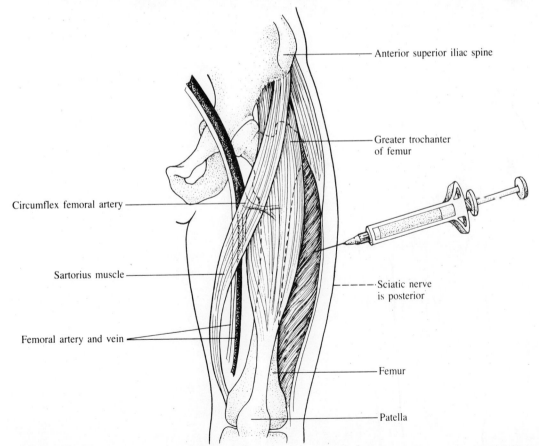

Anterior superior iliac spine

Greater trochanter of femur

Circumflex femoral artery

Sartorius muscle

Sciatic nerve is posterior

Femoral artery and vein

Femur

Patella

FIGURE 14-14 Vastus lateralis IM injection site. (Courtesy of Winthrop-Breon Laboratories, New York. Reprinted with permission from Atkinson, L. D., and Murray, M. E., *Fundamentals of Nursing: A Nursing Process Approach.* Macmillan, New York, 1985.)

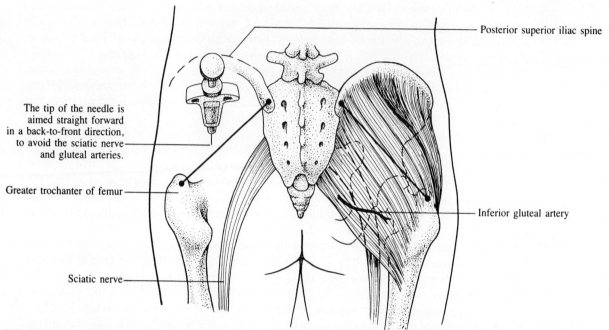

The tip of the needle is aimed straight forward in a back-to-front direction, to avoid the sciatic nerve and gluteal arteries.

Greater trochanter of femur

Sciatic nerve

Posterior superior iliac spine

Inferior gluteal artery

FIGURE 14-15   Gluteus medius/IM injection site. (Courtesy of Winthrop-Breon Laboratories, New York. Reprinted with permission from Atkinson, L. D., and Murray, M. E., *Fundamentals of Nursing: A Nursing Process Approach.* Macmillan, New York, 1985.)

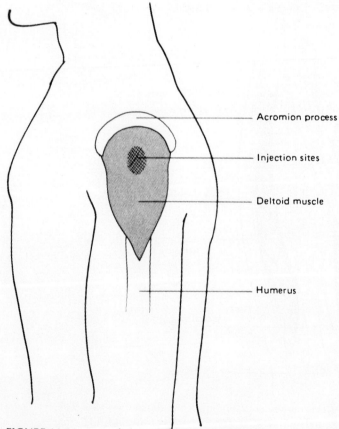

Acromion process

Injection sites

Deltoid muscle

Humerus

FIGURE 14-16   Lateral view of deltoid injection site.

fold. Next, an imaginary vertical line is drawn from the top of the iliac crest to the bottom of the buttock. The injection sites lie in the upper outer quadrant. Another way to locate the gluteus medius is to draw the imaginary line diagonally between the greater trochanter of the femur and the posterior superior iliac spine of the hip (Fig. 14–15). The injection sites lie above and outside the imaginary line.

    D. The *deltoid muscle* may be used for either children or adults in the sitting, standing, or lying position. The sites are limited because there are major blood vessels, nerves, and bones in the area. This site should not be used for repeated injections or amounts of drug greater than 1 ml. The site is located by placing two fingers just below the acromion process and placing the other hand around the upper arm at the point of the axillary fold. The injection sites lie in a small rectangle of the lateral surface between these two points (Fig. 14–16).

  III. Cleanse the site as previously explained. A tip in making the location of injection sites easier is to place an alcohol swab over the injection site as soon as it is located.

  IV. After removing the needle cap, hold the syringe like a pencil. Stretch the skin of the injection site between the thumb and index finger of your free hand.

   V. Inject the needle into the site at a 90° angle.

  VI. Aspirate the plunger to make certain the needle has not entered a blood vessel.

 VII. After the medication has been injected slowly, withdraw the needle, apply pressure to the needle site, and massage it as explained earlier.

USING THE Z-TRACT INJECTION METHOD

The Z-tract injection is a method of administering an IM injection that prevents damage and staining to skin and SC tissue surrounding the injection area. The gluteus medius muscle is the site most often selected when the Z-tract method is used. Two drugs that require the use of the Z-tract method are Imferon and hydroxyzine hydrochloride (Vistaril). The procedure for using the Z-tract method is as follows:

  1. After removing the drug from the vial or ampule, change the needle so that there is no medication remaining in it.

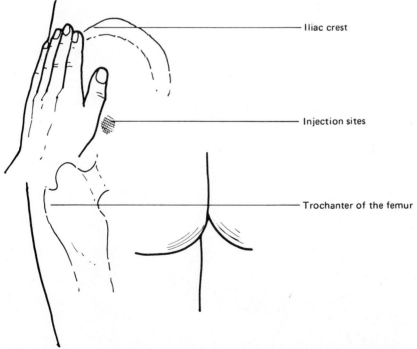

Iliac crest

Injection sites

Trochanter of the femur

FIGURE 14-17   *Z-tract injection. The skin is being stretched laterally and tautly.*

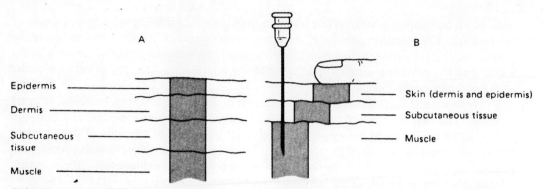

FIGURE 14-18   Z-tract injection. A. Relative position of the skin, SC tissue, and muscle. B. Skin and SC tissue pulled laterally. (Courtesy of Palm Beach County Practical Nursing Program, The School Board of Palm Beach County, Fla.)

2. Add 2 to 3 m. of air to the syringe. This will prevent any drug from being disseminated into the tissues as the needle is being withdrawn.
3. Using the heel of the free hand, retract laterally and tautly the skin of the dorsogluteal area (skin must be held in this position during the entire procedure) (Figs. 14–17, 14–18).
4. After the skin is retracted, select the injection site as described above on pp. 98, 99, 101.
5. Inject the medication.
6. Wait 10 s before removing the needle.
7. Do not massage the site.
8. Use alternate buttocks for subsequent injections.

Chapter 15 | ADMINISTERING DRUG THERAPY BY OTHER ROUTES

EXPECTED BEHAVIORAL OUTCOMES

After completing this chapter, you should return to the expected behavioral outcomes and evaluate your ability to:

1. Instill ear, eye, and nose drops.
2. Insert a suppository.
3. Administer topical drug therapy.
4. Monitor the patient receiving IV drug therapy.
5. Instill medication through a feeding tube.
6. Administer selected drug therapy by inhalation.
7. Monitor the patient following intraspinal or intrathecal injection.

INTRODUCTION

In addition to the oral and parenteral routes, drugs may be administered in many other ways. This chapter provides directions for other routes. Although not repeated here, the rules and procedures described in Chapters 13 and 14 that guide safe and effective administration of drug therapy apply also to these routes.

PROCEDURE FOR INSTILLING EAR DROPS

1. Wash the hands.
2. Position the patient so that the head is tilted to the unaffected side.
3. Draw up the medication in the dropper.
4. For the adult patient, straighten the external auditory canal by pulling the pinna upward and back with the free hand.
5. For the child, straighten the external auditory canal by pulling the earlobe downward and back with the free hand.
6. Instill the number of drops prescribed.
7. Plug the external auditory canal loosely with cotton to prevent the medication from leaking out. Encourage the patient to keep the head in the tilted position for several minutes after instillation. (*Note*: Some physicians do not want cotton placed in the ear.)

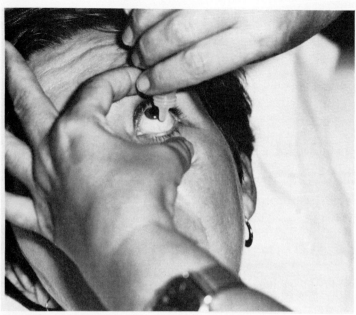

FIGURE 15-1   Instilling eye drops.

8. If drops are prescribed for both ears, wash the hands thoroughly and repeat the procedure. Some experts recommend that separate droppers and medications be used for each ear to prevent the transfer of organisms from one ear to the other.
9. Chart the medication according to hospital procedure.

PROCEDURE FOR INSTILLING EYE DROPS AND OINTMENTS* (Fig. 15–1)

1. Wash the hands thoroughly.
2. Position the patient either on the back, sitting up, or standing with the neck slightly hyperextended.
3. Draw up the prescribed number of drops or uncap the prescribed ointment.
4. Gently grasp the lower lid using the thumb and index finger of the free hand to pull the lower lid out slowly and create a pouch. An alternate method is to pull the lower lid down until the conjunctival sac is visible.
5. Instruct the patient to look upward.
6. Instill the prescribed number of drops into the pouch *without* touching the patient's eye with the dropper at any time. The hand holding the dropper may be rested gently on the patient's forehead or cheek to steady it.
7. Instruct the patient to close the eyes gently and move the eye around in the socket to distribute the medication. At the same time, apply gentle pressure to the inner canthus near the bridge of the patient's nose to prevent overflow and reduce systemic absorption.
8. Wait at least 5 min before instilling additional drops into the same eye. This is because of limited volume in the spaces under the lids.
9. Apply eye ointment as a thin ribbon inside the lower lid. (Ointment and drops are not interchangeable because of differences in concentration in the target tissue of the eye.) Pressure over the bridge of the nose is not used following application of an ointment.
10. If drops are prescribed for both eyes, the hands must be washed thoroughly again. A sepa-

*Adapted from Mason, M. A., and Bates, G. F., *Basic Medical-Surgical Nursing,* 5th ed. Macmillan, New York, 1984.

rate medication container or dropper is used for the second eye to prevent the spread of microorganisms from one eye to the other.

11. Chart the medication.

PROCEDURE FOR INSTILLING NOSE DROPS

1. Wash the hands.
2. Position the patient by hyperextending the neck over a tightly rolled pillow, the edge of the bed, or the back of the chair.
3. Draw up the medication into the dropper if necessary. Push the tip of the patient's nose up toward the forehead to visualize the nares.
4. Instill the prescribed number of drops.
5. Instruct the patient to remain in the same position for 1 to 2 min following the installation.
6. Chart the medication.

PROCEDURE FOR INSERTING SUPPOSITORIES

Drugs may be inserted into the rectum, vagina, or urethra through suppositories. *Suppositories* are cone-shaped semisolid fusible substances containing a drug. When introduced into body cavities, suppositories are melted by body heat that permits the drug to come in contact with mucous membranes for local or systemic effects. Suppositories are stored in a cool place to prevent premature melting.

1. Wash the hands.
2. Position the patient in either the supine or lateral Sims position.
3. Lubricate the suppository if directed.
4. Insert the suppository either with an applicator if directed or a gloved finger.
5. Rectal suppositories should be inserted beyond the sphincter to prevent expulsion from the rectum. One expert has recommended that the *flat* end of the suppository is inserted first. This causes the anal sphincter to close around the rounded edge and prevents premature expulsion of the suppository.
6. Wipe away excess lubricant if necessary.
7. Chart the medication.
8. Some suppositories may cause staining on underclothing. The patient may want to wear a protective pad to prevent this.

ADMINISTERING TOPICAL DRUG THERAPY

Topical drugs are applied to the skin for a variety of reasons. Most topical drugs are lotions, creams, or ointments prescribed to relieve pruritus, or to act as anti-infectives or emollients. A common relatively new drug is nitroglycerin ointment prescribed for long-term relief of angina. There are a variety of procedures for applying topical drug therapy. The nurse locates directions for each medication before application. The following questions help to guide the nurse in getting the correct information.

1. How should the skin be prepared before the application? (Should previous doses be removed? How are previous doses removed? Should the skin be cleansed? Should the skin be dry or moist?)
2. How should the new medication be applied? (Is the medication to be applied in a thin layer, thick layer? Should the medication be rubbed into the skin, patted on the skin, or simply left on the skin?)
3. What supplies are used to administer the topical drug therapy? (Does the nurse use a tongue blade, gloves, cotton-tipped applicator?)

4. What needs to be done following application of topical therapy? (Should the area be left covered or uncovered? Should the clothing be protected from staining?)

PROCEDURE FOR ADMINISTERING DRUG THERAPY BY INHALATION

Drug therapy may be prescribed by inhalation for either local or systemic effects. Inhalation is the process of drawing air, gas, or vapor into the lungs. This route is associated with very rapid absorption because of the many blood vessels and an abundance of target tissue present in the lungs. Typical drugs prescribed by inhalation include antibiotics, bronchodilators, antiinflammatories, and gases such as oxygen. The procedure described in this section is for an inhaler device. An inhaler is a small pressurized container that holds the drug and an attachment called the mouthpiece (Fig. 15–2). Each inhaler comes with manufacturer's directions for use and cleaning. Therefore, the procedure below may need to be modified according to those directions.

1. Wash the hands.
2. Instruct the patient completely before administering the drug.
3. Shake the inhaler well according to the manufacturer's directions.
4. Instruct the patient to exhale completely.
5. Place the mouthpiece fully in the patient's mouth with instructions to close the lips securely. Hold the inhaler in the upright position unless otherwise directed.
6. Instruct the patient to inhale deeply while fully depressing the top of the inhaler.
7. Instruct and encourage the patient to hold the breath as long as possible.
8. Remove the inhaler just before the patient exhales.
9. Wait 1 min and repeat the procedure for each breath prescribed by the physician (the order is sometimes written as 2 puffs tid). Be sure to shake the inhaler before each puff.
10. Clean the inhaler by removing the mouthpiece and rinsing it under warm running water and drying it or according to the manufacturer's directions.
11. Chart the medication.

ADMINISTERING DRUG THERAPY BY INTRAVENOUS INFUSION

A drug may be placed directly into the circulation by injecting it or infusing it into a vein. The dose is drawn up into a syringe using exactly the same procedure as that used for parenteral injections. Dur-

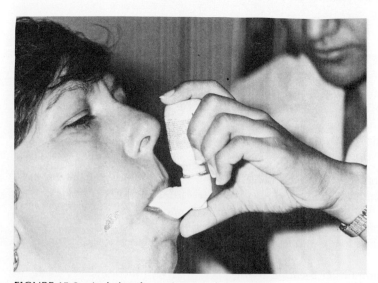

FIGURE 15-2   Assisting the patient in using an inhaler.

ing a direct IV injection, the needle is then inserted into a peripheral vein or into IV administration tubing and the medication is injected over a period of 1 to 5 min. This procedure is often done during an emergency by a physician or registered nurse. *Intravenous infusion* means that the drug is diluted in a volume of liquid. This *admixture* (mixed fluid) drips into the patient's vein through a special needle over a period from 30 min to 24 h. The infusion may be continuous or intermittent. The volume of liquid in which the drug is dissolved may vary from 50 to 1,000 ml.

As with other injections, all medication and equipment that breaks the skin barrier must be sterile. Sterile technique is used to prepare the IV injection or infusion. In some hospitals, all drugs prepared for the IV route are prepared in the pharmacy under laminar air flow that prevents the introduction of microorganisms. In other hospitals, preparation of IV drug therapy is done by registered nurses and/or licensed practical nurses (LPNs) on the nursing unit.

The specific policy that governs preparation and administration of drugs by the IV route is influenced by the Nurse Practice Act in each state, the State Board of Nursing rules and regulations, and community nursing practices. In order to practice legally, safely, and effectively, the LPN/LVN should gather complete and accurate information about state laws, rules and regulations, and policies that affect preparation, administration, and monitoring of drug therapy by the IV route. For example, in some states, only registered nurses and physicians are permitted to prepare and administer IV drug therapy. In other states, LPNs and LVNs may use these procedures.

The following procedures are divided into those associated with preparation, administration, and monitoring drug therapy by the IV route.

PROCEDURE FOR PREPARING INTRAVENOUS ADMIXTURES

1. Prepare a label that includes the patient's name and room number, the date and time the admixture was prepared, the name of drug and dose, and the name of the nurse preparer.
2. Wash the hands.
3. Draw the prescribed dose in a needle and syringe following the usual rules for comparing the label and the physician's order. The procedure is exactly the same as that used to prepare a parenteral injection (Chapter 14). Check the hospital policy about the use of filtered needles to prepare IV admixtures.
4. Change the needle.
5. If the medication is for intermittent infusion, select the appropriate solution and volume.
   a. Some medication may be diluted only with certain kinds of IV fluids. Specific directions may be located in the package insert or by calling the pharmacy.
   b. Small containers made of either glass or plastic may be used for intermittent infusions. Such containers may be called *partial fills* (Fig. 15-3). Other common terms (depending on the specific method of administration) include secondary bottle, or piggyback bottle (see Fig. 15-5). The drug from the syringe is injected into the container and infused over a specified time. Several volumes are available: 50 ml, 100 ml, and 250 ml.
   c. Another way to administer drug therapy by intermittent infusion is to use a volume control device called a *burette* (Fig. 15-4). Several brands are available and the directions for use vary according to the manufacturer. Burettes are calibrated plastic cylinders that attach to the primary IV container and hold up to 150 ml. Fluid from the primary bottle is allowed to flow into the burette to the desired volume and the inflow is then clamped. Medication may be added to the burette through a special port and the cylinder is then gently rotated to mix thoroughly. The outflow is then regulated using the usual roller clamp. When the medication has been administered, most burettes may be adjusted so that a regular amount of fluid from the primary bottle flows into it as the unmedicated IV fluid infuses.
6. Remove the protective cap from the container of IV fluid and cleanse the port with an alcohol swab using rotary motion and friction.
7. Inject the prepared medication through the injection port of the bottle or bag. If a bottle is used, the vacuum inside the bottle draws the medication from the syringe into the bottle. If a

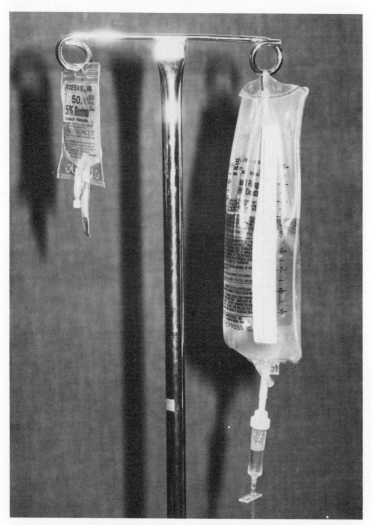

FIGURE 15-3   Examples of containers for IV drug therapy. The container on the left is a partial fill to which medication may be added; the
container on the right may be used to administer large volumes of IV
fluids or an admixture.

bag is used, hold the port securely with one hand while injecting the medication with the
other.

8. Immediately place the prepared label on the bottle or bag.
9. Rotate the bottle or squeeze the bag to mix the drug thoroughly with the IV fluid. Make certain that there are no visible particles in the mixture and that the resulting solution is clear.
10. Attach the appropriate IV tubing if necessary.
    a. Cleanse the port of the IV container with an alcohol swab using rotary motion and fric-
       tion. (Remove the thin, tan rubber disk first if the container is a glass bottle.)
    b. While the alcohol is drying, clamp the tubing of the administration set and remove the
       cover from the spiked end of the drip chamber without contaminating it.
    c. Insert the spiked end of the tubing into the port of the bag or bottle. If a bag is used, it
       should be hung or placed on a flat surface first. Then the port is held firmly with one
       hand while the spike is inserted with the other hand.
11. Prime the IV tubing either according to the manufacturer's direction or using the following
    directions.
    a. Squeeze the drip chamber until it is ⅓ to ½ full.

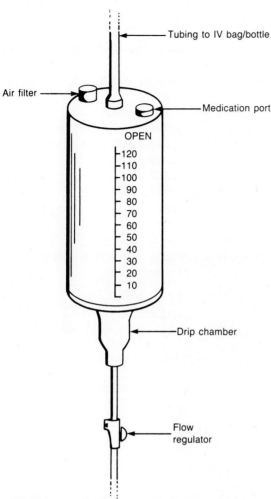

Tubing to IV bag/bottle

Air filter

Medication port

OPEN

120
110
100
90
80
70
60
50
40
30
20
10

Drip chamber

Flow
regulator

**FIGURE 15-4   A volume control device is used to di-
lute medication in small amounts of fluid.** (Reprinted
with permission from Atkinson, L. D., and Murray, M.
E., *Fundamentals of Nursing: A Nursing Process Approach.* Macmillan, New York, 1985.)

b. Remove the cover on the opposite end of the administration set and attach a needle if necessary. Remove the needle cover and hold the end of the administration set over a collecting device such as the sink or a clean container.

c. Open the clamp of the administration set slowly and allow fluid to fill the tubing and the
needle. Avoid loss of more than a drop or two of medicated fluid from the administration
set by watching the priming process carefully.

d. Close the clamp and cover the needle or end of tubing without contaminating it.

12. Calculate the infusion rate using the following formula:

$$\frac{\text{volume to be infused} \times \text{drop factor}}{\text{time to be infused in minutes}} = \text{drops per minute}$$

a. *Volume to be infused* means the amount of admixture containing the medication.

b. *Drop factor* means the number of drops per milliliter according to the manufacturer's
specifications (usually 10, 15, or 60 gtts/ml). The drop factor is printed on every box
containing the IV tubing.

c. *Time to be infused in minutes* means the length of time in minutes that the infusion is to
run.

ADMINISTERING AN INTRAVENOUS ADMIXTURE

1. Bring the prepared drug or admixture to the patient's bedside and carefully identify the patient according to the hospital policy.

2. If a *burette* is used (Fig. 15–4), follow the manufacturer's directions for filling it with the desired amount of fluid and clamping the inflow.

   a. Cleanse the medication port and inject the medication into the burette.

   b. Immediately place the prepared label on the burette without covering the calibrations.

   c. Rotate the cylinder gently between the palms of both hands to mix the medication and IV fluid thoroughly.

   d. Regulate the outflow to the desired flow rate for the medication.

   e. When the burette is empty, open the inflow clamp and fill the burette with primary IV fluid. Adjust the clamp if desired according to the manufacturer's directions to provide a continuous inflow of fluid from the primary container.

   f. Regulate the flow rate again to meet the desired flow rate for the IV fluids prescribed.

3. A *secondary system* may be used when both the primary fluid and the medicated IV fluid need to run at the same time.

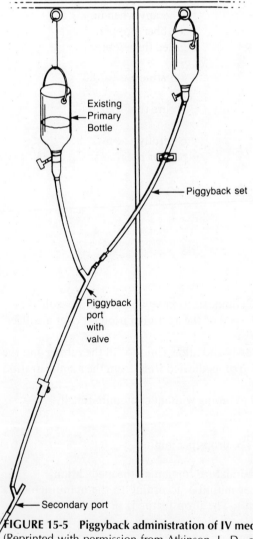

Existing
Primary
Bottle

Piggyback set

Piggyback
port
with
valve

Secondary port

FIGURE 15-5   Piggyback administration of IV medication.
(Reprinted with permission from Atkinson, L. D., and Murray, M. E., *Fundamentals of Nursing: A Nursing Process Approach.* Macmillan, New York, 1985.)

    a. Hang the container at the same height as the primary container.

    b. Connect the secondary set to the secondary port of the IV administration set according to manufacturer's directions.

    c. Adjust the infusion rate to the desired flow rate for the medication.

    d. When the secondary infusion is complete, clamp the secondary administration set and adjust the primary clamp, if necessary, to provide the desired flow rate.

4. A *piggyback system* may be used when only the medicated fluid is to run intermittently with the primary fluid (Fig. 15–5).

    a. Use the hanger in the administration set to lower the primary bottle.

    b. Hang the piggyback bottle higher than the primary bottle.

    c. Use a 1-in. or shorter needle to connect the piggyback tubing to the primary tubing. (Be sure to cleanse the port thoroughly first.)

    d. Tape the needle securely to the port to insure that it does not become disconnected during the infusion.

    e. Adjust the flow rate to the desired number of drops per minute.

    f. When the infusion of the piggybacked medication is complete, clamp the piggyback bottle and readjust the flow rate of the primary bottle according to the physician's order for IV fluids.

5. A *heparin lock system* may be used for intermittent IV drug therapy when no other IV fluid is needed (Fig. 15–6). A heparin lock is a special needle with a rubber stopper. A dilute solution of heparin sodium or sterile normal saline for injection is flushed through the needle regularly to prevent clotting in between doses of medication.

    a. Prepare a secondary system with a 22-gauge, 1-in. needle attached to the administration set.

    b. Aspirate the heparin lock with 3 ml of normal saline to ensure that the needle is still in the vein.

    c. Flush the heparin lock with the same saline, watching carefully for infiltration or resistance that would indicate a clot in the needle. If there is pain or puffiness at the needle site

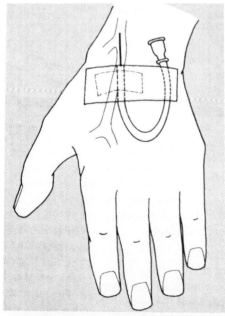

FIGURE 15-6 A heparin lock is used for intermittent infusion of medications. (Reprinted with permission from Atkinson, L. D., and Murray, M. E., *Fundamentals of Nursing: A Nursing Process Approach.* Macmillan, New York, 1985.)

or resistance to flow, stop the procedure and report the observations to the registered nurse. The heparin lock should be removed and a new one inserted.

    d. Cleanse the rubber stopper with an alcohol swab and insert the needle through the rubber stopper, taping it securely.

    e. Start the infusion at the desired rate.

    f. When the infusion is complete, remove the secondary set and cleanse the rubber stopper again.

    g. Flush the needle with either dilute heparin sodium or normal saline according to hospital policy.

MONITORING THE PATIENT DURING INTRAVENOUS DRUG THERAPY

1. Explain the purpose of the particular drug prescribed, using terms the patient can understand.
2. Briefly explain in general terms how the particular administration set works.
3. Ask the patient if there are allergies. Observe the patient for skin rash, dyspnea, or unstable vital signs that may affect later observations.
4. Check the IV site for redness, warmth, tenderness, or swelling. If any of these are present, have the site changed before beginning the medication.
5. During the infusion, check the container regularly to be certain that the solution remains clear. Stop the infusion and check with the registered nurse or pharmacy if the solution turns cloudy or particles appear at any time.
6. Shake the bag or bottle every 15 min or so during the infusion to make certain the drug remains evenly distributed throughout the IV fluid.
7. Check all junction sites to make sure they are intact and not leaking.
8. Check the flow rate during the infusion to make sure it is not running too fast or too slow. Consult the registered nurse before changing the flow rate of infusions that are running too slow.
9. Observe the patient carefully for changes that may indicate an adverse drug reaction. If any changes appear, notify the charge nurse or physician at once to stop the infusion.
10. After the medication has been infused, record the dosage accurately according to hospital policy.
11. Record the intake of IV fluid according to hospital policy.

INSTILLING MEDICATION THROUGH A FEEDING TUBE

Some medications may be instilled through a feeding tube when a patient is unable to swallow. Feeding tubes may be placed either through the nose or by an incision made through the skin into the stomach, duodenum, or jejunum. Only liquids may be instilled into a feeding tube. The nurse must check with a pharmacist before crushing and dissolving tablets, pills, capsules, or any other solid medication. If the pharmacist states that the medication may be safely crushed and dissolved, it must be ground up finely with a mortar and pestle to prevent clogging the feeding tube.

1. Wash the hands.
2. Position the patient in semi-Fowler's position.
3. Unclamp the feeding tube or stop the continuous feeding. Measure residual feeding and notify the registered nurse if the residual exceeds 50 to 100 ml depending upon hospital or agency policy.
4. Verify placement and patency of the feeding tube using the same methods used for a nutritional feeding. (Instill 20 to 30 ml of air quickly into the tube and listen for a loud whooshing sound by placing a stethoscope approximately 2 fingerbreadths below the xiphoid process. Air should pass without resistance if the feeding tube is patent. Aspirate air if possible.)

5. Attach a syringe without a barrel and pour the liquid medication into it. Keep the feeding tube clamped with the other hand to prevent unnecessary air from entering the feeding tube.
6. Raise the syringe so that the liquid medication flows by gravity into the feeding tube.
7. Flush the feeding tube with 50 to 100 ml of water immediately after the medication has been instilled.
8. Clamp the feeding tube or restart the continuous feeding if ordered.
9. Leave the patient in the semi-Fowler's position for approximately 30 min after the dose of medication. Then reposition as desired.

INTRASPINAL OR INTRATHECAL INJECTION

Intraspinal (within vertebral column), intrathecal (within a sheath), or interspinal (between two spinous processes) injections are usually administered by the physician or anesthetist. These methods are frequently employed to administer regional anesthetic drugs in both obstetrics and surgery and occasionally to inject anti-infective agents.

1. *Caudal*—regional anesthesia using the peridural space at the sacral hiatus; single or continuous.
2. *High spinal*—regional anesthesia to thoracic$_5$ and thoracic$_6$ interspaces.
3. *Lumbar epidural*—small catheter is introduced into the epidural space to block nerves; single or continuous.
4. *Midspinal*—regional anesthesia reaching to the tenth thoracic interspace.
5. *Saddle block*—makes use of the subarachnoid space; blocks the sacral segment; "a low spinal."

To monitor the patient following spinal or intrathecal injection, the following procedures are suggested:

1. Observe the patient's respiratory rate and pattern carefully to make sure that the drug has not adversely affected them.
2. Check the patient's blood pressure for early detection and treatment of hypotension.
3. Check the patient's bladder for distention and urinary retention that may develop even after movement and sensation have returned to the lower extremities.
4. Check the lower extremities for the return of movement and sensation.
5. Force fluids if possible to prevent post–spinal–injection headache.

DRUG ADMINISTRATION QUIZ

You are assigned to administer medications to a team of 12 patients on your nursing unit. Answer all of the following questions to evaluate your ability to administer drug therapy safely and effectively. When indicated, circle all the answers that are correct.

1. As the medication nurse, you will have access to medications through:
   a. A key that you carry with you at all times.
   b. A key that is hidden and known only to the nursing staff.
   c. A key held by the head nurse.
   d. A key held by the pharmacist.
2. Which of the follow is (are) essential to know about each drug you administer today.
   a. The name of the drug.
   b. The usual dosage range.
   c. The desired effect on a particular patient.
   d. The main side effects.
   e. The nursing implications.

3. List the five rights of drug administration that you will have to observe to prevent a medication error.

    a. _____.

    b. _____.

    c. _____.

    d. _____.

    e. _____.

4. List at least three kinds of information you will gather at the shift report.

    a. _____.

    b. _____.

    c. _____.

5. Describe the actions you could take to clarify an unclear drug order.

    a. _____.

    b. _____.

    c. _____.

6. When preparing a drug, describe the times you will check the label.

    a. _____.

    b. _____.

    c. _____.

7. List two ways you will identify the patient correctly.

    a. _____.

    b. _____.

8. List the sequence you will use to administer all of the following drugs to the same patient at the same time: lanoxin 0.25 mg IM, Robitussin 10 ml PO, nitroglycerin gr $1/150$ sublingually, furosemide 40 mg PO.

    a. _____.

    b. _____.

    c. _____.

    d. _____.

9. Circle the preparation(s) that may be crushed or broken for a smaller dose.

    a. Enteric-coated tablets.

    b. Spansules.

    c. Tablets.

    d. Capsules.

    e. Suppositories.

10. Circle the part(s) of the needle that you will keep sterile for a parenteral injection.

    a. Needle cover.

    b. Hub of the needle.

    c. Shaft of the needle.

    d. Bevel of the needle.

11. Circle the part(s) of the syringe that you will keep sterile for a parenteral injection.

    a. The plunger.

    b. The flange.

    c. The outside of the barrel.

    d. Syringe tip.

12. Circle your most important responsibility(ies) when administering medications.

    a. To know the name of the physician who ordered the drug.

    b. To be accurate in measuring and giving the drug.

    c. To explain all about the drug to the patient.

    d. To administer an average dose to each patient.

13. Circle what you should do if a patient refuses a drug.
    a. Tell the patient to take it anyway.
    b. Report the information to the charge nurse.
    c. Say nothing if it only happens one time.
    d. Restrain the patient and administer the medication.
14. Circle the correct term(s) for a drug administered into the bloodstream.
    a. Sublingual.
    b. Parenteral.
    c. Intradermal.
    d. Intravenous.
15. Circle the answer(s) that describe(s) when you may leave a medication at the bedside.
    a. If the patient is eating when you bring the medication and tells you he or she will take it after the meal.
    b. If the physician is treating the patient at the bedside when you bring the medication.
    c. If the physician writes an order to leave medication at the bedside and hospital policy permits it.
    d. If the patient's family member promises to give the patient the medication as soon as he/she awakens.
16. Circle the answer(s) that describe(s) what you will do about a very unpleasant-tasting oral medication that has been ordered for a patient.
    a. Explain that the medication tastes awful but must be taken anyway.
    b. Administer the medication rectally instead.
    c. Dilute the medication before administering it.
    d. Offer the medication with juice or an orange slice if the patient's diet permits.
17. When administering medication, you discover a pill on your patient's linens. Circle the action(s) you would take.
    a. Give the medications you have prepared and the one you found on the linens.
    b. Give the medications you have prepared and return the other pill to the nurse's station for further identification. Notify the registered nurse.
    c. Give the medications you have prepared and throw the other pill away.
    d. Hold the medications and notify the pharmacy.
18. Circle all the steps you would take when administering an intramuscular injection.
    a. Select a site on the inner buttock.
    b. Inject the needle at a 45° angle.
    c. Aspirate for blood before injecting the medication.
    d. Massage the site following injection.
19. The physician has ordered meperidine 75 mg IM q4h prn pain. Circle the answer(s) that describe(s) how you would interpret this order.
    a. The patient may have the drug every 4 h routinely.
    b. The patient may have the drug whenever he or she wants it.
    c. The patient may have the drug as little as possible.
    d. The patient may have the drug as needed but no more often than the 4-h intervals.
20. Circle the statement(s) that describe(s) a rule about preparing and administering medication.
    a. The nurse who prepares the medication administers it.
    b. The LPN/LVN may administer any drug provided it has been prepared by a registered nurse or an MD.
    c. The LPN/LVN may prepare a medication for the registered nurse to administer.
    d. The nurse may prepare a medication for another nurse provided that it is done accurately.
21. Circle the answer(s) that describe(s) steps to be taken in administering an intradermal injection.
    a. Select a site on the forearm.
    b. Make sure the bevel of the needle is up.
    c. The needle is injected at a 10 to 15° angle with the skin.
    d. Look for the appearance of a wheal as the medication is injected.

22. Circle the structure(s) to be avoided when administering an IM injection into the gluteus muscles.
    a. Femur
    b. Iliac crest and greater trochanter.
    c. Sciatic nerve and gluteal artery.
    d. Ischial tuberosity and femoral artery.
23. Circle the step(s) you would take to administer a rectal suppository correctly.
    a. Lubricate the suppository.
    b. Insert the suppository above the sphincter flat end first.
    c. Place the suppository in an applicator.
    d. Use sterile technique to insert the suppository.
24. Circle the step(s) you would take to administer a medication by an inhaler.
    a. Instruct the patient completely before administering the medication.
    b. Ask the patient to inhale completely first.
    c. Ask the patient to exhale completely first.
    d. Depress the inhaler as the patient is inhaling.
    e. Ask the patient to hold the breath as long as possible after inhaling the medication.
    f. Instruct the patient to hold the breath for 1 min just before administering the inhaler.
25. Circle the answer(s) that describe(s) what information the LPN/LVN needs before administering medication by IV infusion.
    a. The State Nurse Practice Act that describes what the LPN/LVN must or must not do to practice legally.
    b. The rules and regulations of the State Board of Nursing that pertain to the preparation, administration, and monitoring of medication by the IV route by the LPN/LVN.
    c. The hospital policy and procedure for using this route.
    d. The National Federation of Licensed Practical Nurses position paper on IV administration of drugs.
    e. The National League for Nursing statement on IV administration of drugs.
26. Circle the answer(s) that describe(s) a safety rule to be used in calculating doses.
    a. Use a calculator to obtain the correct dose.
    b. Have another nurse calculate and compare answers as a checkout.
    c. Use several different formulas to be certain you get the same answer each time.
    d. Ask someone who is good in mathematics to do all your dosage calculations for you.
27. Fill in the essential information you would need to administer an IM injection to the deltoid muscle.
    a. Patient position:_____.
    b. Landmarks and their location:_____.
    c. Location of injection sites with respect to landmarks:_____.
    d. Needle angle during injection:_____.
    e. Special precautions if indicated:_____.
28. Fill in the essential information you would need to administer an IM injection in the ventrogluteal site.
    a. Patient position:_____.
    b. Landmarks and their location:_____.
    c. Location of injection sites with respect to landmarks:_____.
    d. Needle angle during injection:_____.
    e. Special precautions if indicated:_____.
29. Fill in the essential information you would need to administer an IM injection in the dorsogluteal site (gluteus medius).
    a. Patient position:_____.
    b. Landmarks and their location:_____.
    c. Location of injection sites with respect to landmarks:_____.
    d. Needle angle during injection:_____.
    e. Special precautions if indicated:_____.

30. Fill in the essential information you would need to administer an IV injection to the vastus lateralis site.
   a. Patient position:_____.
   b. Landmarks and their location:_____.
   c. Injection sites with respect to landmarks:_____.
   d. Needle angle during injection:_____.
   e. Special precautions if indicated:_____.

31. Fill in the essential information you would need to administer a SC injection to the upper outer arm site.
   a. Patient position:_____.
   b. Landmarks and their location:_____.
   c. Injection sites with respect to landmarks:_____.
   d. Needle angle during injection:_____.
   e. Special precautions if indicated:_____.

32. Fill in the essential information you would need to administer an intradermal injection to the inner aspect of the forearm.
   a. Patient position:_____.
   b. Landmarks and their location:_____.
   c. Injection sites with respect to landmarks:_____.
   d. Needle angle during injection:_____.
   e. Special precautions if indicated:_____.

33. Fill in the essential information you would need to administer an IM injection using the Z-tract method.
   a. Patient position:_____.
   b. Landmarks and their location:_____.
   c. Injection sites with respect to landmarks:_____.
   d. Needle angle during injection:_____.
   e. Special precautions if indicated:_____.

34. Fill in the essential information you would need to administer eye drops to a patient.
   a. Patient position:_____.
   b. Landmarks and their location:_____.
   c. Position of eyedropper with respect to landmarks:_____.
   d. Instructions to patient:_____.
   e. Special precautions if indicated:_____.

35. List the actions you will take if you discover that you have made a medication error.
   a. _____.
   b. _____.
   c. _____.
   d. _____.
   e. _____.
   f. _____.

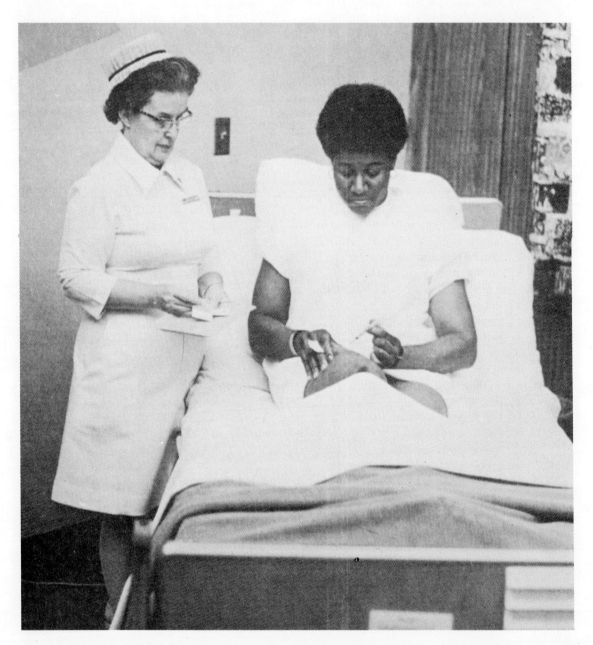
Courtesy of Palm Beach County Practical Nursing Program, The School Board of Palm Beach County, Fla.

Section V

DRUGS AFFECTING BODY SYSTEMS

Chapter 16 | DRUG THERAPY AFFECTING THE PATIENT'S CENTRAL NERVOUS SYSTEM

EXPECTED BEHAVIORAL OUTCOMES

After completing this chapter you should return to the expected behavioral outcomes and evaluate your ability to:

1. Relate the actions of a selected drug to the basic structure and function of the central nervous system.
2. Relate nursing implications associated with narcotic analgesia to the enhancement of pain relief and prevention of adverse responses.
3. List the nursing implications for a postoperative patient who has received general anesthesia.
4. Compare antianxiety agents–antidepressants and antipsychotic agents from the perspective of the patient's condition, intended effects, adverse responses, and nursing implications.
5. Compare anticonvulsant drugs and drug therapy in Parkinson's disease from the perspective of the patient's condition, intended effects, adverse responses, and nursing implications.
6. List nursing actions that enhance effectiveness and prevent adverse responses when the patient is receiving a sedative-hypnotic.

STRUCTURE AND FUNCTION REVIEW

The central nervous system is composed of two major organs: the brain and the spinal cord (Fig. 16-1). Although composed of only a few organs, the central nervous system plays a critical part in regulating and coordinating body functions including:

- Information processing, retrieval, and storage.
- Voluntary and involuntary motor activities.
- Intellectual functions such as thinking, learning, and reasoning.

The brain and spinal cord are composed of special nerve cells called *neurons*. The work of the central nervous system is accomplished mainly through the interactions of billions of neurons with each other and with smooth and voluntary muscle.

Neurons are stimulated by chemical and electrical activity that occurs at the receiving end of the cell. This produces an electrical impulse that travels to the transmitter end of the cell. At the transmitter end, a chemical known as a *neurotransmitter* is released. The neurotransmitter travels across the space between two neurons known as the *synapse*. The neurotransmitter reaches the receiving end of the next neuron and may either excite (cause it to produce a new impulse) or inhibit it (prevent the production of a new impulse). Some important neurotransmitters include acetylcholine, dopamine, epinephrine and norepinephrine, and the endorphins and enkephalins.

The brain is a large organ composed of distinct areas each with different functions:

1. Cerebral cortex.
   a. Highest level of somatic motor control.
   b. Processes information.
   c. Provides high-level integration of various autonomic functions.
   d. Concerned with abstract thought, consciousness, memory, associations.
2. Limbic system.
   a. Provides integration of emotional state with behavior.
   b. Contains the *hypothalamus*, a part of the brain believed to integrate various autonomic activities such as body temperature, sleep cycles, certain metabolic activities, hormone regulation.

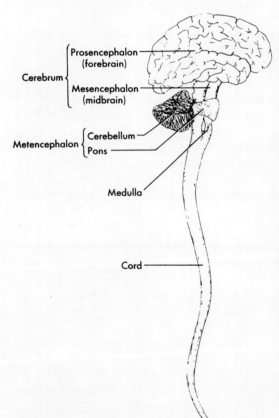

Cerebrum—memory, association, personality. Synthesizes sensory impressions into perceptions. Highest level of somatic motor control. Receives impulses from and sends impulses to all lower levels.

Midbrain—contains many nuclei for control of ocular reflexes, eye movement, higher postural reflex actions. Motor nuclei of cranial nerves III and IV. Nuclei for control of many visceral activities.

Cerebellum—vestibular and postural reflexes, equilibrium and orientation in space. Helps to maintain muscle tone and regulate muscle coordination.

Pons—relay station from lower to the higher centers. Contains nuclei for cerebrocerebellar relay of impulses. Nuclei and pathways for regulation of skeletal muscle tones. Contains nuclei for cranial nerves V, VI, VII, and VIII. Connects both halves of the cerebellum.

Medulla—contains nuclei of many cranial nerves. Location of many vital centers. Contains nuclei for relaying sensory impulses to higher centers. Contains fiber tracts for all ascending and descending impulses.

Cord—only means by which impulses from the periphery can reach higher centers and impulses from higher centers can reach the periphery. Contains neurons which form ascending sensory pathways. Receives incoming sensory fibers and their impulses. Centers for intersegmental and segmental reflexes.

FIGURE 16-1 **Central nervous system, showing cerebrum, midbrain, cerebellum, pons, medulla, and spinal cord.** (From Miller, M. A., and Leavell, L. C.: *Kimber–Gray–Stackpole's Anatomy and Physiology*, 16th ed. Macmillan, New York, 1972.)

   c. Contains the *extrapyramidal tract*, a collection of nerves that act as complements to the voluntary motor system.
   d. Contains the *thalamus*, a relay station for impulses related to heat and cold, pain, position of muscles.
3. Midbrain and brain stem.
   a. Connects cerebral hemispheres to spinal cord.
   b. Contains most of cranial nerves.
   c. Provides integration of various reflex acts such as swallowing, vomiting.
   d. Provides central integration for respiratory and cardiovascular function.
4. Cerebellum.
   a. Maintains body posture in space.
   b. May regulate blood flow and heart rate according to postural changes.

The spinal cord, the other organ of the central nervous system, also has several specialized functions:

1. Transmits impulses from the periphery to higher brain centers.
2. Transmits impulses from the brain to the periphery.
3. Provides local coordination of incoming information from skin, muscles, and joints with motor neurons and higher brain centers.

The *blood–brain barrier* has not yet been anatomically located but has several important functions that influence drug therapy:

1. Serves as the boundary between the central nervous system and the peripheral nervous system (see Chapter 17).
2. Prevents certain substances in the blood (including many drugs) from entering areas of the brain.

The brain and spinal cord require a continuous supply of oxygen and nutrients to function. Even a short temporary disruption to the circulation may cause permanent irreversible damage to the neurons. The circulation to the central nervous system can be summarized as follows:

1. Vertebral arteries originating from the subclavian artery and the carotid arteries, branching from the aorta supply most of the arterial circulation to the brain.
2. Circulation to the spinal cord is provided by the anterior and posterior spinal arteries and their branches.
3. Venous drainage in the brain is provided by sinuses that empty into the jugular veins.
4. Venous drainage for the spinal cord is provided by a network of drainage vessels that are located in the abdomen, neck, and, thorax.
5. *Cerebrospinal fluid* is a clear liquid formed in the ventricles of the brain. This fluid bathes, lubricates, and protects the brain and spinal cord.

ALCOHOLS

Alcohols are drugs that depress the central nervous system. Occasionally, alcohols are prescribed to improve appetite and digestion in elderly debilitated patients. However, most of the alcohol used in the United States is consumed as a beverage for social use. Because of its frequent use and interactions with many other prescribed drugs, the nurse administering medications needs to know the actions and uses, adverse effects, and nursing implications.

I. Actions and uses.
   A. Depresses neurons of the cerebral cortex first; produces depression of the cerebellum and medulla in larger doses.
   B. Initial behavioral changes include increased talkativeness, impulsive behavior, and feelings of enhanced confidence.

    C. Produces initial increase of heart and respiratory rates followed by respiratory depression as the dose increases.

    D. May produce a fall in internal body temperature when dose is large enough to affect temperature regulation centers in the body.

    E. Initial stimulation of gastric secretions may be followed by inhibition of secretions; alcohol is detoxified in the liver.

    F. May be used locally on the skin either to cleanse it or to reduce fever by creating superficial dilatation.

II. Adverse responses.

    A. Allergy may be present when a person is allergic to substances used to make alcohol.

    B. Acute intoxication causes a gradually diminishing level of consciousness to the point of coma, nausea and vomiting, loss of muscle coordination, and symptoms of withdrawal known as a *hangover*.

    C. Excessive chronic use is associated with nutritional and vitamin deficiencies, neurologic and mental disorders, cardiomyopathy, cirrhosis of the liver and other liver disorders, cancers of the mouth, pharynx, esophagus, lungs, liver, and increased accidents and injury.

    D. Excessive chronic use leads to alcohol dependence also called *alcoholism* during which withdrawal of alcohol may trigger a life-threatening withdrawal syndrome known as *delirium tremens*. Delirium tremens is characterized by mental confusion, auditory and/or visual hallucinations (see p. 139), dangerous tachycardia, and/or hypertension, seizures.

    E. The use of alcohol during pregnancy is associated with an increased incidence of birth defects. Excessive chronic alcohol use during pregnancy is associated with *fetal alcohol syndrome* in which the newborn is mentally retarded, has typical facial abnormalities, other birth defects, and symptoms of withdrawal.

    F. Drug interactions include:

      • Exaggeration of effects when combined with sedatives, hypnotics, anticonvulsants, antidepressants, analgesics, and antianxiety agents (tranquilizers).

      • Unpredictable fluctuations of blood sugar when combined with oral hypoglycemics (see Table 22–4).

      • Increased risk of bleeding in gastrointestinal tract when combined with aspirin or other salicylate compounds.

      • Interference with the therapeutic effects of anticoagulants (see Table 18–8).

III. Nursing implications.

    A. Complete a life-style assessment on patients that includes information about usual patterns of alcohol consumption. A minimum assessment includes the usual amount, type, and frequency of drinking, and when the last drink was taken. This information may be collected when the drug history is obtained (see Table 4–1).

    B. Avoid administering other depressants when the patient is known to be under the influence of alcohol. Instead, report the facts to the professional nurse or physician and wait for specific instructions.

    C. Observe and report early signs of alcohol withdrawal in hospitalized patients. Symptoms usually appear within 72 h after the last drinks were consumed. However, this may be delayed if the patient has had anesthesia or narcotics associated with an accident, injury, or surgery. Early symptoms include increasing anxiety and tremulousness, developing mental confusion, tachycardia, increased respiratory rate.

    D. Anticipate delayed healing in patients when there is evidence of frequent and extensive alcohol use.

    E. For the patient whose alcoholism is arrested, be sure to check with the professional nurse or physician before administering any elixirs or tinctures. Even the small amounts of alcohol used to mix these preparations may cause a relapse in a patient who is recovering from alcohol dependency. Anticipate a change in the form of drug prescribed when this information is presented to the physician.

    F. For the patient taking disulfiram (Antabuse) for chronic alcoholism, avoid all forms of alcohol including sauces, fermented vinegar, aftershave lotions, tinctures, elixirs, backrub lotions. These will produce a serious syndrome known as the *aldehyde syndrome* (hot flushed skin, nausea and vomiting, headache, sweating, chest pain, weakness, dizziness, confusion).

G. Have referrals available for patients, friends, and family members who are directly or indirectly involved with alcohol-dependent patients.

H. Teach the patient to avoid driving and other activities requiring physical coordination and judgment after consuming alcohol.

I. Teach the patient taking other drugs not to mix them with alcohol without checking with the physician or nurse first.

ANALGESICS AND NARCOTICS

Analgesics are drugs that prevent, control, or relieve pain without a loss of consciousness (Tables 16–1, 16–2). The patient in pain has a complex subjective experience of hurt that includes physical sensations, thoughts and feelings, and behavior. Several types of pain have been identified. For example, acute pain is a temporary event that begins immediately, usually in response to a known stimulus and is accompanied by anxiety. Chronic pain has a more gradual onset from a cause that may or may not be known. Chronic pain may persist or recur for months or even years. The patient with chronic pain usually experiences feelings of depression. *Intractable pain* is a term used to describe persistent pain that cannot be relieved.

Effective pain relief is built upon several principles:

• Careful assessment of the patient's pain before selecting a pain-relieving intervention.
• Early intervention and prevention before the pain becomes severe.
• Selection of a variety of pain-relieving methods that are known to affect physical sensation, thoughts and feelings, and behavior.
• Selection of methods that encourage the patient's participation and control and are individualized to the patient's experience and specific pain.

Drug therapy is one kind of intervention for pain relief. Other kinds of pain-relieving interventions include massage, pressure and other forms of therapeutic touch, repositioning, planned distraction, breathing exercises, heat and cold applications, relaxation techniques, physical therapy, radiotherapy, psychotherapy, electrical stimulation, biofeedback, and surgery.

I. Actions and uses.
   A. Narcotic analgesics depress central neurons by binding to special receptors on the cell membranes of neurons located in the brain (Table 16–1).
   B. Narcotic analgesics are generally prescribed for the patient with acute severe pain of short duration or severe progressive pain associated with painful fatal illnesses.
   C. Narcotic analgesics may also be prescribed to produce a state of relaxation before the induction of anesthesia.
   D. Narcotics may be prescribed to depress the cough center in the brain and thus relieve a patient's severe nonproductive cough.
   E. Narcotics decrease peristalsis and may be prescribed to relieve severe diarrhea.
   F. Narcotics cause a reduction of heart and respiratory rates as well as blood pressure. Thus narcotics may be prescribed for the patient with congestive heart failure.
   G. Narcotics may be mixed with other drugs to ehhance pain relief (Table 16–1).
   H. Narcotic overdosage may be reversed by drugs called *narcotic antagonists* (see Table 16–2).
II. Adverse responses.
   A. Allergies are unusual but may occur.
   B. Drug tolerance, physical dependence, and drug addiction may develop with any narcotic analgesic.
   C. Side effects include disturbances in perception and coordination, a reduction in the level of consciousness, pupil constriction, nausea and vomiting, constipation, hypotension, and respiratory depression.
   D. Toxicity may cause death from paralysis of respiratory centers in the brain.

TABLE 16–1   Narcotic Analgesics

Nonproprietary Name	Trade Name	Adult Dose Range	Notes
alphaprodine	Nisentil	0.4–1.2 mg/kg SC, IV	Pain-relieving effects short (1.5–2 h)
buprenorphine	Temgesic	0.3–0.6 mg PO, SC, IM	25–50 times more potent than morphine
codeine phosphate and codeine sulfate		20–60 mg PO, SC, IM	
ethoheptaine	Zactane	75–100 mg PO	Instruct patient to take with food or fluids; not for patients who are narcotic dependent
fentanyl	Sublimaze	0.05–0.1 mg IM, IV	50–100 times more powerful than morphine; rapid onset and short duration; generally used during surgery; watch for and report muscle rigidity, hypotension, respiratory depression
hydrochlorides of opium alkaloids	Pantopon	5–20 mg SC, IM	Generally prescribed for surgical pain
hydrocodone	Hycodan	5–10 mg PO	Generally prescribed as an antitussive
hydromorphone hydrochloride	Dilaudid	1–2 mg PO, SC, IM, IV 3-mg suppository	
levorphanol tartrate	Levo-Dromoran	2–3 mg PO, SC	Longer duration of action (6–8 h)
meperidine	Demerol	50–150 mg PO, SC, IM, IV	One of the most widely used analgesics; potentially fatal interaction when combined with monoamine oxidase inhibitors (see Table 16–6)
methadone hydrochloride	Dolophine	2.5–10 mg PO, SC, IM Dosage individualized for opiate detoxification to prevent withdrawal	SC route may result in local irritation; longer duration of action (6– 8 h); also prescribed as therapy for patients addicted to narcotics
morphine sulfate		8–15 mg SC, IM 2.5–15 mg IV Also available as suppository and oral liquid	Increased doses may be prescribed as continuous IV infusion for the patient with terminal cancer
	Roxanol 100		Oral liquid available as 20 mg/ml; teach patient how to use calibrated spoon to measure dose
oxymorphone hydrochloride	Numorphan	1–1.5 mg SC, IM 5-mg suppositories	
pentazocine hydrochloride	Talwin	30–50 mg PO, IM, SC, IV; total daily oral dose should not exceed 600 mg; total daily parenteral dose should not exceed 360 mg	IM route is preferred over SC route; may produce symptoms of withdrawal in patients addicted to narcotics; cannot be mixed in the same syringe as barbiturates
propoxyphene hydrochloride	Darvon	65 mg PO	
propoxyphene napsylate	Darvon N	100 mg PO	
Narcotic Antagonists			
levallorphan tartrate	Lorfan	Dose individualized to patient—SC, IM, IV routes can be used	Used to treat patients for narcotic overdosage; may be used to diagnose physical dependence or treat narcotic addicts
naloxone hydrochloride	Narcan	As above	As above
naltrexone	Trexan	50 mg PO per day	New drug for patients with drug addiction; may initiate acute withdrawal in patients who have not been detoxified

TABLE 16–2 Narcotic Analgesic Mixtures*

Ingredients	Trade Name	Notes

aspirin, <u>codeine</u>, phenacetin, caffeine	APC with codeine
	   No. 2 contains 15 mg codeine
	   No. 3 contains 30 mg codeine
	   No. 4 contains 60 mg codeine	

<u>propoxyphene napsylate</u>, acetaminophen	Darvocet N 100	
<u>propoxyphene hydrochloride</u>, aspirin, phenacetin, caffeine	Darvon compound 65	

<u>codeine</u>, aspirin	Empirin compound
	   No. 1 contains 7.5 mg codeine
	   No. 2 contains 15 mg codeine
	   No. 3 contains 30 mg codeine
	   No. 4 contains 60 mg codeine	

<u>ethoheptazine citrate</u>, aspirin, meprobamate	Equigesic	
<u>oxycodone</u>, aspirin	Percodan	
<u>oxycodone</u>, acetaminophen	Percocet, Tylox	

<u>codeine phosphate</u>, acetaminophen	Phenaphen with codeine
	   No. 2 contains 15 mg codeine
	   No. 3 contains 30 mg codeine
	   No. 4 contains 60 mg codeine
	Tylenol with codeine
	   No. 1 contains 7.5 mg codeine
	   No. 2 contains 15 mg codeine
	   No. 3 contains 30 mg codeine
	   No. 4 contains 60 mg codeine	

<u>morphine or other narcotic analgesic</u>, alcohol, stimulant such as cocaine or amphetamine, flavorings	Brompton's mixture	Primarily used for chronic severe pain in patients who are terminally ill
<u>tincture of opium</u>, benzoic acid, camphor, anise oil	Paregoric	5–10 ml for severe diarrhea

*Narcotic ingredients are underlined.

    E. Drug interactions include:
- Exaggeration of central nervous system depression when combined with other depressants such as alcohol, anesthetics, antianxiety agents, antidepressants, phenothiazines.
- Increased likelihood of hypotension when combined with diuretics, rauwolfia drugs such as rauwolfia and reserpine (see Table 18–9).
- Potentially fatal interaction when combined with monoamine oxidase inhibitors (MAOIs) such as those listed in Table 16–6.
- Exaggerated effects of meperidine when combined with oral contraceptives.
- Increased side effects of isoniazid (see Table 24–7) when it is combined with meperidine.
- Decrease of therapeutic effects of methadone when combined with rifampin (see Tables 24–5 and 24–7).

   III. Nursing implications.
    A. Assess the patient's pain carefully before and after administering narcotic analgesics. Assessment includes a minimum of location and duration of pain, respiratory rate, time since last dose, and extent of pain relief.
    B. Sign out for all narcotics according to hospital policy.
    C. Keep narcotics stored under double lock at all times.
    D. Count narcotics at the beginning and end of each shift. Follow hospital policy in reporting inaccuracies of the narcotic count.
    E. Use safety measures to prevent accidents and injury after administering a narcotic. Safety measures include raising the siderails, placing the call bell and other needed items close at

hand, removing cigarettes from the bedside, and cautioning the patient not to get up without assistance.

F. Use a combination of methods including drug therapy to relieve the patient's pain.

G. Medicate the patient early before the pain becomes severe.

H. Pain that returns before the patient can have more analgesia indicates ineffective relief. Avoid making the patient wait until the next dose is due. Instead notify the physician that the patient's pain has returned and anticipate a change in the order for analgesia.

I. Avoid administering narcotic analgesia to a patient with known or suspected head or spinal cord injury, known or suspected respiratory illness. Instead, seek additional information first from either the registered professional nurse or the patient's physician.

J. Teach the patient nondrug measures for pain relief.

K. Know where narcotic antagonists are located on the nursing unit in case of severe respiratory depression.

L. Use nursing measures known to prevent addiction such as thorough assessment, early medication, selection of a variety of pain-relieving measures, communication of a confident, caring attitude.

M. Offer additional fluids and a high-fiber diet to prevent side effects such as constipation and retained secretions in the tracheobronchial tree.

N. Check the preoperative consent form to be sure it has been signed before administering narcotic analgesia as a preanesthetic medication.

O. When narcotic analgesia is needed in the hours before surgery, seek additional information before administering the preanesthetic narcotic. Anticipate a possible dosage adjustment.

P. Teach the patient to report pain early before it becomes severe.

ANTIPYRETICS AND NONNARCOTIC ANALGESICS

Antipyretics and nonnarcotic analgesics are drugs that relieve mild to moderate pain and/or fever (Table 16–3). Pain was discussed in Analgesics and Anesthetics, above. Fever is a symptom associated with inflammation and disturbances in temperature regulation in the hypothalamus. The person with a fever may experience chills, a feeling of being cold, and/or shivering. These sensations result in heat conservation by constricting blood vessels. This initial experience may be followed by a sensation of heat, restlessness, tachycardia, and increased respiratory rate. When vasodilatation occurs, the person with a fever is able to lose heat by sweating. Some antipyretics such as local applications of alcohol reduce fever by producing local vasodilation and evaporation. An important related fact is that the person with a fever has an increased metabolic rate (rate at which the body uses fuel). This in turn causes an increase in the rate at which the body breaks down and eliminates drugs. Thus the nurse may notice that the patient's pain medication does not relieve the pain as long as anticipated when fever is present. This is true of other drugs also.

Many antipyretics and nonnarcotic analgesics are purchased and taken by persons without professional medical knowledge treating themselves or their children for minor ailments. A special nursing responsibility is the need for teaching hospitalized patients, family members, neighbors, and others about how to use nonprescribed drugs safely.

In learning about nonprescription drugs and teaching others, it is important to remember that commercial advertising of these products is designed to improve sales. The facts about the products may be omitted, enhanced, or minimized as they are explained to television viewers or radio listeners. One way for the beginner to become familiar with nonprescription drugs is to examine the major ingredients. Most preparations contain some combination of the following ingredients: acetaminophen, aspirin, caffeine, and phenacetin. Buffered products contain some form of antacid such as those described in Table 21–3. Acetaminophen, aspirin, and phenacetin have analgesic and antipyretic effects described in this chapter. Caffeine is a stimulant discussed on pp. 146–147. Understanding basic facts about these ingredients and reading the labels on nonprescribed preparations will enable most persons to improve their skill in selecting and using nonprescribed products safely.

TABLE 16–3   Antipyretics and Nonnarcotic Analgesics

Nonproprietary Name	Trade or Popular Name	Adult Dose Range	Notes
acetaminophen	Tempra, Tylenol, Panadol	325–650 mg PO or by suppository every 4 h	Also available as a liquid; aspirinlike adverse effects; potentially fatal liver damage results from toxicity
mefanamic acid	Ponstel	500 mg PO for initial dose; thereafter 250 mg every 6 h	Adverse effects similar to aspirin. Not recommended during pregnancy
methotrimeparazine	Levoprome	10–20 mg IM every 4 h for analgesia	Adverse effects include orthostatic hypotension, dizziness, blurred vision, dry mouth, dysuria, chills, pain at injection site
phenacetin	Available only as mixture with other drugs	300 mg average single oral dose; total daily dose should not exceed 2.4 g	
Salicylates			
aspirin		325–650 mg orally or by suppository	
methyl salicylate	Oil of wintergreen, sweet birch oil, betula oil		Used only for local applications to the skin
salicylic acid	Zinc oxide and salicylic acid, benzoic and salicylate acids and ointments		Used only as a component for ointments and pastes applied to the skin

I. Actions and uses.
   A. Current research indicates that most nonnarcotic analgesics and antipyretics act by preventing the manufacture and release of *prostaglandins*, hormones associated with pain, fever, and inflammation.
   B. This group of drugs is usually effective for pain of low to moderate intensity and dull throbbing pain rather than sharp stabbing pain.
   C. Drugs may be prescribed for fever and anti-inflammatory effects instead of or in addition to pain relief.
II. Adverse responses.
   A. Allergy is common with aspirin like drugs, especially if a person is already sensitive to other allergens. Symptoms may range from mild nasal congestion to skin eruptions to complete cardiovascular and respiratory collapse with anaphylaxis.
   B. Side effects include gastrointestinal (GI) irritation that can progress to ulceration, disturbances in coagulation, disturbances in fertility in susceptible men, nausea and vomiting, changes in acid-base balance, increased bleeding time, unfavorable liver changes that can lead to permanent damage.
   C. Analgesic abuse syndrome may develop in persons who take large doses of nonprescribed analgesics over a period of years. The drug does not have to be a narcotic for this syndrome to develop.
   D. Toxicity with aspirin is common and may be fatal. Accidental overdosage is common especially in children. Symptoms of toxicity include headache, dizziness, ringing in the ears, decreased auditory and visual perception, mental confusion, drowsiness, disturbances of acid-base balance, convulsions, respiratory failure.
   E. Toxicity with acetaminophen and phenacetin results in symptoms such as skin rashes, oral lesions, anemias, nephritis, mental confusion, dyspnea, delirium, fever, and fatal liver or kidney damage.
   F. Some studies show an increased incidence in Reyes' syndrome in children under 18 years

old when aspirin or its derivatives are given for fever associated with chicken pox or influenza.

G. Children with chronic asthma may develop adverse pulmonary response after taking aspirin.

H. Drug interactions include:
- Enhancement of anticoagulation effects when combined with anticoagulants (see Table 18-8).
- Reduction of therapeutic effects when combined with antacids.
- Greater reduction of blood glucose when combined with oral hypoglycemics or insulins.
- Increased possibilities for gastric ulceration when combined with alcohol, antirheumatics (see Table 22-2), corticosteroids (see Table 22-2), nonsteroidal anti-inflammatory agents (see Table 22-3).
- Decrease in therapeutic effects of spironolactone.

III. Nursing implications.

A. Check all new patients for aspirin allergy and record allergy prominently at the bedside, on the chart, and on the drug administration profile.

B. Administer nonnarcotic analgesics with a full glass of water and/or food to minimize gastric irritation. Maintain adequate fluid intake.

C. Instruct the patient to report signs of toxicity such as auditory or visual disturbances, bruising, bleeding from the nose, gums, urine, stools, skin rashes, oral lesions.

D. When collecting a drug history, be sure to ask the patient about nonprescribed drugs.

E. Anticipate a longer bleeding time when removing IV needles, administering IM injections, drawing blood, or checking a dressing when the patient has received an aspirinlike drug.

F. Teach patients who are allergic to aspirin to wear an allergy identification band at all times.

G. Teach patients and families to store aspirin and other analgesics away from the reach of children.

H. Teach parents about the increased risk of Reye's syndrome in children under 18 who receive aspirin for fevers associated with chicken pox or influenza. Avoid recommending aspirin to friends and neighbors with sick children. Instead, advise parents to check with their pediatrician.

I. Tell patients that phenacetin may color the urine a dark brown or wine color.

J. Advise persons on a sodium restriction to check with the physician before taking buffered analgesic compounds.

K. Teach patients to read labels on all nonprescribed drugs to look for ingredients that may be harmful.

L. Instruct patients receiving anticoagulants not to use aspirin products without first checking with the physician. Seek additional information from a registered nurse or physician before administering aspirin products to a patient receiving anticoagulants.

GENERAL ANESTHETICS

General anesthetics are drugs given by inhalation or intravenous routes to remove sensation, produce muscle relaxation, produce unconsciousness, and prevent pain associated with surgery (Table 16-4). The patient having surgery has an illness or symptom that is being diagnosed or treated by a planned manipulation of body structures. Most surgical procedures activate three important mechanisms: the patient's stress response, psychological and physiologic body defenses, and body image. A unique feature of surgery and the need for a general anesthetic is the extent to which the patient's defenses are penetrated at a time when they are needed the most. Thus, many nursing implications are related to protecting the patient whose defense system is weakened by three factors: the underlying condition or illness, the surgical procedure, and the anesthetic.

A characteristic of most general anesthesia is the use of preanesthetic medication to relieve anxiety and to produce drowsiness and muscle relaxation before the general anesthesia is administered. Another kind of anesthesia, discussed in Chapter 17, is known as *local anesthesia*.

Also included in this section (Table 16-5) is a list of drugs known as *neuromuscular blocking agents*. These drugs work by interfering with the transmission of nerve impulses at the junction between a neuron and skeletal muscle. Neuromuscular blocking agents produce relaxation and actual paralysis of skeletal muscles. These agents are used primarily during major surgical procedures to relax skeletal muscles making operative manipulation easier for the surgeon and less traumatic for the patient. The patient whose muscles are more relaxed requires a lighter level of anesthesia. This, in turn, reduces the risk of cardiovascular and respiratory depression associated with general anesthetics.

I. Actions and uses.
   A. Depresses the central nervous system producing unconsciousness, absence of sensation and perception, muscle relaxation, and preventing pain.
   B. Develops in stages that are described by the changes that occur in respiration, muscle tone, and reflexes.
      1. Stage 1: analgesia. Begins with induction of anesthesia and lasts until the patient loses consciousness.

TABLE 16-4   General Anesthetics

Nonproprietary Name	Trade Name	Route of Administration	Notes
enflurane	Ethrane	Inhalation	Deep anesthesia produces more respiratory and circulatory depression than other agents; not used for patients with a history of seizures
etomidate	Amidate	IV	New ultra-short-acting hypnotic used to produce rapid induction of anesthesia; resembles thiopental in actions and uses; especially useful for patients with chronic heart and lung diseases; hypertension
halothane	Fluothane	Inhalation	May produce fatal elevation of body temperature; most common agent currently in use
isoflurane	Forane	Inhalation	
methoxyflurane	Penthrane	Inhalation	Used mainly during first stage of labor because it does not inhibit uterine contractions; may produce kidney damage
midazolam	Versed	IV, IM	New sedative/anesthetic drug from benzodiazepine family; may be given IM for preoperative sedation or IV for short diagnostic procedures and induction of general anesthesia; produces amnesia during and after surgery, see p. 143 for adverse responses to benzodiazepines
nitrous oxide		Inhalation	Used primarily to supplement other agents during major surgery; also used alone for dental procedures; there are reports of patients who recall events that occurred during surgery while affected by this drug
*Methohexital	Brevital	IV	* Very short-acting barbiturates administered IV to produce a rapid and pleasant induction of anesthesia; fast recovery with little nausea or vomiting. May be used for very short minor procedures or to produce sleep before administering a more powerful agent by inhalation.
*Thiamylal sodium	Surital		
*Thiopental sodium	Pentothal (most common agent used)		
†Droperidol	Inapsine	IV	† These drugs are used to produce a state of quietness and relaxation for minor diagnostic or surgical procedures; may also be used with other inhalation agents to produce a more powerful anesthesia. Useful for elderly or debilitated patients.
†Droperidol fentanyl citrate	Innovar	IV	
Ketamine hydrochloride	Ketaject Ketalar	IV, IM	Produces a rapid onset of sedation, immobility, amnesia, analgesia, indifference to surroundings, and unconsciousness; awakening is slow and often associated with nightmares that persist for several weeks; useful as an induction agent and for minor procedures in children

2. Stage 2: delirium. Begins with a loss of consciousness and lasts until the period of excitement, restlessness, respiratory irregularity, and involuntary activity stops.
3. Stage 3: surgical anesthesia. Begins with the cessation of involuntary behavior described in stage 2; lasts until spontaneous respirations stop; contains four planes of increasing depth of anesthesia that are described by the quality of respiration, pupillary and eyeball movements, and reflexes.
4. Stage 4: medullary depression. Begins with the end of spontaneous respiration and ends with circulatory failure.

II. Adverse responses.
   A. Vary with the specific agent used, the patient's condition, and the duration of anesthesia.
   B. Cardiovascular system: hypotension, a reduction of cardiac output, and cardiac arrhythmias.
   C. Respiratory system: a reduction of normal body mechanisms that influence respirations; some drugs produce coughing and airway spasm.
   D. Nervous system: shivering from heat loss; lengthy recovery time needed for return of mental functions.
   E. Muscles: some drugs produce seizurelike muscle activity.
   F. Kidneys: may result in postoperative urinary retention.
   G. Liver: occasionally, hepatitis develops as a result of anesthesia.
   H. Gastrointestinal system: postoperative nausea and vomiting may occur.
   I. Other: some drugs are flammable and/or explosive.

III. Nursing implications.
   A. Provide preoperative instruction about measures that will be used postoperatively to assist the patient's recovery from anesthesia. Such measures include periods of rest interspersed with periods of planned activity for coughing, turning, deep breathing, leg exercises, and ambulation. Have the patient practice and demonstrate these measures.
   B. Instruct the patient not to eat, drink, or smoke for 6 to 12 h before surgery according to the physician's preoperative orders.
   C. Give preanesthetic medication on time so that the patient's anesthesia experience will be more relaxed.
   D. Call the patient by name in the operating room. Speak slowly in low tones. Avoid whispering or confidential communication that does not include the patient.
   E. Wear nonstatic shoes and clothing in the operating room as directed. Follow smoking and other safety regulations.
   F. Check all electrical equipment to be used during surgery before the procedure begins. Follow operating room (OR) policies for equipment maintenance.
   G. Position the patient carefully for the surgical procedure. Check frequently during the surgery for pressure areas, impaired circulation to extremities.
   H. Prevent chilling from unnecessary exposure of body parts not in the operating field during surgery.
   I. Provide extra blankets to reduce shivering when the patient is recovering from anesthesia.

TABLE 16–5 Neuromuscular Blocking Agents Used During Surgery

Nonproprietary Name	Trade Name
atracurium besylate	Tracrium
gallamine triethiodide	Flaxedil
hexafluorenium bromide	Mylaxen
metocurine iodide	Metubine iodide
pancuronium bromide	Pavulon
succinylcholine chloride	Anectine and others
turbocurarine chloride	Tubarine
vecuronium bromide	Norcuron

J. Develop a postoperative plan that includes a regular sequence of turning, coughing, deep breathing, leg exercises, and ambulation to reduce adverse effects of anesthesia.

K. Check the anesthesia record postoperatively to note the duration of anesthesia, particular agent used, and the patient's response.

L. Observe the patient for gagging or choking when the first oral fluids are taken postoperatively.

M. Report a urine output that falls below 30 ml/h in the postanesthetic period.

N. Check the vital signs carefully postoperatively and report tachycardia, pulse irregularities, or slowing respirations.

ANTIANXIETY AGENTS AND ANTIDEPRESSANTS

Antianxiety agents (tranquilizers) and antidepressants are drugs prescribed for the patient with an emotional disorder involving moods (Table 16–6). Such a patient may experience anxiety, depression, or a combination of symptoms.

The patient with *anxiety* experiences persistent feelings of apprehension, uncertainty, and worry without a known cause. There are corresponding physical changes such as tachycardia, sweating, tremors, and increased activity.

The patient with *depression* experiences overwhelming feelings of worthlessness, sadness, hopelessness, and a lack of energy and enthusiasm for living. There are corresponding physical changes such as insomnia, anorexia, constipation, loss of sexual interest, and decreases in activity and productivity. One form of depression is known as *bipolar disorder* or *manic-depression*. The person with this illness experiences wide mood swings characterized by cycles of hyperactivity, elation, and uncontrolled thoughts and speech (manic phase), alternating with symptoms of depression. The individual with a severe depression may withdraw completely from others or may attempt to commit suicide.

Patients hospitalized for other reasons may experience temporary feelings of anxiety or depression as part of a normal response to illness. Drug therapy for these patients helps to relieve unpleasant symptoms. However, for some patients, anxiety or depression becomes so intense that it interferes with normal functioning. In some cases, the patient may also have a psychosis (see pp. 139–140). In this situation, drug therapy may be one part of a comprehensive treatment plan that includes hospitalization, psychotherapy, recreational therapy, and other forms of treatment.

I. Actions and uses.
  A. *Tricyclic antidepressants* are a group of chemically related drugs that are believed to block certain activities of the neurotransmitters norepinephrine, serotonin, and acetylcholine.
  B. Tricyclic antidepressants may be prescribed for patients with alcoholism, certain mood disorders, chronic pain syndromes, neuralgias, and migraine.
  C. *Monoamine oxidase inhibitors* are another chemical group of antidepressants that form a second line of therapy for the depressed patient. Because of their many serious side effects, MAOIs are usually limited to depressed patients who do not respond to tricyclic antidepressants.
  D. *Lithium salts* are drugs prescribed for the patient with bipolar disorder. Because of serious side effects, the patient should have a normal sodium intake and normal cardiac and renal function.
  E. *Antianxiety agents*, also called *tranquilizers*, are believed to work by helping certain inhibitory neurotransmitters in the brain. Antianxiety agents produce depression in the limbic system, believed to be the center of emotional activities in the brain.
II. Adverse responses.
  A. Antidepressants.
    1. Central nervous system: blurred vision, fatigue, dizziness.
    2. Cardiovascular system: tachycardia, arrhythmias, orthostatic hypotension, myocardial infarction, congestive heart failure.
    3. Genitourinary system: urinary retention, edema, and polyuria (lithium only), distur-

TABLE 16–6   Antianxiety Agents and Antidepressants

Nonproprietary Name	Trade Name	Adult Dose Range	Notes
Antianxiety Agents			
alprazolam	Xanax	0.25–0.5 mg PO 3×/day	Used for patients with anxiety; anxiety with depression; caution patient not to stop taking drug abruptly (may produce symptoms of withdrawal)
barbiturates	See Tables 16.7 and 16.9		Rarely used for anxiety; used more often as hypnotics, anticonvulsants
chlordiazepoxide	Libritabs	15–60 mg/day PO in divided doses	
chlordiazepoxide hydrochloride	Librium	15–60 mg/day PO, IM in divided doses	May be used to prevent or treat delirium tremens resulting from alcohol withdrawal; parenteral solution should be clear without sediment
clorazepate potassium	Tranxene	30 mg/day PO in divided doses	
diazepam	Valium	4–40 mg/day PO, IM 2–20 mg/IV per dose	Also used as skeletal muscle relaxant, anticonvulsant, hypnotic, preanesthetic
halazepam	Paxipam	60–100 mg/day PO	
lorazepam	Ativan	2–6 mg/day PO	
meprobamate	Equanil, Miltown	400 mg/day PO in divided doses	
oxazepam	Serax	30–60 mg/day PO	
prazepam	Centrax	20–40 mg/day PO	
Tricyclic Antidepressants			
amitriptyline hydrochloride	Elavil, Endep, Amitril	75–200 mg/day PO	
amoxapine	Asendin	200–300 mg/day PO	May produce agranulocytosis
desipramine hydrochloride	Norpramin, Pertofrane	75 mg–200 mg/day PO	
doxepin hydrochloride	Adapin, Sinequan	75–100 mg/day PO	
imipramine hydrochloride	Tofranil and others	100–200 mg/day PO, IM	May be prescribed for enuresis in children over 7 years in lower doses
maprotiline hydrochloride	Ludiomil	75–300 mg/day PO	
nortriptyline hydrochloride	Aventyl, Pamelor	75–100 mg/day PO	
protriptyline hydrochloride	Vivactyl	15–40 mg/day PO	
trimipramine maleate	Surmontil	5–150 mg/day PO	
trazodone hydrochloride	Desyrel	150–200 mg/day PO in divided doses	
Combination Products			
Amitryptyline and chlordiazepoxide	Limbitrol		Contains tricyclic antidepressant and antianxiety agents; used for patients with depression and coexisting anxiety
amitryptyline and perphenazine	Triavil		Contains tricyclic antidepressant and antipsychotic agents; used for patients with anxiety, agitation, and depression
Antidepressants—Monoamine Oxidase Inhibitors			
isocarboxazid	Marplan	10–30 mg/day PO	Drug and food interactions may be fatal; review adverse responses before administering MAO inhibitors

TABLE 16–6   (*cont.*)

Nonproprietary Name	Trade Name	Adult Dose Range	Notes
phenylzine	Nardil	15–30 mg/day PO	
tranylcypromine sulfate	Parnate	20–30 mg/day PO	
Other Antidepressants			
lithium carbonate	Eskalith, Lithane, Lithotabs	1,200–2,700 mg/day PO in hospitalized patients; 900–1,500 mg/day PO for outpatients	Drug of choice for bipolar disorders; dosage adjustments are made according to plasma drug levels; therapeutic range for most patients lies between 0.8 and 1.5 mEq/L. Lithium toxicity produces vomiting, diarrhea, fine tremors, confusion, convulsions, coma, and death.
nomifensine	Merital	100–200 mg/day PO in divided doses	New drug that resembles tricyclic antidepressants; adverse responses include dry mouth, bad taste, nervousness, restlessness, insomnia and sleep disturbances, headache, nausea, vomiting, constipation; less toxic to heart; doses should be administered in the morning and early afternoon; bedtime doses not recommended

bances in sexual performance, albuminuria and kidney damage (lithium only), increased birth defects.

4. Gastrointestinal system: dry mouth, constipation, weight gain, jaundice, polydipsia and liver damage (MAOI and lithium), sour metallic taste, epigastric distress.
5. Musculoskeletal system: joint pains, fine tremors.
6. Skin: rashes, dermatitis and other types of hypersensitive skin reactions, diaphoresis.
7. Acute toxicity with tricyclic antidepressants is marked by symptoms of hyperexcitement which may include seizures followed by coma, depressed respirations, hypoxia, hypothermia, hypotension, flushed dry skin.
8. Acute lithium toxicity produces vomiting, diarrhea, ataxia, mental confusion, coma and convulsions, gross tremors.
9. Acute toxicity from MAOI produces agitation, hallucination, hyperreflexia and high fever, abnormally high or low blood pressure, convulsions. Irreversible damage may occur to the brain, liver, and/or cardiovascular system.
10. Drug interactions include:
    • Tricyclic antidepressants increase the effects of alcohol and other hypnotics-sedatives; block the effects of some antihypertensives such as guanethidine; may produce toxicity when combined with MAOIs; have more powerful effects when combined with cimetidine, phenytoins, phenylbutazone, aspirin, aminopyrine, scopolamine, phenothiazines, steroids, oral contraceptives, methylphenidate; have less powerful effects when combined with barbiturates and certain sedatives.
    • Monoamine oxidase inhibitors generally prolong and intensify effects of other central nervous system depressants; produce agitation and hypertension when combined with dopamines, reserpine; produce potentially fatal hypertensive crisis when combined with foods that contain amines (beer and wine, cheeses, yeast products, cream, coffee and chocolate, pickled herring, snails, chicken livers, citrus fruits, canned figs, broad beans).

B. Antianxiety agents (tranquilizers).
1. Central nervous system: headache, vertigo, light-headedness.
2. Cardiovascular system: increased heart rate, decreased blood pressure.
3. Respiratory system: decreased respiratory rate.

    4. Genitourinary system: menstrual irregularities, impaired sexual function.

    5. Gastrointestinal system: weight gain, nausea.

    6. Skin: hypersensitive rashes.

    7. Blood: agranulocytosis.

    8. Behavior: paradoxical increases in anxiety, increased irritability and hostility, nightmares, oversedation.

    9. Withdrawal symptoms may appear following abrupt discontinuation.

III. Nursing implications.

  A. Observe and document the patient's behavior completely and accurately. Minimum observations of the patient with anxiety or depression include: food and fluid intake, weight gain or loss, urinary and fecal elimination pattern, menstrual cycle in women, patterns of speech and activity, interactions with others.

  B. Immediately report verbal and nonverbal behavior that indicates the patient may be considering suicide. Even if the patient seems to be joking, not serious, or later denies such behavior, the specific behavior or words should be reported.

  C. Initiate a relationship with the patient that conveys warmth, acceptance, and caring. Identify and support the patient's strengths.

  D. Check the mouth of the severely depressed patient to be certain the prescribed oral antidepressant has been swallowed.

  E. When administering IM injections of antianxiety or antidepressant drugs, use the following guidelines:

    1. Do not mix with other drugs in the same syringe.

    2. Change the needle before administering the IM injection.

    3. Choose an injection site that provides a large muscle mass.

    4. Aspirate the plunger to prevent accidental injection into the circulation.

  F. When permitted by the physician, administer lithium on a full stomach to prevent gastric irritation and upset.

  G. When permitted by the physician, administer larger doses of antianxiety agents at bedtime to promote rest and reduce daytime side effects.

  H. Use nondrug nursing measures such as backrubs and shared activities to convey caring when the patient is nonverbal.

  I. Use some or all of the following safety measures to prevent accidents and injury after antianxiety agents have been administered:

    1. Place siderails up for the hospitalized patient.

    2. Restrict cigarette smoking unless the patient can be observed.

    3. Observe ambulation to make sure the patient's gait is steady.

    4. Encourage appropriate footwear and clothing to prevent falls.

    5. Make sure rooms, bathrooms, and corridors are free from obstacles and objects that may cause falls.

  J. Teach the patient taking antianxiety drugs the following:

    1. Avoid excessive use of stimulants such as cigarette smoking, colas, coffee and tea, chocolate, highly sugared substances.

    2. Do not drive or operate machinery after taking antianxiety drugs until dosage is well established.

    3. Avoid alcohol and nonprescribed drugs.

    4. Carry drug identification information at all times.

    5. Avoid abrupt discontinuation of drugs.

  K. Teach the patient taking antidepressant drugs the following:

    1. Avoid abrupt withdrawal or discontinuation of antidepressant drugs; this may produce adverse drug responses.

    2. Wear drug identification information at all times.

    3. Avoid alcohol and nonprescribed drugs.

  L. Teach women of childbearing age to consult the physician as a part of planning a pregnancy. Some drugs are associated with an increase in birth defects.

M. Provide a list of foods to be avoided for the patient taking MAOIs. Order a tyramine-free diet for hospitalized patients.

N. Encourage the patient with anxiety or depression to maintain a daily schedule that includes exercise and rest periods.

O. Encourage the patient to participate fully in other therapies.

P. Do not force medication on an acutely ill patient who refuses it. Instead, report the patient's refusal to the registered nurse and wait for further instructions. In some cases, a court order is needed before medication can be administered to a patient who refuses it. Record the patient's refusal and the nursing action taken in response.

ANTICONVULSANTS

Anticonvulsants are drugs administered to prevent, control, or relieve seizures or a seizure disorder (Table 16–7). The patient with seizures has a sudden episode of excessive electrical discharge from neurons in the brain. This causes the patient to experience abnormal sensory and motor activity and/or changes in the level of consciousness. Several kinds of seizures have been identified. The person with *generalized seizures* usually experiences a loss of consciousness, tonic-clonic contractions of major muscle groups throughout the body. Urinary and/or fecal incontinence may also be present. Another type of generalized seizure activity is known as *absence seizures*. The patient with absence seizures experiences a brief loss of consciousness lasting no more than 15 s. During this period, there may be blinking of an eyelid or jerking movement of a body part.

The person with a *partial or focal seizure* experiences contractions of an isolated muscle group without a loss of consciousness. Another type of partial seizure, known as *psychomotor seizure*, involves a change of behavior that may seem bizarre, and impairment of consciousness. The person having this type of seizure may act very peculiar for a short time but does not remember what happened during that episode. *Status epilepticus* is an emergency condition in which the patient has continuous seizures that interfere with vital functions.

Spontaneous seizures may develop from a variety of conditions such as head injury, alcoholism, drug toxicity, electrolyte imbalance. When there is periodic seizure activity with characteristic changes on the electroencephalogram (EEG), a person may be diagnosed as having *epilepsy*, a seizure disorder.

Whenever an anticonvulsant is prescribed for a patient, the nurse should anticipate and prepare for possible seizures. In addition to administering drug therapy as prescribed, the nurse has several other important responsibilities when the patient is having a seizure, including:

• Observation of the onset, progression, duration, and aftermath of a seizure.
• Maintenance of the patient's airway during a seizure.
• Protection of the patient from injury during a seizure.

I. Actions and uses.

A. Anticonvulsants act by preventing excess neuron discharge and reducing the spread of impulses from seizure-producing neurons in the brain.

B. Multiple drug therapy is common for the patient with a seizure disorder.

C. Plasma concentration levels assist the physician to adjust the dosage as needed.

D. Barbiturate anticonvulsants are believed to control seizures by competing with naturally occurring neurotransmitters for receptor sites on the cell membrane.

E. The specific prescription for anticonvulsants depends upon the type of seizures and the patient's response to drug therapy.

II. Adverse responses.

A. Skin and mucous membranes: rashes, exfoliative dermatitis, urticaria, hirsutism, overgrowth of gum tissue (phenytoins only), systemic lupus erythematosus, Stevens–Johnson syndrome (potentially fatal bullous blistering rash of the oropharynx and anogenital areas that includes fever and inflammations of the conjunctiva, urethra, and other body organs).

B. Behavior: hyperactivity and increased irritability in children and confusion in elderly (barbi-

TABLE 16–7   Anticonvulsants

Nonproprietary Name	Trade Name	Adult Dose Range	Notes
Hydantoins			
ethotoin	Peganone	2–3 g/day in divided doses PO	Used mainly as an adjunct with other agents to control tonic-clonic and other generalized seizures
mephenytoin	Mesantoin	300–600 mg/day in divided doses PO	Used mainly as an adjunct with other drugs; useful for all kinds of seizures except absence type
phenytoin sodium	Dilantin	300 mg/day in divided doses PO, IV	Principal agent for tonic-clonic seizures; useful for all kinds of seizures except absence type; also prescribed to control cardiac arrhythmias, trigeminal neuralgia
Barbiturates, (see Table 16.9)			
mephobarbital	Mebaral	120–400 mg/day PO	Anticonvulsant barbiturates are helpful agents for generalized tonic-clonic seizures, focal seizures, and febrile seizures.
metharbital	Gemonil	100 mg 2–3 ×/day PO	
phenobarbital		60–200 mg/day PO	
primidone	Mysoline	50–1,500 mg/day in divided doses	Related to barbiturate family
Other Anticonvulsants			
carbamazepine	Tegretol	Initial dose 400 mg/day in divided doses PO; gradual increase to 600–1,200 mg/day PO	May be prescribed for partial seizures; temporal lobe epilepsy; may also be prescribed for the patient with manic-depression who does not respond to lithium (see Table 16–6). Monitor laboratory work for renal, hepatic, and bone marrow function.
clonazepam	Klonopin	1.5 mg/day in three divided doses; maximum recommended dose 20 mg/day PO	Useful for absence seizures
diazepam	Valium	5–10 mg/dose *slowly* IV for emergency control of seizures; no more than 100 mg/24 h	Drug of choice for status epilepticus but cardiovascular and respiratory collapse may occur following IV administration
ethosuximide	Zarontin	Initial dose of 500 mg PO is gradually increased until seizures stop or toxicity develops	Useful for absence seizures
methsuximide	Celontin	600–1,200 mg daily PO	Useful for absence seizures
paramethadione	Paradione	900–2,100 mg/day PO	
phenacemide	Pheneurone	1.5–5 g/day PO	
phensuximide	Milontin	2–4 g/day PO	Useful for absence seizures
trimethadione	Tridione	900–2,100 mg/day PO	Useful for absence seizures
valproic acid	Depakene	1,000–3,000 mg/day PO	Useful for absence seizures

turates only), drowsiness and oversedation, inability to concentrate, inappropriate behavior.

C. Gastrointestinal system: anorexia, nausea, vomiting, epigastric pain, liver damage.

D. Genitourinary system: kidney damage, edema.

E. Central nervous system: fever, unsteady gait, increased frequency of seizures, blurred vision, peripheral neuropathy, hiccough.

F. Blood: various anemias, some of which can be fatal.

G. Musculoskeletal system: osteomalacia.

H. Drug tolerance and dependence may develop with barbiturates; poisoning from accidental or intentional overdose is a major problem.

I. Drug interactions.

    1. Phenytoins:

      a. Plasma concentration increases when combined with chloramphenicol, cimetidine dicumerol, disulfiram, isoniazid, certain sulfonamides, phenylbutazone.

      b. Plasma concentration decreases when combined with carbamazepine, folate.

      c. Toxicity may develop when combined with miconazole (Monistat) or when changing brands of a phenytoin.

      d. Decreases effects of corticosteroids and oral contraceptives by causing them to be metabolized more quickly.

      e. Has variable effects when combined with barbiturates.

   2. Barbiturates (see Table 16–9).

      a. Greatly enhanced effects when combined with valproic acid, alcohol.

      b. Greatly decreases effects of drugs such as corticosteroids, oral anticoagulants, digitoxin, oral contraceptives, testosterone, tricyclic antidepressants (see Table 16–6).

III. Nursing implications.

   A. Administer phenytoins in divided doses and with meals if permitted by the physician.

   B. When phenytoin is prescribed IV, use the following guidelines:

      1. The concentration should be no stronger than 1,000 mg/130 ml *normal saline.*

      2. The infusion rate should not exceed 40 mg/min.

      3. A piggyback setup should be used to stop or adjust the dose if necessary.

      4. The drug should not be mixed with other drugs to prevent physical incompatibilities.

   C. Instruct and assist the patient receiving phenytoins to use good oral hygiene.

   D. Instruct the patient receiving anticonvulsants to avoid alcohol, nonprescribed drugs. Furthermore, all physicians who care for the patient should be informed about the patient's drug therapy with anticonvulsants.

   E. Instruct the patient to wear a drug identification tag at all times.

   F. Anticipate and prepare for seizures in the hospitalized patient.

   G. Instruct the patient receiving barbiturates not to leave them at the bedside or where they may be reached by children. This is recommended to prevent accidental overdosage.

   H. Observe the patient and related laboratory studies for the effects of anticonvulsants on liver, bone marrow, and kidney function.

   I. Check laboratory reports for drug plasma levels when appropriate.

   J. Ask all female patients about possible pregnancy before administering the first dose of an anticonvulsant. If pregnancy is known or suspected, seek additional information and instruction from the physician before administering anticonvulsants.

   K. Instruct patient receiving phenytoin not to switch brands when renewing prescriptions. The drug concentration may vary across brand names and interfere with seizure control and prevention of toxicity.

   L. Shake anticonvulsant suspensions well and administer with the same measuring utensil for each dose.

   M. Review drug interactions before administering anticonvulsants.

ANTIPSYCHOTICS

Antipsychotics are drugs prescribed for treatment of the patient with a psychosis (Table 16–8). Such a patient has a mental illness that is characterized by a loss of contact with reality, inability to think clearly, and lack of insight or awareness of abnormal symptoms. The patient may experience symptoms such as *hallucinations* or *delusions.* Hallucinations are sensory perceptions that have no source in the external environment. The patient may hear, see, smell, taste, or feel things that are not present in the environment. The patient with a delusion has a false belief that cannot be corrected by logical reasoning or contrary evidence. For example, a person who has a delusion may believe he or she is Jesus Christ or some other well-known person like the president.

    The person with a psychosis experiences disturbances in thoughts, feelings, behavior, and body functions. Several kinds of psychoses have been identified. *Organic psychosis* may develop as a result of deterioration of brain cells from brain tumor, electrolyte imbalance, or drug withdrawal. *Func-*

TABLE 16–8   Antipsychotics

Nonproprietary Name	Trade Name	Adult Dose Range	Notes
Phenothiazines			
acetophenazine hydrochloride	Tindal	60–120 mg/day PO	
chlorpromazine hydrochloride	Thorazine	300–800 mg/day PO, IM; 25–50 mg per IM dose	Orthostatic hypotension and sedation are frequent.
fluphenazine	Prolixin	2.5–20 mg/day PO; 25–50 mg IM every 1–3 weeks	Has frequent side effects, especially in CNS; intramuscular route is often used
mesoridazine besylate	Serentil	75–300 mg/day PO, IM; 25 mg per IM dose	
perphenazine	Trilafon	8–32 mg/day PO, IM; 5–10 mg per IM dose	CNS side effects are frequent.
piperacetazine	Quide	20–160 mg/day PO	
thioridazine hydrochloride	Mellaril	200–600 mg/day PO	Sedation is a frequent side effect.
trifluoperazine	Stelazine	6–20 mg/day PO; 1–2 mg per IM dose	CNS side effects are frequent.
triflupromazine hydrochloride	Vesprin	100–150 mg/day PO, IM	CNS side effects are frequent.
Other Antipsychotics			
chlorprothixene	Taractan	50–400 mg/day PO, IM	Sedation is frequent.
haloperidol	Haldol	6–20 mg/day PO, IM; 2.5–5 mg per IM dose	CNS side effects are frequent.
loxapine succinate	Daxolin, Loxitane	60–100 mg/day PO	
molindone hydrochloride	Lidone, Moban	50–225 mg/day PO	
thiothixene hydrochloride	Navane	6–30 mg/day PO, IM; 2–6 mg per IM dose	Sedation is a frequent side effect.
Drug Therapy for Extrapyramidal Symptoms			
amantidine hydrochloride	Symmetrel	100–300 mg PO/day	See Table 16–10. These drugs are also prescribed for the patient with Parkinson's disease (see pp. 145–146).
antihistamines	See Table 23–3		Antihistamines such as those listed in Table 23–3 may also be prescribed for the patient with extrapyramidal symptoms.
benztropine mesylate	Cogentin	1–6 mg/day PO	
biperiden hydrochloride	Akineton	2–6 mg/day PO	
cycrimine hydrochloride	Pagitane	3.75–15 mg/day PO	
ethopropazine hydrochloride	Parsidol	50–60 mg/day PO	
procyclidine hydrochloride	Kemadrin	5–20 mg/day PO	
trihexyphenidyl hydrochloride	Artane	2–15 mg/day PO	

Abbreviations: CNS, central nervous system.

tional psychoses are not associated with physical causes. Examples of functional psychoses are bipolar disorders (also known as manic-depressive illness) and schizophrenia.

A psychosis may start with one episode and progress to a chronic disabling illness. Hospitalization may be needed when the patient is acutely ill. If the psychosis is organic, every effort is made to treat the underlying cause. However, in most cases, the cause of the patient's psychosis is not known. Because the psychotic patient has difficulty thinking clearly, a very important role of the nurse is observing and recording the patient's behavior.

I. Actions and uses.

    A. Antipsychotic drugs are believed to antagonize the activities of dopamine, a neurotransmitter.

    B. Antipsychotic drugs are more likely to be prescribed for the patient with a functional psychosis.

    C. Certain antipsychotics (the phenothiazines) may also be prescribed for other conditions such as nausea and vomiting, hiccoughs, and shivering. However, the dosage for these conditions is markedly different from that indicated for the patient with a psychosis. See Table 16–8 for additional information.

D. Antipsychotic drugs control symptoms such as agitation, hallucinations, delusions, and hyperactivity, hostility, combativeness.

E. The acutely ill patient may require 3 or more weeks of drug therapy before symptoms subside.

F. Intramuscular therapy is common during initial treatment when the acutely psychotic patient may refuse to swallow oral preparations.

G. Additional drugs are frequently ordered to control side effects (see Table 16–8).

II. Adverse responses.

A. Musculoskeletal system: may produce parkinsonian symptoms such as tremors, muscle rigidity, disturbances in posture and gait; patient may experience a compelling need to be in motion; there may be typical repetitive involuntary movement, facial grimacing. These responses are usually called *extrapyramidal side effects.*

B. Central nervous system: blurred vision, increased reaction time, decreased sweating and salivation, changes in ejaculation in males, increased sensitivity to heat and cold, increased sedation.

C. Endocrine system: changes in hormone production, distribution, and excretion may lead to galactorrhea, gynecomastia, changes in glucose tolerance, weight gain, peripheral edema, menstrual irregularities.

D. Cardiovascular system: postural hypotension.

E. Gastrointestinal system: dry mouth, elevation of plasma cholesterol, obstructive jaundice, constipation.

F. Urinary system: urinary retention.

G. Skin: increased pigmentation, urticaria, petechiae, greatly increased sensitivity to sunlight, leading to sunburn.

H. Blood: agranulocytosis, blood dyscrasias.

I. Behavior: may reduce patient's initiative.

J. Drug tolerance and physical dependence may develop but addiction (drug-seeking behavior) is rare.

K. Drug interactions.

1. Enhanced sedation when combined with central nervous system depressants such as alcohol, hypnotics and sedatives, antihistamines, analgesics.

2. May block therapeutic lowering of blood pressure when combined with guanethidine (see Table 18–9). May produce unpredictable results when combined with other antihypertensives (see Table 18–9).

3. May block therapeutic effects of digitalis derivatives (see Table 18–15).

4. May enhance undesirable side effects of tricyclic antidepressants (see Table 16–6).

5. Therapeutic effects may be shortened considerably when combined with phenobarbital and similar hypnotics-sedatives.

III. Nursing implications.

A. Observe and record details of the patient's behavior as a departure point for assessing the effects of drug therapy.

B. When permitted by the physician, administer a larger dose of oral agents at bedtime to avoid daytime sedation.

C. Monitor blood pressure and caution the patient to change positions slowly.

D. Mix liquids with fruit juice or other liquids as directed by the manufacturer to disguise unpleasant taste.

E. When administering oral preparations, be sure the patient has actually swallowed the drug. Some acutely ill patients may hide tablets or capsules, believing them to be poisons.

F. Do not mix parenteral injections with other drugs.

G. Change the needle before IM injection; inject into a large muscle in the ventrogluteal or gluteal site.

H. Check the patient explicitly for less obvious side effects such as urinary retention, constipation. The acutely ill psychotic patient may not report skin rashes, menstrual irregularities, fevers, sore throat, and other symptoms of serious adverse responses.

I. Assist and encourage the patient to participate in other therapies such as psychotherapy, exercise, recreation.

J. Assist and encourage the patient with self-care activities; encourage oral hygiene and sugarless gum to relieve dry mouth.

K. Encourage adequate fluids and fresh fruits and vegetables, whole grains to prevent urinary retention and constipation.

L. Do not force medication on a patient who refuses it. Instead, report the patient's refusal to the registered nurse and wait for further instructions. In some cases, a court order is needed before medication can be administered under these circumstances. Record the patient's refusal and the nursing action taken in response.

HYPNOTICS AND SEDATIVES

A *hypnotic* is a drug that induces the patient to become drowsy (Table 16–9). Hypnotics encourage the onset of a sleep state that resembles natural sleep. Sleep is a series of regularly occurring cycles lasting from 70 to 90 min. Each cycle has distinct parts that can be recorded on the EEG. For example, *non-rapid eye movement* (NREM) sleep is a part of the cycle that lasts about 60 min. During NREM sleep, a person falls asleep and is believed to reach a state of physical rest. Non–rapid eye movement sleep is

TABLE 16–9   Hypnotics and Sedatives

Nonproprietary Name	Trade Name	Adult Dose Range for Hypnotic Effect Only	Notes
Barbiturates			
amobarbital	Amytal	100–200 mg PO	IM route is usually avoided
hexobarbital	Sobulex	250–500 mg PO	Accumulation of barbiturates in plasma with repeated doses favors the development of tolerance, and abuse aftereffects are common.
pentobarbital	Nembutal	90–180 mg PO	
secobarbital	Seconal	100 mg PO	
Benzodiazepines			
chlordiazepoxide	Librium	25 mg PO	
diazepam	Valium	5–10 mg PO	May also be prescribed as antianxiety agents, and as muscle relaxants, preanesthetic medication
flurazepam	Dalmane	15–30 mg PO	
lorazepam	Ativan	2–4 mg PO	
oxazepam	Serax	10–30 mg PO	
prazepam	Centrax	10–20 mg PO	
quazepam	Dormalin	7.5–15 mg PO	
temazepam	Restoril	15–30 mg PO	
Triazolam	Halcion	0.25–0.5 mg PO	Doses for the elderly patient may be lower (0.125–0.25 mg)
Other Drugs			
chloral betaine	Beta-Chlor	870–1000 mg PO	
chloral hydrate	Chloral Hydrate	500–2,000 mg PO	
ethchlorvynol	Placidyl	500–1,000 mg PO	
ethinamate	Valmid	500–1,000 mg PO	
glutethimide	Doriden	250–500 mg PO	
meprobamate	Equanil Miltown	800 mg PO	
methyprylon	Noludar	200–400 mg PO	

followed by rapid eye movement (REM) sleep, which is another part of the cycle lasting from 10 to 30 minutes. Rapid eye movement sleep is associated with dreams and nightmares.

Patients under nursing care often experience a condition known as *sleep deprivation*. Depriving a person of sleep leads to increased feelings of irritability, impaired learning and performance, and increased sensitivity to pain. *Insomnia* is a state of being unable to sleep. Because sleep deprivation is common in hospitalized patients, the nurse can expect to administer hypnotics frequently.

Sedatives are drugs that decrease activity, alleviate excitement and produce a sense of calm (see Table 16-9). Many drugs have both hypnotic and sedative effects depending upon the dosage.

I. Actions and uses.
  A. Hypnotics and sedatives produce widespread depression of the central nervous system.
  B. Most hypnotics-sedatives lose their effectiveness in promoting sleep with several weeks of daily use.
  C. Hypnotics-sedatives may also be prescribed for short periods of insomnia or sedation before certain diagnostic or surgical procedures.
  D. Benzodiazepines (see Table 16-8) increase total sleep time, decrease REM sleep, and help the individual fall asleep faster. They affect the production and breakdown of various neurotransmitters involved in the sleep cycle.
  E. Barbiturates (see Table 16-8) decrease REM sleep, help the person to fall asleep faster, and may also increase total sleep time.
II. Adverse responses.
  A. Respiratory system: benzodiazepines depress ventilation in patients with chronic obstructive lung disease; barbiturates depress respiration in all patients.
  B. Cardiovascular system: benzodiazepines decrease systolic blood pressure; barbiturates decrease blood pressure and cardiac output.
  C. Musculoskeletal system: benzodiazepines cause increased reaction time and motor incoordination, ataxia, joint pains; barbiturates produce impairment of fine motor coordination.
  D. Central nervous system: benzodiazepines produce lassitude, mental confusion, thought disorganization, light-headness, paradoxical excitement, paranoia, and blurred vision. In addition to these symptoms, barbiturates may also produce joint pain.
  E. Gastrointestinal system: benzodiazepines produce nausea, vomiting, and epigastric distress; barbiturates also depress secretions of the GI tract and reduce peristalsis.
  F. Skin: barbiturates may produce localized swelling of lips, eyelids, cheeks in hypersensitive persons; urticaria and dermatitis may also occur.
  G. Drug abuse, tolerance, and physical dependence may occur with all sedatives and hypnotics. Cross-tolerance of benzodiazepines to other sedatives, hyponotics, and alcohol is not unusual.
  H. Toxicity: barbiturate poisoning may occur with overdosage; symptoms include coma, constricted pupils that may dilate in later stages, respirations either very slow or rapid and shallow, hypotension, shock, and renal failure.
  I. Drug interactions include:
    • Increased side effects, tolerance, and central nervous system depression when combined with other central nervous system depressants such as alcohol.
    • Unfavorable depression of central nervous system when barbiturates are combined with alcohol, antihistamines, isoniazid, methylphenidate, and MAOIs (see Table 16-6).
    • Barbiturates decrease the therapeutic effects of corticosteroids, oral anticoagulants, digitoxin, oral contraceptives, certain hormones, phenytoin, zoxazolamine.
    • Chloral hydrate affects oral anticoagulants unpredictably.
    • Chloral hydrate and furosemide interaction may cause vasodilation, flushing, tachycardia, diaphoresis, elevated or decreased blood pressure.
III. Nursing implications.
  A. Assess the patient's need for a hypnotic by collecting data about usual sleep habits.
  B. Use nondrug measures to set the stage for natural sleep such as hygiene, backrub, temperature and lighting adjustment, reduction of noise in the environment, improved ventilation, positioning.

C. When appropriate, use pain-relieving measures to prevent sleep disruption.
D. Encourage the patient to avoid substances, food, and fluids that may interfere with normal sleep such as coffee, tea, cigarette smoking, large late meals, large alcohol intake.
E. Organize nursing care to avoid disruptions of the patient's sleep whenever possible.
F. When the prescribed dose is a range, administer the smallest dose possible and observe the patient's response.
G. Encourage the patient to maintain a pattern of daily physical activity.
H. Whenever possible, administer hypnotics intermittently to decrease the development of tolerance, dependence, and abuse syndrome.
I. Raise siderails and place needed items close at hand after administering hypnotics-sedatives to hospitalized patients.
J. Use more frequent observation when the patient has prn orders for hypnotics and/or analgesics, antihistamines, antidepressants because of added depression of the central nervous system when these drugs are combined.
K. When administering barbiturates by injection, use the following guidelines:
  1. Do not use solutions that are cloudy or contain sediment.
  2. Do not mix barbiturates in the same syringe as other drugs.
  3. Inject medication deeply into a large muscle in the gluteal or ventrogluteal sites.
  4. Aspirate the plunger to make certain the needle is not in a blood vessel.
L. Teach patients not to store barbiturates or other hypnotics at the bedside when drug tolerance and nighttime confusion may lead to accidental overdose.
M. Teach patients not to drive, operate machinery, or drink alcohol after taking a hypnotic.
N. Store hypnotics-sedatives safely because of high abuse potential.

DRUG THERAPY FOR PARKINSON'S DISEASE

The patient with *Parkinson's disease* has a chronic progressive condition that involves muscle tremors, muscle rigidity, slow voluntary movements, and postural changes. In the early stages, the patient may experience trembling and stiffness of muscles in one body part. Symptoms then spread to other body parts. As the disease progresses, the patient develops an expressionless face because of muscle rigidity. Movements become slow and stiff. Postural changes and muscle rigidity cause the patient to lean forward and take increasingly shorter faster steps when walking. Fine movement is lost but the patient's intelligence is generally not affected. Symptoms become more intense when the patient is tired or excited.

The exact cause of Parkinson's disease is not known but in most cases, a deficiency of the neurotransmitter dopamine is present. Other factors associated with the appearance of Parkinsonism include cerebral arteriosclerosis, viral encephalitis, and drug therapy with reserpine (see Table 18–9) or phenothiazines (see Table 16–8).

Drug therapy is an important part of the treatment plan (Table 16–10). Dopaminelike drugs replace the neurotransmitter that is usually deficient. Other drugs known as *anticholinergics* inhibit the actions of acetylcholine, another neurotransmitter. In addition, muscle relaxants such as those in Table 16–12 may be prescribed. Antihistamines such as those listed in Table 23–1 may also be prescribed to relieve symptoms of drooling that may occur in later stages of the patient's illness.

I. Actions and uses.
  A. Dopaminelike drugs and anticholinergic drugs act on basal ganglia in the brain.
  B. Muscle relaxants depress the activity of neurons that control muscle tone.
  C. Dopaminelike drugs help to alleviate symptoms and also produce a feeling of well-being.
  D. Drug therapy usually begins at the low end of the dose range. The dose is gradually increased until symptoms subside.
II. Adverse responses.
  A. Cardiovascular: tachycardia, orthostatic hypotension, cardiac arrhythmias.
  B. Gastrointestinal system: nausea and vomiting, constipation.
  C. Behavior: anxiety, hallucinations, insomnia, inappropriate sexual behavior, oversedation.

TABLE 16–10   Drug Therapy for the Patient with Parkinson's Disease

Nonproprietary Name	Trade Name	Adult Dose Range	Notes
Dopaminelike Drugs			
amantidine	Symmetrel	100 mg twice daily PO	Fewer side effects than other dopaminelike drugs
bromocriptine	Parlodel	1.25 mg twice daily PO with meals	
carbidopa	Lodosyn		
carbidopa, levodopa	Sinemet	Each tablet contains 10 mg carbidopa and 100 mg levodopa; several combinations are available ($^{10}/_{100}$, $^{25}/_{100}$, $^{25}/_{250}$)	Combination therapy that may reduce or prevent side effects of levodopa.
levodopa	Bendopa, Dopar, Larodopa	Initial dose of 0.5–1 g/day PO in three to four divided doses; maintenance dose 3–8 g/day PO in at least four divided doses	1–6 months of drug therapy may be needed to relieve symptoms; smaller doses at more frequent intervals may reduce side effects.
Anticholinergic Drugs			
benztropine mesylate	Cogentin	1–6 mg/day PO, IM	May be prescribed alone to control mild symptoms or as combination therapy with dopaminelike drugs
biperiden hydrochloride	Akineton	2–10 mg/day PO	
cycrimine hydrochloride	Pagitane	3.75–15 mg/day PO	
ethopropazine hydrochloride	Parsidol	50–600 mg/day PO	
procyclidine hydrochloride	Kemadrin	6–20 mg/day PO	
trihexyphenidyl hydrochloride	Artane	1–10 mg/day PO	Most commonly used
Antihistamines			
See Table 23–1			May be prescribed to reduce anxiety, drooling in advanced stages
Muscle Relaxants			
See Table 16–12			May be prescribed to reduce muscle spasm and related pain

    D. Central nervous system: facial tics, grimacing, head bobbing, rocking movements of trunk or extremities.

    E. Genitourinary system: urinary retention with anticholinergics.

    F. Abnormal laboratory tests: false-positive ketoacidosis using dipstick method (dopaminelike drugs only), changes in urine color (red then black when urine is exposed to air).

    G. Drug interactions include:
- Reduction of therapeutic effects when dopaminelike drugs are combined with pyridoxine (an ingredient in multivitamins and high-protein foods such as meat, poultry, milk, fish, cheese, eggs, and nuts).
- Reduction of therapeutic effects when combined with drugs that produce parkinsonian symptoms (phenothiazines, reserpine, haloperidol).
- Undesirable exaggeration of effects when combined with drugs such as phenelzine, isocarboxizad, and other MAOIs (see Table 16–6).
- Enhancement of desirable therapeutic effects when dopaminelike drugs are combined with anticholinergics (see Table 17–4).

III. Nursing implications.

    A. Administer dopaminelike drugs with foods to prevent nausea and vomiting.

B. Check blood pressure during initial therapy and teach the patient to change positions slowly.

C. Teach patients to increase intake of water and fresh fruits, vegetables, and whole grains to prevent urinary retention and constipation, respectively.

D. Use and teach safety measures appropriate to the patient with disturbance in ambulation (avoid rushing, wear nonskid shoes, avoid flowing robes, gowns, and dresses, keep halls and floors free from obstacles).

E. Teach patients to report irregular heartbeat that develops while taking dopaminelike drugs.

F. Observe and record changes of mood that occur while the patient is taking antiparkinsonian drugs.

G. Teach the patient to store dopaminelike drugs in light-resistant containers.

H. Increase observations for adverse responses as the dose is increased.

CENTRAL NERVOUS SYSTEM STIMULANTS

Central nervous system stimulants are drugs that increase activity in the brain and spinal cord (Table 16–11). The use of stimulants has declined in recent years with the corresponding increase in more selective drug therapy.

At the present time, most stimulants used in the United States are consumed as beverages such as coffee, tea, or colas. Occasionally, a stimulant is prescribed for the patient who is oversedated and/or has respiratory depression. However, mechanical ventilation with a respirator is used more frequently.

Stimulants may be prescribed for the patient with *narcolepsy*, an uncontrollable urge to sleep at frequent intervals during the day. Children with hyperkinetic syndrome may be treated with stimulants. Stimulants are also part of a variety of nonprescribed drugs to promote wakefulness and delay sleep, relieve pain, and/or suppress appetite.

TABLE 16–11   Central Nervous System Stimulants

Nonproprietary Name	Trade Name	Adult Dose Range	Notes
Amphetamine Stimulants			
amphetamine	Benzedrine	5–10 mg/dose PO	Used for narcolepsy
dextroamphetamine	Dexedrine	5–60 mg/day PO	Used for narcolepsy, Parkinson's disease, epilepsy
methamphetamine	Desoxyn, Fentamin	2.5–15 mg/day PO	Used for narcolepsy
Xanthine Stimulants			
aminophylline	Aminophylline, Aminodur, many others	Available for PO, IM, IV administration; dosage rectal individualized	See Table 20–2; used primarily for the patient with asthma, chronic obstructive lung disease, infant apnea syndromes
caffeine	Caffeine and sodium Benzoate injection	Available in ampules of 500 mg/2 ml for IM injection	
theophylline	Accurbron, Elixophyllin, Theobid, many others	Same as aminophylline	Same as aminophylline; see Table 20–2
Other Stimulants			
doxapam hydrochloride	Dopram	0.5–1.5 mg/kg IV	Limited use for the patient with oversedation from a sedative-hypnotic
methylphenidate	Ritalin	10 mg PO 2–3 ×/day	Used for narcolepsy, hyperkinesis
nikethamide	Coramine	1–15 ml of a 25% solution IV	Limited use for the patient with oversedation from a sedative-hypnotic
pemoline	Cylert	1 tablet/day PO	Used for narcolepsy, hyperkinesis

I. Actions and uses.

  A. Stimulants are believed to act at all levels of the brain and spinal cord to produce increased alertness and wakefulness.

  B. Stimulants also suppress appetite and the sense of smell.

  C. Some stimulants act as bronchodilators and respiratory stimulants by their actions on the medulla.

  D. Certain stimulants reduce activity in hyperkinetic children but the mechanism of action is unknown.

  E. Amphetamine stimulants are occasionally used for epilepsy, and absence seizures (see pp. 138–39).

  F. Amphetamine stimulants may be used with other drugs to relieve symptoms of Parkinson's disease when the patient cannot tolerate levodopa (see p. 145).

II. Adverse responses.

  A. Cardiovascular system: palpitations, tachycardia or bradycardia, abnormally high or low blood pressure, angina.

  B. Respiratory system: increased respiratory rate.

  C. Central nervous system: overstimulation, restlessness, insomnia, headache, agitation, euphoria, seizures, fatigue, fever.

  D. Gastrointestinal system: metallic taste, anorexia, nausea, vomiting, diarrhea, abdominal cramps, weight loss, epigastric pain.

  E. Genitourinary system: difficulty in urinating, diuresis.

  F. Skin: urticaria, sweating, chills.

  G. Musculoskeletal system: muscle tension and tremors.

  H. Blood: anemias.

  I. Drug tolerance physical dependence and abuse develop with repeated use of amphetamine stimulants.

  J. Tolerance develops with stimulant beverages such as coffee, tea, or colas.

  K. Drug interactions include:

    1. Increase of stimulant effects when amphetamine stimulants are combined with acetazolamide, levarterenal, sodium bicarbonates, urinary antiseptics, tricyclic antidepressants.

    2. Decrease of stimulant effects when amphetamine stimulants are combined with ammonium chloride, ascorbic acid, haloperidol, lithium, phenothiazines.

    3. Inteference of antihypertensive effects when amphetamine stimulants are combined with guanethidine, methyldopa.

    4. May produce hypertensive crisis when amphetamines are combined with MAOIs such as those listed in Table 16–6.

III. Nursing implications.

  A. When permitted by the physician, administer the last dose of the day at least 6 h before bedtime to prevent insomnia.

  B. Encourage and assist the patient with effective oral hygiene to relieve dry mouth.

  C. Teach patients to avoid drinking stimulant beverages before bedtime.

  D. Teach patients, friends, family members, neighbors to avoid self-medication with nonprescribed stimulants. Students, long-distance drivers, and athletes are more likely to use stimulants to promote wakefulness, delay sleep, and increase the sense of well-being. However, stimulants may impair performance.

  E. Encourage others to avoid using nonprescribed stimulants for weight loss. Instead, suggest calorie restriction, increased exercise, and mutual support groups.

  F. Weigh patients regularly to detect abnormal weight loss.

SKELETAL MUSCLE RELAXANTS

  I. Actions and uses.

  A. Skeletal muscle relaxants relieve painful muscle spasms that may occur in the patient with musculoskeletal injury, neuromuscular diseases, spinal cord injury (Table 16–12).

TABLE 16–12   Skeletal Muscle Relaxants

Nonproprietary Name	Proprietary Name	Adult Dose Range	Notes
baclofen	Lioresal	5 mg PO 2–3×/day initially; gradually increased to a maximum of 20 mg PO 4×/day	Useful for the patient with muscle spasms associated with multiple sclerosis, spinal cord disease and injury; abrupt withdrawal not recommended
carisoprodol*	Soma	350 mg PO 4×/day	
chlorphenesin carbamate*	Maolate	800 mg PO 3×/day for no longer than 8 weeks	
chlorzoxazone*	Paraflex	250–500 mg PO 3–4×/day up to a maximum of 750 mg PO 3–4×/day	Advise patient that drug turns urine color orange or reddish-purple.
cyclobenzaprine hydrochloride*	Flexeril	20–40 mg PO per day in two to four divided doses; total daily dose should not exceed 60 mg	
dantrolene sodium	Dantrium	25 mg PO per day initially gradually increased every 4–7 days to a maximum of 400 mg PO per day in four divided doses	Acts directly on skeletal muscle; relieves muscle spasm for patients with paraplegia, hemiplegia, cerebral palsy, multiple sclerosis, may also be used IV for the patient with malignant hyperthermia
diazepam	Valium	5–10 mg PO 3–4×/day gradually increased to avoid oversedation	Central nervous system depressant that relieves muscle spasms in patients with spinal cord lesions, cerebral palsy
methocarbamol	Robaxin	1.5 g PO 4×/day 0.5–1 g IM and repeat every 8 h if needed 1–3 g IV once per day	
orphenadrine citrate	Norflex	100 mg PO 2×/day	Not recommended for patients with glaucoma, prostate hypertrophy, myasthenia gravis, urinary retention; has anticholinergic effects

*Older drugs that act primarily by depressing the central nervous system; not helpful for muscle spasm associated with neurologic disease; other drugs listed on this table are gradually replacing these agents.

    B. Most skeletal muscle relaxants act as depressants on the transmission of nerve impulses in the nervous system.

  II. Adverse responses.

    A. Central nervous system: drowsiness, insomnia, weakness, ataxia, mental confusion, euphoria, light-headedness.

    B. Liver toxicity with dantrolene.

    C. See p. 143 for possible adverse responses to diazepam.

    D. All of the central nervous system depressants listed in Table 16–12 may produce oversedation. Short-term use (no longer than 3 weeks) is recommended.

    E. Hypersensitivity reactions may occur.

 III. Nursing implications.

    A. Assist in the collection of appropriate information from the patient. Seek additional information from the pharmacist, physician, or registered nurse before administering a skeletal muscle relaxant to a patient with liver disease.

    B. Administer with food or milk if drug causes gastrointestinal symptoms.

    C. Use safety measures that prevent accidents and injury caused by drowsiness or oversedation.

    D. Tell the patient with muscle spasms in advance when you are going to handle his or her body.

    E. Assist the patient with appropriate self-care if muscle spasms prevent independent eating, dressing, toileting.

    F. Handle the patient's body gently and place extremities in functionally correct positions when possible.

    G. Prevent personal musculoskeletal muscle spasm by using good body mechanics to lift, turn, and move.

    H. Instruct the patient not to drive, drink alcohol, or engage in other activities requiring coordination and judgment while taking a muscle relaxant.

    I. Seek additional information before administering a skeletal muscle relaxant to pregnant women, children under 12 years, or persons taking MAOIs.

CASE STUDY 5

Ronald Najita is a 36-year-old man admitted to the hospital with severe abdominal pain in the right upper quadrant. The physician has diagnosed appendicitis and has scheduled surgery in 6 h at 8 PM.

    The preoperative orders include:

- NPO.
- Consent for exploratory laporotomy, possible appendectomy under general anesthesia.
- D5 .45NS IV at 125 cc/h.
- Meperidine hydrochloride (Demerol) 75 mg IM q3h prn pain.
- Preoperative medication at 7 PM tonight:
  1. Meperidine hydrochloride 75 mg IM.
  2. Atropine 0.4 mg IM
  3. Hydroxyzine hydrochloride 50 mg IM.
- To OR at 7:30 PM.

    Mr. Najita received meperidine 75 mg IM at 3 PM. At 6 PM Mrs. Najita requests another "pain shot" for Mr. Najita and tells the nurse, "he says the pain is back."

Questions

    1. Underline the narcotic analgesics in the case study.

    2. Explain the effects of narcotic analgesia in the central nervous system.

    3. Identify the type of pain Mr. Najita is experiencing.

    4. List at least five nursing actions that will prevent Mr. Najita from developing an adverse response to narcotic analgesia.

    5. List at least five nursing actions that will enhance the effectiveness of narcotic analgesia for Mr. Najita.

    6. How should the nurse respond to Mrs. Najita's request for another pain shot for her husband?

    7. What nursing implications are related to narcotic analgesia and operative consent?

    8. From the labels on drugs listed below, determine how much solution will be injected IM. Show all work.

       a. Meperidine hydrochloride 50 mg/ml.

       b. Atropine sulfate 0.5 mg/ ml.

       c. Hydroxyzine hydrochloride 50 mg/ml.

    9. Explain the essential factors you would consider to prepare the preanesthetic medication for Mr. Najita.

    10. List the essential nursing implications to be considered for Mr. Najita during and after general anesthesia.

CASE STUDY 6

Mrs. Dolly Mason is a 68-year-old woman admitted to the hospital with Parkinson's disease. The physician's orders include:

- Bedrest with bathroom privileges.
- Force fluids.
- Levodopa 1 g PO qid pc and hs with snack.
- Flurazepam (Dalmane) 15 mg PO hs prn.

Questions

1. How does levodopa affect the central nervous system?
2. How will levodopa affect the symptoms of Parkinson's disease?
3. What adverse responses to levodopa should you look for in Mrs. Mason?
4. What kind of drug is flurazepam?
5. What nursing implications should be considered when administering flurazepam to Mrs. Mason?

EXERCISES

1. Compare diazepam (Valium) and amitriptyline hydrochloride (Elavil) to chlorpromazine hydrochloride (Thorazine) and haloperidol (Haldol) from the perspective of the patient's conditions, intended effects, adverse responses, and nursing implications. Space is provided below to help you organize the information.

2. Compare phenytoin (Dilantin) to trihexyphenidyl hydrochloride (Artane) from the perspective of the patient's condition, intended effects, adverse responses, and nursing implications. Space is provided below to help you organize the information.

Chapter 17 | DRUG THERAPY AFFECTING THE PATIENT'S AUTONOMIC NERVOUS SYSTEM

EXPECTED BEHAVIORAL OUTCOMES

After completing this chapter, you should return to the expected behavioral outcomes and evaluate your ability to:

1. Compare the effects of sympathetic and parasympathetic nerves on major body systems including the central nervous system, respiratory system, cardiovascular system, gastrointestinal system, and genitourinary system.
2. Explain the actions, uses, effects and at least five nursing implications for drug therapy with epinephrine or its relatives.
3. Describe the effects of cholinergic drugs on the autonomic nervous system.
4. Given an example of a cholinergic drug, explain its actions and uses, adverse responses, and at least five nursing implications.
5. Explain the effects of anticholinergic drugs on the autonomic nervous system.
6. Explain the actions and uses, adverse responses, and at least five nursing implications of administering atropine.
7. Define at least four methods for producing local anesthesia and describe at least two nursing implications for each method.

STRUCTURE AND FUNCTION REVIEW

The autonomic nervous system is composed of nerves, ganglia, and plexuses distributed throughout the body to regulate involuntary activities of the heart, blood vessels, glands, smooth muscle, and internal organs. A key feature of the autonomic nervous system is that it does not depend upon awareness, decision making, or conscious control. For this reason, the autonomic nervous system may also be called the *involuntary* or *visceral nervous system*.

Ganglia are collections of nerve fibers that lie outside the central nervous system and act as relay centers. Preganglionic nerve fibers enter the ganglia from various points in the brain or spinal cord. Postganglionic nerve fibers exit the ganglion and go to all the various target organs regulated by the autonomic nervous system. Thus there are many more postganglionic fibers than preganglionic fibers.

151

Plexuses are large collections of ganglia and fibers located in each of the body cavities. Plexuses are closely connected to each other and provide integration and coordination of various body functions.

There are two distinct subdivisions within the autonomic nervous system based on the origin and functions of the specialized nerves in each division. *Sympathetic nerves* originate in the thoracolumbar area of the spinal cord. The primary neurotransmitters of sympathetic nerves are *norepinephrine* and *epinephrine* (see Fig. 17–1). The specific nerve fibers involved with these neurotransmitters are known as *adrenergics*. The specialized effects of epinephrine and norepinephrine on target organs are listed in Table 17–1.

The other subdivision of the autonomic nervous system contains *parasympathetic nerves* that originate in the midbrain, medulla, and sacral area of the spinal cord. The primary neurotransmitter of parasympathetic nerves is *acetylcholine*. Nerve fibers releasing acetylcholine are known as *cholinergic*. The specialized effects of this neurotransmitter are listed in Table 17–1.

Most body organs contain both sympathetic and parasympathetic nerves. The two subdivisions tend to complement each other. Where one subdivision may increase activity in a target organ, the other subdivision frequently decreases activity in the same organ. These complementary functions enable humans to respond effectively to the infinite variety of internal and external conditions.

It is interesting to note that all preganglionic nerve fibers in both subdivisions manufacture and use acetylcholine as a neurotransmitter. It is the postganglionic sympathetic nerve fibers that use epinephrine and norepinephrine. It is the postganglionic parasympathetic nerve fibers that use acetylcholine as a neurotransmitter. Remembering that postganglionic fibers end on target organs enables the nurse to understand the different effects of each subdivision.

Most drugs affecting the autonomic nervous system act primarily on either the sympathetic or parasympathetic subdivision. A few drugs act on both subdivisions.

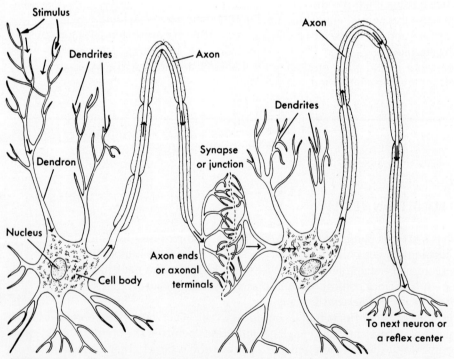

FIGURE 17-1   Illustration showing synapse between two neurons. The synapse is the point at which a nerve impulse passes from one neuron to another. Acetylcholine or norepinephrine is released as the "impulse transmitter" at the axonal terminals.

TABLE 17–1   Subdivisions of the Autonomic Nervous System

Target Organ	Effect of Sympathetic Nerves (Epinephrine, Norepinephrine)	Effect of Parasympathetic Nerves (Acetylcholine)
Eye	Pupil dilation	Pupil constriction, stimulates lacrimal secretions
Lungs	Dilates bronchi	Constricts bronchi
Heart	Increases heart rate, strengthens myocardial contraction	Slows heart rate, constricts coronary arteries
Blood vessels	Produces vasoconstriction	Little effect
Glands	Produces sweating	
	Decreases saliva	Increases saliva
	Decreases gastric secretions	Increases gastric secretions
	Increases adrenal secretions	
Liver	Releases glycogen, glucose	Little effect
Gallbladder	Decreases bile flow	Increases bile flow
Kidneys	Decreases urine flow	Little effect
Bladder	Relaxes muscle tone and constricts sphincter	Increases muscle tone and relaxes sphincter
Intestines	Decreases peristalsis and constricts sphincter	Increases peristalsis and relaxes sphincter
Sexual organs	Increases uterine contraction in women; constricts ductus deferens, seminal vesicles in men	Produces vasodilation and erection in men
Blood	Increases coagulation	Little effect
Skin	Excites piloerector muscles so that hair stands up and "goose flesh" develops	Little effect

ADRENERGICS (SYMPATHOMIMETICS)

Adrenergics, also known as *sympathomimetics*, are drugs that mimic activities of sympathetic nerves (Table 17–2). The adrenergic drugs have effects that are similar to norepinephrine and epinephrine. Some adrenergics occur naturally, such as norepinephrine, epinephrine, and dopamine. Other adrenergics are prepared synthetically.

Adrenergics act by attaching to special receptors on cell membranes. Two kinds of receptors have been identified: alpha and beta. Since receptors are scattered throughout the body, adrenergics may be prescribed for a variety of clinical conditions involving the heart, blood vessels, bronchi, and the immune system. Most adrenergics have one or more of the following effects: central nervous system stimulation, metabolic stimulation, endocrine influences, stimulation of smooth muscle, inhibition of smooth muscle.

In this section, only adrenergics that have general effects will be discussed. These include epinephrine, norepinephrine, dopamine, and their relatives. Adrenergics having selective effects for specific clinical conditions are discussed elsewhere in this book. For example, amphetamines are described in Chapter 16, bronchodilators in Chapter 20.

I. Actions and uses.
   A. Adrenergics may be used to control hemorrhage by producing vasoconstriction.
   B. Adrenergics may be used as decongestant for mucous membranes and to dilate bronchi (see Chapter 20).
   C. Some adrenergics may be combined with local anesthetics to slow absorption.
   D. Adrenergics may be used to raise blood pressure in certain emergencies by producing vasoconstriction.
   E. Adrenergics may be used to treat the patient with cardiac arrhythmias or to stimulate the heart in cardiac arrest (see Chapter 18).
   F. Adrenergics may be prescribed for the patient having an allergic response (see Chapter 23).
   G. Adrenergics may be prescribed to dilate the pupil so that a person's eyes may be examined.

TABLE 17–2 Adrenergic Drugs

Nonproprietary Name	Trade Name	Adult Dose Range	Notes
Catacholamines			
dobutamine	Dobutrex	Administered IV only; dosage adjusted according to patient's response	Used as emergency treatment to improve cardiac output for patients with congestive heart failure; also used for certain kinds of shock
dopamine	Intropin	Administered IV only; dosage adjusted to patient's response	Increases systolic blood pressure and blood flow to kidneys; produces few CNS effects because it does not cross blood–brain barrier
epinephrine	Epinephrine Adrenalin	May be administered SC, IV, inhalation, intracardiac, topically, suppository	Used as emergency treatment for bronchospasm, reverse allergic responses, stimulate the heart in cardiac arrest; adjunct to local anesthesia
ethylnorepinephrine hydrochloride	Bronkephrine	1–2 mg SC, IM	Used as a bronchodilator or to stimulate heart
norepinephrine (levarterenol) bitartrate	Levophed bitartrate	Administered IV only; dosage adjusted according to patient's response	Limited to emergency treatment of hypotension in certain kinds of shock; produces necrosis and sloughing of tissue if accidentally introduced outside of veins
Other Drugs			
Amphetamines—for additional information, see pp. 146–147			
ephedrine sulfate		15–50 mg PO, SC; 20 mg IV; 1–3% nasal solution	Used mainly for bronchospasm, Stokes-Adams syndrome, allergy, decongestant
hydroxyamphetamine hydrobromide	Paradrine	1% ophthalmic solution	Used to dilate pupil
mephentermine sulfate	Wyamine	10–30 mg IM; may also be administered by slow IV infusion	Used as emergency treatment for hypotension
metaproterenol sulfate	Alupent Metaprel	20 mg PO 3–4×/day 2–3 inhalations every 4 h (not to exceed 12 inhalations per day)	Used as bronchodilator
metaraminol bitartrate	Aramine	2–10 mg IM; may also be given by slow IV infusion	Used for emergency treatment of hypotension; produces necrosis and sloughing if given SC
methoxamine hydrochloride	Vasoxyl	10–20 mg IM, 3–5 mg IV	Used for emergency treatment of hypotension; may also be used for paroxysmal atrial tachycardia
methoxyphenamine hydrochloride	Orthoxine	50–100 mg PO every 3–4 h if necessary	Used to relieve asthma and selected allergies
phenylephrine	Isoprine Neosynephrine	250 mg PO; 5–10 mg SC, IM; 0.8 mg IV, available as nasal and ophthalmic solutions	PO absorption not reliable; used to relieve nasal congestion, dilate pupils, raise blood pressure in hypotensive states
terbutaline sulfate	Brethine Bricanyl Brethaire	2.5–5 mg PO 3×/day; 0.25 mg SC, may be repeated in 15–30 min	Used primarily as bronchodilator; may also be administered by IV infusion to delay delivery of premature infant

Abbreviations: CNS, central nervous system.

II. Adverse responses.

  A. Central nervous system: headache, dizziness, tenseness, anxiety, restlessness, cerebral hemorrhage, photophobia.

  B. Cardiovascular system: palpitations, tachycardia, cardiac arrhythmias, chest pain, overly elevated blood pressure.

  C. Respiratory system: dyspnea.

  D. Musculoskeletal system: tremors, weakness.

  E. Skin: pallor, necrosis of tissue if IV infiltration of norepinephrine occurs.

  F. Gastrointestinal system: vomiting.

  G. Drug tolerance may develop with long-term use of ephedrine and isoproterenol as bronchodilators.

  H. Drug interactions include:

   • Potential for hypertensive crisis when adrenergics are combined with doxapram, tricyclic antidepressants, MAOIs, antihistamines, methylphenidate.

   • Increased potential for cardiac arrythmias when adrenergics are combined with general anesthetics, cocaine, digitalis drugs, thyroid drugs, xanthine drugs including coffee, tea, cola beverages.

   • Decreased therapeutic effects when adrenergics are combined with anticholinesterases (see Table 17–4), antihypertensives (see Table 18–9), antipsychotics (Table 16–8), and adrenergic blocking agents.

III. Nursing implications.

  A. Assess the newly admitted patient carefully for allergies, respiratory difficulties, and use of nonprescribed adrenergics such as nasal decongestant sprays, cold remedies, asthma remedies, coffee, tea, or cola beverages.

  B. Anticipate and prevent emergencies that require adrenergics whenever possible.

   1. Develop a method for observing patient completely and systematically. Report early changes in patient's condition.

   2. Display allergies prominently in several places such as on the patient's wristband, on the front of the chart, and on the medication administration record.

   3. Encourage patients and others to decrease exposure to known allergens.

  C. Monitor the blood pressure and pulse carefully on patients receiving adrenergics. Report pulse irregularities and rapidly rising blood pressures.

  D. Encourage, suggest, and provide decaffeinated beverages for the patient on long-term therapy with adrenergic drugs.

  E. Teach the patient how to use and clean inhalers containing adrenergic drugs.

  F. Use the following guidelines to administer adrenergics by the SC route:

   1. Use a 1-ml tuberculin syringe to draw the dose up.

   2. After injecting the needle into SC tissue, aspirate the plunger to prevent accidental injection into a blood vessel.

   3. Massage the site well following injection.

  G. Use the following guidelines when administering adrenergics via the IV route:

   1. Stay with the patient until a transfer to the intensive care unit is arranged.

   2. Use only clear solutions of adrenergics to prepare an IV solution.

   3. Double-check the dosage with another nurse before preparing the IV solution.

   4. Use a piggyback setup so that dosage can be regulated or stopped according to changes in the patient's condition.

   5. During a cardiac arrest, do not administer epinephrine and sodium bicarbonate through the same IV tubing. This will cause precipitation in the tubing. The tubing must be flushed thoroughly with IV solution before epinephrine is injected.

   6. Use an infusion pump to regulate flow rate of continuous IV infusions of adrenergics. This will prevent wide fluctuations of flow rate that could cause adverse drug responses.

   7. Monitor the IV site frequently and report possible infiltration immediately. Some adrenergics cause tissue necrosis if accidentally introduced into SC tissue.

8. Monitor the patient's intake and output carefully. Adrenergics will worsen the patient's condition if dehydration is present.

H. Know where emergency adrenergics are stored on the nursing unit, in the doctor's office, and in the clinic. Keep emergency supplies needed to administer these drugs in the same location. Check drugs and supplies regularly to make sure the supply is complete and not expired.

I. Learn and practice cardiac arrest procedures used in your agency and retrain at regular intervals.

CHOLINERGIC AGENTS

Cholinergics, also known as *parasympathomimetics*, are drugs that mimic activities of parasympathetic nerves (Table 17–3). Thus cholinergics have effects that resemble those of acetylcholine.

TABLE 17–3 Cholinergic Drugs

Nonproprietary Name	Trade Name	Adult Dose Range	Notes
acetycholine chloride	Miochol	Ophthalmic solution	Used to produce rapid myosis during cataract extractions and similar eye surgery
ambenonium chloride	Mytelase	Available as 10-mg tablets; dosage adjusted to patient's response	Used for patients with myasthenia gravis
bethanechol chloride	Myotonachol, Urecholine	10–100 mg PO 2–5 mg SC 3–4×/day	Used to stimulate voiding and peristalsis; should not be administered IM or IV
carbachol	Isoptocarbachol	Ophthalmic solution only	Used to reduce intraocular pressure in patients with wide-angle glaucoma
demecarium bromide	Humorsol	Ophthalmic solutions in several strengths (0.125% and 0.25%)	Used to reduce intraocular pressure, in patients with glaucoma; longer acting
echothiophate	Echodide Phospholine	Available as powder to be mixed with diluent for ophthalmic use only	Used to reduce intraocular pressure in patients with glaucoma; longer acting; keep refrigerated
edrophonium chloride	Tensilon	For parenteral injection only	Used only to diagnose patients with myasthenia gravis; have atropine and emergency equipment available
isofluorophate	Floropryl	Ophthalmic solution available in several strenghts	Used to reduce intraocular pressure in patients with glaucoma
metoclopramide	Reglan	10 mg qid PO, IV	Used to stimulate peristalsis and as antiemetic
neostigmine bromide	Prostigmin	15 mg PO, 0.5–1 mg SC 7.5 mg PO	Used to reduce gastric disention, relieve urinary retention, relieve symptoms of myasthenia gravis.
physostigmine salicylate or sulfate	Antilirium	Available for PO, parenteral injection, ophthalmic solution	Used to reduce intraocular pressure in acute glaucoma
pilocarpine hydrochloride or pilocarpine nitrate	Ocusert PV Carpine Isoptocarpine Pilocar	One elliptical-shaped unit placed in the eye every 7 days; ophthalmic solution available in several strengths	Used to reduce intraocular pressure in patients with glaucoma
pyridostigmine bromide	Mestinon	Available for oral, subcutaneous, intramuscular, intravenous administration; dosage adjusted to patient's response	Used for patients with myasthenia gravis

Cholinergics may act in one of several ways. Some drugs act directly on cholinergic fibers stimulating them to release acetylcholine. Other cholinergics act by slowing the breakdown of acetylcholine by an enzyme called *acetylcholinesterase*. This group of drugs may also be called *anticholinesterases*.

I. Actions and uses.
  A. Cholinergics increase the tone and force of peristalsis in the gastrointestinal tract; gastric secretions also increase. For these effects they may be prescribed to relieve abdominal distention, adynamic ileus.
  B. Cholinergics decrease the holding capacity of the urinary bladder; the rhythmic movements of ureters are increased; voiding pressure is increased; the trigone muscle and sphincter become relaxed. For these effects they may be prescribed for the patient with urinary retention.
  C. Cholinergics produce pupillary constriction and reduce intraocular pressure. For these effects, they may be prescribed for the patient with glaucoma.
  D. Cholinergics produce increased skeletal muscle contraction through anticholinesterase actions. For this effect, they may be prescribed for the patient with a neuromuscular disorder such as myasthenia gravis.
II. Adverse response.
  A. Cardiovascular: hypotension, bradycardia, heart block, substernal chest pain.
  B. Respiratory system: bronchospasm, retained secretions in tracheobronchial tree, dyspnea.
  C. Gastrointestinal system: increased salivation, abdominal cramps, colic, diarrhea, nausea and vomiting, epigastric distress, belching.
  D. Urinary system: tight sensation over the bladder.
  E. Central nervous system: fainting, headache, visual disturbances
  F. Skin: characteristic flush, sweating
  G. Drug interactions include:
    • All therapeutic or adverse effects of cholinergics are blocked by anticholinergics (see Table 17–4) and antihistamines (see Table 23–1).
III. Nursing implications.
  A. Collect a careful nursing history on all newly admitted patients because cholinergics are not indicated for those with asthma, hyperthyroidism, coronary insufficiency, or peptic ulcer.
  B. Observe the postoperative patient for positive bowel sounds and urine output. Measure and record intake and output.
  C. Use nondrug nursing measures that prevent abdominal distention, urinary retention, retained secretions in the tracheobronchial tree. Nondrug measures include coughing, turning, deep breathing, early ambulation, sufficient fluid intake.
  D. Teach patients with myasthenia gravis to take drugs correctly and report adverse drug responses.
  E. Know where atropine is stored on your nursing unit in case an antidote for cholinergic toxicity is needed.
  F. Instruct patients to avoid eating wild mushrooms because certain varieties contain enough natural cholinergic substances to produce fatal poisoning.

ANTICHOLINERGICS

Anticholinergics are drugs that block the effects of acetylcholine on parasympathetic nerves (Table 17–4). Anticholinergics act primarily by competing with acetycholine receptor sites in salivary, bronchial, and sweat glands, muscle in the gastrointestinal system, and cardiac muscle. The drug most commonly used for its anticholinergic effects is atropine.

  I. Actions and uses.
    A. Anticholinergics produce pupil dilation (mydriasis) and paralyze the muscle of eye accommodation. For these effects, anticholinergic ophthalmic solutions may be used before examination of the retina.

TABLE 17–4   Anticholinergic Drugs

Nonproprietary Name	Trade Name	Adult Dose Range	Notes
Atropinelike drugs			
atropine sulfate		0.5 mg PO, SC, IV; ophthalmic doses vary with patient's response	Used mainly as preanesthetic, for gastrointestinal disorders, bradyarrythmias, as mydriatic
belladonna extract		15 mg PO 3×/day	Fluid extract contains alcohol; used for antispasmodic effects on gastrointestinal system
cyclopentolate hydrochloride	Cyclogyl	Opthalmic solution 0.5%, 1%, 2%	Mydriatic
homatropine methylbromide	Sed-Tens, Ru-Spas, Homapin Ophthalmic	2.5–10 mg PO 4×/day, ophthalmic solutions in 2%, 5%	Occasionally used for gastrointestinal conditions; used more often as a mydriatic
methscopolamine bromide	Pamine	2.5 mg PO	Used occasionally for the patient with a peptic ulcer
scopolamine hydrobromide		0.6 mg PO, parenteral injection; also available as ophthalmic solution, transdermal patch	Used for prevention of motion sickness; also used during labor and delivery to produce amnesia; mydriatic
tropicamide	Mydriacyl	Ophthalmic solutions in 0.5%, 1%	Mydriatic
Anticholinergics for gastrointestinal conditions			
anisotropine methylbromide	Valpin	50 mg PO	For additional information about drug therapy for the patient with a gastrointestinal condition, see Chapter 21.
clidinium bromide	Quarzan	2.5–5 mg PO	
dicyclomine hydrochloride	Bentyl	10–20 mg PO	
diphemanil methylsulfate	Prantal	100–200 mg PO	
glycopyrrolate	Robinul	1–2 mg PO	
hexocyclium methylsulfate	Tral	25 mg PO	
isopropamide iodide	Darbid	5 mg PO	
mepenzolate	Cantil	25–50 mg PO	
methantheline bromide	Banthine	50–100 mg PO	High doses may produce impotence.
methixene hydrochloride	Trest	1–2 mg PO	
oxyphencyclimine hydrochloride	Daricon	5–10 mg PO	
oxyphenonium bromide	Antrentyl	5–10 mg PO	
propantheline bromide	Pro-Banthine	15 mg PO	
thiphenamil hydrochloride	Trocinate	400 mg PO	
tridihexethyl chloride	Pathilon	25–50 mg PO	
Anticholinergics for Parkinson's Disease			
benztropine	Cogentin	0.5–6 mg PO daily, also available for IM, IV administration	For additional information about drug therapy for the patient with Parkinson's disease, see pp. 145–146; also used to treat extrapyramidal side effects from antipsychotic drugs (see pp. 139–140).
biperiden	Akineton	2 mg PO 3–4×/day; also available for IM administration	
cycrimine	Pagitane	1.25–5 mg PO 2–4×/day	
procyclidine	Kemadrin	5 mg 2–4×/day	
trihexyphenidyl	Artane	2–15 mg PO daily in divided doses	

    B. Anticholinergics reduce secretions in the nose, mouth, pharynx, and tracheobronchial tree. Smooth muscle of the bronchi relax and widen slightly. For these effects, atropine is often prescribed as part of preanesthetic medication.

    C. Anticholinergics slow the heart rate in very small doses. As the dosage increases, heart rate increases with little effect on central blood vessels. For these effects, atropine may be prescribed for the patient with bradycardia or certain kinds of heart block.

    D. Anticholinergics decrease salivation, slightly decrease the amount of gastric acid, and reduce peristalsis. For these effects, anticholinergics may be prescribed to relieve abdominal pain associated with spasms and hyperactivity in the gastrointestinal system.

    E. Anticholinergics decrease bladder tone and relax smooth muscle in the ureters. For these effects, anticholinergics may be prescribed for spasm and pain associated with urinary tract infections or neurogenic bladder.

    F. Anticholinergics inhibit activities of the salivary glands and reduce muscle spasms and tremors. For these effects, certain anticholinergics may be prescribed for the patient with Parkinson's disease. For additional information about drug therapy for this condition, see pp. 145–146.

    G. Certain anticholinergics have central nervous system effects and may be prescribed to prevent motion sickness.

    H. Atropine may be prescribed as a specific antidote for poisoning from certain mushrooms or from cholinergic agents.

II. Adverse responses.

    A. Eyes: photophobias and blurred vision from paralysis of eye muscle that controls accommodation.

    B. Gastrointestinal system: dry mouth, thirst, dysphagia, constipation. At higher doses, nausea and vomiting, abdominal distention may develop.

    C. Cardiovascular system: increase in blood pressure and heart rate, weak pulse, palpitations and cardiac arrhythmias.

    D. Genitourinary system: urgency and difficulty in urinating.

    E. Central nervous system: temperature elevation, restlessness, excitement, giddiness, headache, hallucinations, delirium, memory disturbances.

    F. Respiratory system: thickened secretions in tracheobronchial tree.

    G. Skin: characteristic facial flush.

    H. Musculoskeletal system: weakness and muscle uncoordination.

    I. Drug interactions include:
- Increased therapeutic or adverse responses when anticholinergics are combined with antihistamines (see Table 23–1), disopyramide, phenothiazines and thioxanthenes (see Table 16–8), or tricyclic antidepressants.
- Decreased or blocked effects when anticholinergics are combined with cholinergics (see Table 17–3).

III. Nursing implications.

    A. Collect a careful drug history on newly admitted patients. Many nonprescribed drugs contain small amounts of anticholinergics that may have additive effects when combined with prescribed drugs.

    B. When anticholinergics are prescribed for gastrointestinal disorders, administer ½ h before meals if permitted by the physician.

    C. Mix parenteral injections of atropine with other kinds of preanesthetic medications including meperidine, morphine, and promethazine.

    D. When anticholinergics are prescribed as ophthalmic solutions, use measures that prevent the drug from entering tear ducts and becoming absorbed systemically.
- Apply gentle pressure to the bridge of the patient's nose after instillation.
- Wait at least 5 min before instilling additional drops into the same eye.

    E. Instruct the patient to wear sunglasses in strong light.

    F. Offer sugarless gum or candy to relieve dry mouth if permitted by the physician.

    G. Assist and encourage good oral hygiene to prevent dental caries that may develop from decreased saliva production.

   H. Teach the patient not to take nonprescribed drugs without checking with the physician.

    I. Do not administer belladonna tincture or elixir to patient known to have alcoholism. Instead, report the facts to the physician and request a substitute prescription.

    J. Know where atropine and related supplies are located for emergency use.

LOCAL ANESTHETICS

Local anesthetics are drugs that block the transmission of sensory and/or motor impulses only in the area to which they are applied (Table 17–5). These drugs stabilize local cell membranes to prevent both the formation and transmission of nerve impulses. The duration of action of a local anesthetics is usually brief and directly affected by the length of time a drug remains in contact with the nerve. For this reason, some local anesthetics are mixed with small amount of epinephrine. The adrenergic effects of epinephrine produce vasoconstriction that helps to prolong and intensify the action of locally applied agents. However, this mixture is never used to anesthetize hands, fingers, feet, toes, the nose, or the penis. In these body parts, vasoconstriction may result in severe hypoxia to the tissues and irreversible damage.

    Other factors that affect local anesthesia include the volume of drug applied or injected, the site of injection or application, the patient's position, and the specific drug used. Local anesthesia is pre-

TABLE 17–5 Local Anesthetics

Nonproprietary Name	Proprietary Name	Adult Dose Range	Notes
benoxinate hydrochloride	Dorsacaine	Ophthalmic solution 0.4%; 1–2 drops in the eye	May be used to remove a foreign body from the eye; measure intraocular pressure
benzocaine	Americaine Hurricaine	Available as a dusting powder, ointment, suppository	Used topically on skin or mucous membranes; also can be applied to airways, scopes, catheters, and specula before insertion into a body cavity
bupivacaine hydrochloride	Marcaine	Available for injection in 0.25%, 0.5%, 0.75% solutions	Also available with epinephrine; used for infiltration, nerve block, caudal anesthesia
butamben	Butesin	Available as a dusting powder, ointment, suppository	Used topically
chloroprocaine hydro-chloride	Nesacaine	Available only for injection in 1%, 2%, 3% solutions	Used mainly for infiltration and nerve block anesthesia
cocaine		Available in 1–10% solutions	Used mainly for topical applications to skin and mucous membranes; solutions usually contain epinephrine; high abuse potential
cyclomethycaine	Surfacaine	Available as cream (0.5%), ointment (1%), urethral jelly (0.75%), suppository (10 mg)	Cream or ointment may be applied to damaged skin; jelly or suppository used for urethral or anogenital lesions; may be applied to some equipment before insertion into a body cavity
dibucaine hydrochloride	Nupercaine and others	Available in solution for spinal anesthesia; cream, ointment, spray	
dimethisoquin hydrochloride	Quotane	Available as lotion or ointment (0.5%)	Used to relieve pain and itching in skin conditions
dyclonine hydrochloride	Dyclone	Available as 0.5%, 1% solutions	Used for topical anesthesia of mucous membranes for procedures involving the ear, nose, and throat

ferred when possible because it does not depress the central nervous system or respirations. Preanesthetic medication and/or neuromuscular blocking agents may be used in some patients.

Only physicians and registered nurses with advanced training in anesthesia may administer most local anesthetics. Other nursing personnel provide care that includes observation of the patient's response, prevention of injury and complications. An exception to this rule is the application of selected topical anesthetics to the skin or certain mucous membranes using sprays, ointments, suppositories, or lozenges.

I. Actions and uses.

   A. *Topical anesthesia* is produced by applying a specific drug to the skin or mucous membranes of the nose, mouth, pharynx, tracheobronchial tree, esophagus, or genitourinary tract. This application may be used to relieve pain, soreness, itching. Peak effects usually appear within 2 to 8 min and last for 36 to 60 min depending on the specific drug used.

   B. *Infiltration anesthesia* is produced by injecting a solution of local anesthetic directly into the tissue to be affected. The duration of anesthesia is usually 45 to 60 min but this may be prolonged in certain conditions by adding epinephrine to the agent used.

   C. *Field block anesthesia* is produced by injecting a solution of local anesthetic SC into an area proximal to the site to be anesthetized. This method produces a larger area of anesthesia than can be achieved with infiltration.

   D. *Nerve block anesthesia* is produced by injecting a local anesthetic into or around individual

TABLE 17–5 (cont.)

Nonproprietary Name	Proprietary Name	Adult Dose Range	Notes
etidocaine hydrochloride	Duranest	Available in injectable 0.5%, 1% solutions	Also available with epinephrine; used for all types of local anesthesia *except* topical and spinal anesthesia
hexylcaine hydrochloride	Cyclaine	Available as topical solution (5%), injectable solution (1%)	Used mainly as topical anesthesia for procedures in the respiratory, gastrointestinal, or urinary tracts
lidocaine hydrochloride	Xylocaine	Available as cream (3%), jelly (2%), ointment, spray, and topical solutions from 1 to 4%. Also available in solutions for injection.	Used for all forms of local anesthesia; also used for arrhythmias (see p. 176). Toxicity and side effects of sleepiness, dizziness are not uncommon. Also available with epinephrine. Read label carefully.
mepivacaine hydrochloride	Carbocaine	Available as injectable solution in 1%, 1.5%, 2%, 3%	Also available with levonordefrin for vasoconstriction
pramoxine hydrochloride	Tronothane	Available as 1% cream or jelly	Used on skin and less delicate mucous membranes; too irritating for eye or nose
prilocaine hydrochloride	Citanest	Available as injectable 1%, 2%, 3% solution	Used for all types of local anesthesia except topical; may produce sleepiness; may produce a rare but serious anemia as a complication
procaine hydrochloride	Novocain and others	Available as injectable 0.5%, 1%, 2%, 5%, 10%, 20% solutions	Used for all forms of local anesthesia. Also available with epinephrine
proparacaine hydrochloride	Alcaine and others	Available as 0.5% ophthalmic solution	Less irritating than other topical anesthetics
tetracaine hydrochloride	Amethocaine, Pontocaine, and others	Available as topical solution (0.5%), ointment (0.5%), injectable solution, ophthalmic solution	Used for all forms of local anesthesia

nerves or nerve plexuses. This method can produce anesthesia in a larger area. For example, injecting a brachial plexus produces anesthesia of an upper extremity. The duration of anesthesia varies from 20 min to 6 or 7 h depending upon the specific drug used.

E. *Intravenous regional anesthesia* is produced by injecting a local anesthetic into the vein of an extremity to which a tourniquet has been applied. This method is used primarily for short surgical procedures distal to the elbow of the arm.

F. *Spinal anesthesia* is produced by injecting a local anesthetic mixed with concentrated glucose into the lumbar subarachnoid space at the level of the second lumbar vertebrae. After injection, the patient is gradually tilted to a head down position. This causes the drug to move upward in the subarachnoid space to produce anesthesia to the area below it.

G. *Epidural anesthesia* is produced by injecting a local anesthetic into the epidural space usually at the level of the lumbar vertebrae. A variation of this method is known as *caudal anesthesia*. The local anesthetic is injected through the sacral area into the caudal canal.

H. Local anesthesia may be used for a variety of diagnostic or surgical procedures. Most procedures are relatively short. For example, dental surgery, certain eye, ear, nose, or throat procedures, labor and delivery, and suturing may be done under local anesthesia.

I. Spinal anesthesia is preferred whenever possible for the surgical patient with a cardiovascular or respiratory condition.

J. Local anesthetics may be used for certain procedures such as bronchoscopy, tissue biopsy, cystoscopy.

K. Local anesthetic preparations may also be prescribed to relieve pain, soreness, itching. For example, lozenges, sprays, or ointments containing a local anesthetic may be prescribed for the patient with a sore throat. Sprays, ointments, and suppositories are available for application to the perineal area.

II. Adverse responses.

A. Toxicity develops after local anesthetic agents are absorbed systemically from the local site.

B. Central nervous system: persistent headache may follow spinal anesthesia; dizziness and drowsiness are reported following lidocaine; stimulant effects with early toxicity include euphoria, restlessness, and tremor that may progress to convulsions. As toxicity increases, depression of the nervous system develops; death may occur from paralysis of vital centers in the brain.

C. Cardiovascular system: a decrease in heart rate, force of contraction and conduction of heart beats; cardiac arrest is a rare complication; decreased blood pressure caused by dilation of blood vessels may occur.

D. Allergic responses to local anesthetics are rare.

E. Drug abuse with cocaine has led to serious problems on a national and international scale.

F. Drug interactions include:
- A reduction of therapeutic effects of sulfonamides when combined with procaine.
- An increase of effects of local anesthetics when combined with cardiovascular depressants, general anesthetics, propranolol (see Table 18–4), central nervous system depressants, epinephrine, succinylcholine.
- Succinylcholine may be administered for convulsions associated with toxicity.

III. Nursing implications.

A. Collect a careful drug history that includes information about allergies and nonprescribed drugs that may contain a local anesthetic. Additive effects may produce toxicity.

B. Check to see that a permit has been signed before administering preanesthetic medication.

C. Check the labels of all local anesthetics carefully when assisting a physician with local anesthesia. Do not supply solutions with epinephrine unless specifically requested by the physician. Call out the name and concentration of the drug when holding a vial for the physician.

D. Know where emergency equipment, supplies, and drugs are located before assisting with local anesthesia on your nursing unit.

E. Protect the area under local anesthesia from injury.

F. Teach the patient to use local anesthetics exactly as prescribed: for the body part, for the condition, and at the tissues directed. Loaning, donating, or otherwise using local anesthetics for some other purpose can be dangerous.

G. Cleanse the skin before each application of topical anesthesia. A sitz bath may be needed if the perineum is the affected area.

H. Check the gag reflex and remain with the patient when the first food and fluids are taken after topical oral anesthesia.

I. Record the patient's pulse and blood pressure as a baseline before local anesthetic is administered. This is especially important in clinics and doctors' offices.

J. Avoid inhalation of local anesthetic sprays during application. Hold the container away from the face when spraying.

K. Follow the postanesthetic orders carefully after spinal anesthesia.
   Anticipate some or all of the following orders:
   • Bedrest with the patient in a flat position for 6 to 8 h.
   • Force fluids.
   • Monitor vital signs frequently during the recovery period.
   • Observe for return of movement and sensation in affected part.
   • Palpate the bladder frequently for urinary retention.

L. Store local anesthetics in tightly covered containers away from light. Many preparations are adversely affected by light.

M. Monitor fetal heart rate frequently when local anesthetics are used during labor. Report fetal bradycardia at once.

N. Check with the pharmacy about the length of time unused solutions containing local anesthetic may be stored.

O. Store local anesthetics containing preservatives separately from those without preservatives after initial use. Preservatives are not used in preparations injected into the spinal or caudal canal.

P. Store local anesthetics containing epinephrine separately from those without it. Epinephrine is not used in local anesthesia for the nose, hands, fingers, penis, feet, or toes. This is because epinephrine is a powerful vasoconstrictor that may compromise circulation to these body parts.

Q. Teach patients, families, neighbors and friends to use nonprescribed preparations containing local anesthetics with caution. Persistent soreness, pain, or itching may indicate a condition that needs medical attention. For example, persistent sore throat is one of the seven warning signals of cancer. Continued use of anesthetic lozenges may prevent a person from seeking early medical attention.

ADRENERGIC BLOCKING AGENTS

Adrenergic blocking agents are drugs that interfere with the release of norepinephrine by sympathetic nerves. The primary uses of such drugs are for patients with hypertension or other cardiac disorders. Therefore, a complete description of these drugs can be located in Chapter 18; pp. 182, 185–187; see also Table 18–9.

CASE STUDY 7

Mr. Jones is a 55-year-old man who is recovering from an emergency appendectomy that was done under spinal anesthesia early this morning. He received meperidine 75 mg, atropine sulfate 0.4 mg IM as a preanesthetic medication. The postoperative orders include:

• NPO nasogastric tube to low suction.
• Bedrest until 10 AM today—keep flat.
• Xylocaine viscous 3 ml PO prn for sore throat.
• If unable to void by noon, give bethanechol (Urecholine) 5 mg SC ×1 dose. Report if no results.

- Cefoxitin 1 g IV/q 6h.
- Meperidine 75–100 mg IM q3–4h prn pain.

Questions

1. Underline all the drug orders that directly affect the autonomic nervous system.
2. For each drug underlined, identify whether it is adrenergic, cholinergic, anticholinergic, or local anesthetic.
3. What kind of anesthesia is produced by Xylocaine viscous as ordered for Mr. Jones? What are the nursing implications?
4. Why do you think spinal anesthesia might have been selected for Mr. Jones?
5. What local anesthetics may be used to produce spinal anesthesia? Where would the specific drug administered to Mr. Jones be recorded?
6. Why has the surgeon ordered bedrest with a flat position for Mr. Jones?
7. What are the nursing implications associated with spinal anesthesia for Mr. Jones?
8. What is the intended effect of the order for bethanechol chloride?
9. What nursing actions should be taken before you administer bethanechol to Mr. Jones?

CASE STUDY 8

Irene Forte, age 18, has come to the emergency room with a laceration on the right foot. She says she cut her foot while walking on the beach. The LPN/LVN has cleaned the patient's foot and is preparing a suture tray for the physician. The physician requests procaine hydrochloride (Novocain) 1% as a local anesthetic.

Questions

1. What kind of anesthesia is produced by injecting the local anesthetic directly into the affected tissue?
2. What information should you collect before a local anesthetic is administered?
3. How should procaine hydrochloride (Novocain) be stored?
4. What are the adverse responses associated with procaine hydrochloride (Novocain)?
5. Would you offer procaine hydrochloride (Novocain) 1% with epinephrine to the physician? Explain your answer.

MATCHING EXERCISE

Match the drugs in Column A to the descriptive statements in Column B.

1. epinephrine
2. carbachol (Isoptocarbachol)
3. pyridostigmine (Mestinon)
4. cyclopentolate hydrochloride (Cyclogyl)
5. trihexyphenidyl (Artane)
6. methoxamine hydrochloride (Vasoxyl)
7. scopolamine hydrobromine
8. dimethisoquin hydrochloride (Quotane)
9. atropine sulfate
10. bethanechol chloride (Urecholine)

A. An adrenergic that may be administered to reverse allergic response
B. An adrenergic administered intramuscularly, intravenously for emergency treatment to raise blood pressure
C. Cholinergic that stimulates voiding and reduces intestinal peristalsis
D. Cholinergic that reduces intraocular pressure in patients with glaucoma
E. Cholinergic for the patient with myasthenia gravis
F. Anticholinergic used to dilate the pupil for examination
G. Anticholinergic used as part of preanesthetic medication to reduce secretions
H. Anticholinergic used to prevent motion sickness
I. Anticholinergic for Parkinson's disease
J. Local topical anesthetic that relieves pain and itching

Chapter 18 | DRUG THERAPY AFFECTING THE PATIENT'S CARDIOVASCULAR SYSTEM

EXPECTED BEHAVIORAL OUTCOMES

After completing this chapter you should return to the expected behavioral outcomes and evaluate your ability to:

1. Relate a specific cardiovascular drug to its intended effects on the heart, blood vessels, or blood.
2. Describe at least five observations that would indicate an adverse response to an anticoagulant.
3. Create a list of instructions to be given to the patient who has nitroglycerin tablets at the bedside. The list should be written as you would explain it to the patient.
4. Relate the effects of antiarrhythmic drugs to the four characteristics of the heart.
5. Describe at least five nursing implications to be considered when administering a hypertensive agent.
6. List at least five actions to be taken when assisting with the administration of blood components of volume expanders.
7. Develop a list of questions you would ask a patient to detect digitalis toxicity before administering a digitalis glycoside.

STRUCTURE AND FUNCTION REVIEW

The *cardiovascular system* is a closed system composed of the heart, blood vessels, and blood. These organs work together to provide every body cell with oxygen and nutrients and to remove waste from the cells.

Heart

I. A four-chambered pump that has the following characteristics:
   A. the ability to contract (contractility).
   B. the ability to generate a heartbeat (automaticity).

    C. the ability to beat rhythmically (rhythmicity).

    D. the ability to transmit an electrical impulse (conductivity).

II. Contraction is made possible by the several-layered walls of the heart muscle. The *myocardium* or middle layer is the main substance of heart muscle.

    A. During systole, blood from the right atrium is pushed through the tricuspid valve to the right ventricle. At about the same time, blood is pushed from the left atrium through the mitral valve into the left ventricle.

    B. Also during systole, blood is pushed from the right ventricle through the pulmonic valve to the pulmonary arteries to the lungs where it becomes oxygenated. From the lungs, blood is returned to the left atrium via the pulmonary veins. At about the same time, blood is pushed through the aortic valve to the aorta and distributed through a network of blood vessels to body cells.

    C. The cardiac cycle includes three phases: systole (contraction), diastole (relaxation and filling), and the resting phase.

    D. *Cardiac output* is an important result of the cardiac cycle. This is the amount of blood squeezed out of the ventricles each minute. Cardiac output is influenced by the volume of blood in the heart and the heart rate.

III. Contraction of the heart occurs in response to electrical impulses generated in specialized cells known as *pacemakers*. The characteristic cells and patterns of electrical impulses that occur in the heart is known as the *conduction system*.

    A. Normally, an electrical impulse begins in the sinoatrial (SA) node located in the right atrium. The impulse spreads from the SA node throughout other cells in the atria and results in atrial depolarization and contraction.

    B. The electrical impulse reaches the atrioventricular (AV) node located in the muscle wall that separates the atria and ventricles.

    C. The impulse is delayed slightly in the AV node before spreading to the ventricles through specialized tissues that include the bundle of His, right and left bundle branches, and Purkinje fibers.

IV. The heart muscle is nourished by its own system of arteries and veins.

    A. The right and left coronary arteries and their branches arise from the aortic notch to supply the heart muscle.

    B. Cardiac veins begin at the apex (pointed part) of the heart and empty into the coronary sinus.

Blood Vessels

I. The heart receives and delivers blood through a network of hollow tubes called blood vessels.

II. There are three basic kinds of blood vessels: arteries, veins, and capillaries. (See Figures 18–1 through 18–4.)

    A. Arteries are highly elastic vessels that carry blood from the heart through progressively smaller vessels (arterioles) to the capillaries. The walls of arteries contain three thicker layers with a middle layer that is much thicker than that of the veins.

    B. Capillaries are the smallest vessels—only one cell thick. The thin wall allows substances to pass through it to and from cells. The capillary network also serves as the link between arteries and veins.

    C. Veins are thinner, less elastic vessels that carry blood from capillaries back to the heart. Veins have valves to prevent backflow.

    D. Products from the cell flow through the capillary network into the smallest veins (venules) and into progressively larger veins that eventually return to the right atrium of the heart. Flow is made possible by differences in pressure between arteries, capillaries, and veins.

    E. *Blood pressure* is the force exerted by blood against arterial walls.

        1. *Systolic blood pressure* represents the force exerted during systole, when the ventricles are contracting and squeezing blood out. Normal systolic pressure is below 140 mm Hg (mercury). It is recorded as the top number of the blood pressure reading.

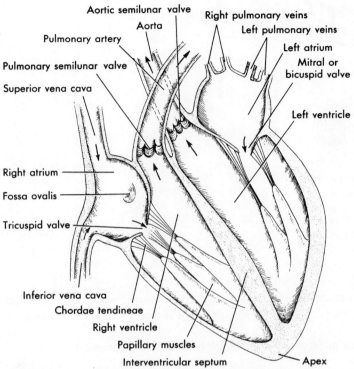

FIGURE 18–1   Longitudinal section of heart showing chambers and valves. Arrows indicate direction of blood flow. (From Miller, M. A., and Leavell, L. C.: *Kimber–Gray–Stackpole's Anatomy and Physiology,* 16th ed. Macmillan, New York, 1972.)

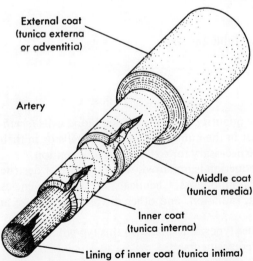

FIGURE 18–2   Schematic drawing of an artery showing the comparative thickness of the three coats. Note that the lining of the inner coat (tunica interna) differs from the other tissue. The different lining facilitates the smooth flow of blood. (Reprinted with permission from Mason, M. A., and Bates, G. F., *Basic Medical-Surgical Nursing,* 5th ed. Macmillan, New York, 1984.)

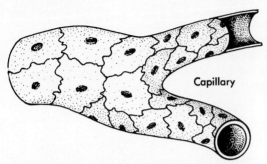

FIGURE 18–3 Schematic drawing of a capillary, which consists of a single layer of endothelial cells. This single layer permits movement of substances between blood and interstitial fluid. The capillary has no muscle coat and no outer coat. (Reprinted with permission from Mason, M. A., and Bates, G. F., *Basic Medical-Surgical Nursing*, 5th ed. Macmillan, New York, 1984.)

2. *Diastolic blood pressure* represents the force exerted during diastole, when the heart is filling. Normal diastolic pressure is below 85 to 90 mm Hg. It is recorded as the bottom number.

3. *Pulse pressure* represents the difference between systolic and diastole pressure.

Blood

1. *Blood* is a liquid sticky substance containing cells, fluid, and materials that are transported to and from cells via blood vessels (Table 18–1). In adults, blood volume represents about $1/13$ of the total body weight.

2. The main functions of blood are to:
   a. Carry material to and from cells.
   b. Assist to maintain normal body temperature.
   c. Provide a defense against microorganisms.
   d. Prevent blood loss through a clotting process (Table 18–2).

ANTIANEMIC AGENTS

Antianemic agents (Table 18–3) are drugs that affect the quantity or quality of red blood cells *(erythrocytes)*. The patient with *anemia* has a deficiency either in the number of red blood cells or in their ability to carry oxygen. Iron, Vitamin B_{12}, and folate are necessary for red blood cell formation.

A person develops anemia when red blood cell production is impaired, when the rate of destruction is faster than the rate of production, or when there is blood loss. Chemicals, dietary deficiencies, drugs, endocrine deficiencies, heredity, infection, lead, radiation, and other diseases may cause an anemia.

Iron deficiency anemia occurs more often than other types. Patients with this type of anemia do not take in, store, or absorb enough iron to meet body requirements.

Pernicious anemia develops when a person does not produce intrinsic factor, a substance secreted by the stomach that is necessary for oral absorption of vitamin B_{12}. Folate deficiency may cause anemia in patients with small bowel disease, alcoholism, and certain drug regimens (anticonvulsants, oral contraceptives, certain anticancer agents).

A person with anemia generally feels weak and tired. The skin may be pale and bruised and there may be dyspnea with exertion. Mucous membranes may look pale and small ulcerations may develop

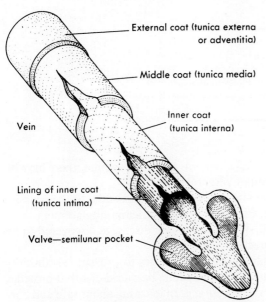

External coat (tunica externa or adventitia)

Middle coat (tunica media)

Inner coat (tunica interna)

Vein

Lining of inner coat (tunica intima)

Valve—semilunar pocket

FIGURE 18–4 Schematic drawing of a vein showing the comparative thickness of the three coats. The outer coat and middle coat are thinner in veins than in arteries. A diagram of a valve is also shown. (Reprinted with permission from Mason, M. A., and Bates, G. F., *Basic Medical-Surgical Nursing*, 5th ed. Macmillan, New York, 1984.)

TABLE 18–1   Substances Present in Blood

Substance	Description
Albumin	A large plasma protein that helps to keep blood within blood vessels by exerting a pulling pressure
Dissolved gases	Oxygen, carbon dioxide, and nitrogen present in plasma
Electrolytes	Electrically charged particles in plasma formed from chemical reactions in the body: sodium, potassium, calcium, magnesium, chlorides, sulfates, phosphates, bicarbonates
Erythrocytes	Red blood cells formed in bone marrow; carry oxygen, carbon dioxide to and from cell; maintain acid-base balance, blood viscosity
Fibrinogen	A plasma protein manufactured in the liver that is part of the clotting process.
Heparin	A natural anticlotting substance formed by special cells in connective tissue and present in plasma
Nutrients	Amino acids, cholestrol, glucose, neutral fats present in plasma
Plasma proteins	Antibodies and other protein substances formed in the liver to fight infection
Platelets	Type of white blood cell formed in bone marrow; seal leaks in blood vessels and promote clotting
White blood cells	Lymphocytes, monocytes, granular leukocytes, eosinophils, neutrophils, basophils; formed in bone marrow, lymph nodes, spleen; protect body from pathogens and promote tissue repair and regeneration

TABLE 18–2   Major Steps in Clotting

1. Thromboplastin and serotonin are released from injured tissue.
2. Thromboplastin and serotonin stimulate the conversion of prothrombin to thrombin.
3. Thrombin acts as an enzyme to convert fibrinogen, a plasma protein, into threads of fibrin.
4. Fibrin threads are deposited to form network that includes red cells, platelets, plasma (a clot).
5. Thromboplastin also neutralizes natural anticlotting substances such as heparin and antithromboplastin.

in the mouth. Bleeding may be obvious or hidden, especially in stool. In severe anemia, there may be congestive heart failure, cardiac arrhythmias, or inadequate cerebral blood flow.

Drug therapy may be prescribed to replace missing vitamins or minerals essential to the production of erythrocytes. Diet therapy may also be needed. For some types of anemia, replacement therapy is not effective. Blood transfusions may be needed. When underlying disease is discovered to be the cause of a patient's anemia, medical treatment is directed to the cause.

The nurse plays an important role in assisting individuals and families to prevent certain anemias. For example, the nurse may provide important information about a balanced diet that provides all of the nutrients to prevent anemia from inadequate dietary intake. In teaching about safe and correct use of prescribed and nonprescribed drugs, the nurse helps to prevent anemias that develop from drug toxicity.

I. Actions and uses.
  A. Iron replacement is prescribed when anemia results from iron deficiency.
  B. Parenteral vitamin B_{12} is prescribed when anemia results from a lack of intrinsic factor secreted by the stomach. This may develop in patients with small bowel disease, surgical procedures involving the stomach, and/or small intestine.
  C. Folic acid may be prescribed for a patient with a disease of the small intestine, alcoholism, or when a drug therapy regimen produces folate deficiency.
II. Adverse responses.
  A. Iron preparations.
    1. Heartburn, nausea, epigastric distress, constipation, dark stools, or diarrhea with oral preparations.
    2. Iron poisoning from accidental or intentional overdose may cause vomiting, abdominal pain, diarrhea, pallor or cyanosis, drowsiness and lassitude, hyperventilation, and cardiovascular collapse.
    3. Parenteral administration of iron may cause headache, malaise, fever, joint pains, urticaria, lymph gland swelling, anaphylaxis, local reaction at IM injection site (pain, skin discoloration, malignant changes).
    4. Antacids reduce oral iron absorption if given together.
  B. Vitamin B_{12} preparations.
    1. Adverse responses are rare and usually related to hypersensitivity to parenteral injections.
  C. Folate preparations.
    1. Adverse responses are extremely rare and usually confined to parenteral routes.
    2. Large doses may reduce theraputic effects of certain anticonvulsants (phenobarbital, phenytoin, primidone).
III. Nursing implications.
  A. Assess newly admitted patients for the presence of factors known to be associated with anemia. A minimum of information would include eating practices, previous illness and surgery involving the gastrointestinal system, alcohol intake, and drugs taken.
  B. When an overview of the patient's eating practices indicates inadequate diet, ask the dietitian for a nutritional assessment.
  C. Administer oral iron preparations when the patient's stomach is empty to encourage greater absorption. If gastrointestinal side effects develop, report them to the physician and anticipate a possible reduction of dosage.

D. Administer IM iron preparations using the following guidelines:
1. Draw up an additional 0.1 to 0.2 ml of air into the syringe after the dosage has been measured. Position the air at the plunger end of the syringe.
2. Replace the needle.
3. Select a large IM injection site such as the buttock.
4. Use the Z-tract injection method.
5. Follow directions in package insert provided by manufacturer.
6. Observe the patient for a hypersensitive reaction up to 24 h after injection. Report any unusual symptoms.
E. Question oral administration of vitamin B_{12} for any patient with known or suspected pernicious anemia. Oral preparations are not absorbed because patients with these conditions do not secrete intrinsic factor.
F. Store parenteral solutions of vitamin B_{12} away from sunlight.
G. Store parenteral preparations of folic acid in the refrigerator and away from light.
H. Encourage patients, families, friends, and neighbors to eat a balanced diet with a sufficient number of servings from each of the basic food groups.
I. Encourage pregnant women to seek early prenatal care. Provide a list of foods and servings that must be increased in order to meet the changed nutritional requirements of pregnancy.

TABLE 18–3 Antianemic Agents

Nonproprietary Name	Proprietary Name	Adult Dose Range	Notes
Folic Acid Preparations			
Folic acid	Folvite	1–5 mg PO, IM dosage adjusted to patient's specific condition and response	Parenteral preparations should be stored in refrigerator and kept in dark
Leucovorin calcium injection		Available in ampules and vials; dosage adjusted to patient's specific condition	Used only for deficiencies that result from drugs such as methotrexate; reconstituted solution should be used as soon as possible (will precipitate if left standing)
Iron Preparations			
Ferrous gluconate		2–3 mg/kg/day PO (200 mg PO per day)	Dosage for iron deficiency anemia
		15–30 mg PO per day	Prevention of iron deficiency anemia during pregnancy
Ferrous sulfate	Feosol	Same as above	Same as above
Iron dextran injection	Imferon	1–10 ml IM	Z-tract method must be used; test dose of 25 mg (0.5 ml) may be ordered 1h before first IM dose
		1–2 drops IV over 5 min initially; then 500 mg IV over 5–10 min; dosage repeated until total amount required has been administered	IV route preferred when possible
Vitamin B_{12} Preparations			
Cyanocobalamin injection	Redisol Rubramin	100 mg SC, IM every 2–4 weeks for maintenance in pernicious anemia; dosage varies for other conditions	Should never be administered IV; used for patients with pernicious anemia
	Betalin and others	10–250 mg PO per day	Not absorbed unless the patient is producing intrinsic factor; used mainly when dietary intake insufficient

TABLE 18–4   Antianginal Agents

Nonproprietary Name	Proprietary Name	Adult Dose Range	Notes
Adrenergic Blockers			
metoprolol	Lopressor	Dose individualized 100–450 mg/day PO	See also Table 18–9. Adrenergic blockers also used for patients with hypertension; see pp. 185–186 for adverse responses and nursing implications.
nadolol	Corgard	40 mg/day PO initially; gradually increased over 3–7 days until maintenance dose of 80–240 mg is established	Must be tapered slowly
propranolol	Inderal	Dose individualized; 10 mg PO 3–4×/day initially; may be increased to 160–240 mg PO per day if no adverse responses	May also be prescribed to prevent recurrence of myocardial infarction
Calcium Antagonists			
diltiazem	Cardizem	30–60 mg PO 3–4×/day	
nifedipine	Procardia	10 mg PO tid initially; 10–30 mg PO—total daily dosage should not exceed 100 mg	May cause reflex increase in heart rate; calcium channel blocker; decrease dosage gradually
verapamil	Calan, Isoptin	320–480 mg PO per day	May also be prescribed for certain ventricular arrhythmias
Organic Nitrates			
amyl nitrate		0.18–0.3 ml by inhalation	
erythrityl tetranitrate	Cardilate	5–15 mg sublingually 30–90 mg PO every 8 h	
isosorbide dinitrate	Isordil Sorbitrate	2.5–10 mg sublingually 5–30 mg PO every 6 h 40 mg PO sustained release capsules every 6–12 h	
nitroglycerin	Nitrobid Nitrol	0.15–0.6 mg sublingually 2.5–6.5 mg PO sustained release capsules every 6–12 h	Instruct patient to get transportation to the nearest emergency room if three sublingual tablets do not relieve a sustained attack of angina within 15 min.
	Nitrostat	1.25–5 cm (1½–2 in) 2% ointment to skin q4h IV 5 mg/min–20 mg/min by infusion pump	IV administration requires a glass bottle and special administration set; dosage may be increased by 10–20 μg/min until the patient responds. IV route may also be used for emergency treatment to reduce high blood pressure.
	Nitro-Disc, Nitro-Dur, Transderm-Nitro	2.5 to 15-mg patches applied to skin every 24 h	
pentaerythritol	Peritrate	30–80 mg PO sustained release capsules every 12 h	
tetranitrate	Duotrate	10–40 mg PO chewable tablets every 6 h	
Other			
dipyridamole	Persantine	50 mg PO 3×/day	Should be administered at least 1 h before meals

J. Encourage patients with pernicious anemia to continue therapy in order to prevent irreversible damage to the nervous system.

ANTIANGINAL AGENTS

Antianginal agents (Table 18–4) are drugs that dilate coronary blood vessels to relieve pain from *angina pectoris.* The patient with angina pectoris experiences sudden substernal pain that may radiate to the left shoulder or arm. Pain is often brought about by exercise or intense emotions and relieved by rest. The underlying cause of angina is usually atherosclerosis of coronary arteries. *Atherosclerosis* is a narrowing and hardening of blood vessels by deposits of fatty plaques. As coronary arteries narrow and harden, they are less able to increase blood flow to the heart when its need for oxygen is increased by exercise.

Antianginal drugs work in one or more of the following ways:

1. By relaxing smooth muscle and causing dilation of blood vessels in the heart.
2. By decreasing venous return to the heart causing a reduction of the workload.

One group of drugs commonly prescribed is organic nitrates such as nitroglycerin. Another group of drugs is adrenergic blocking agents like propranolol. A third group is calcium antagonists such as nifedipine.

I. Actions and uses.
   A. Antianginal agents relax smooth muscle of blood vessels and reduce the need for oxygen by the myocardium. For these effects, they may be prescribed to prevent or relieve angina.
   B. Adrenergic blocking agents block the vasoconstricting effects of sympathetic nerves.
   C. Calcium blockers reduce the muscle tone of blood vessels by interfering with the movement of calcium across the cell membrane.
   D. Organic nitrates also relax smooth muscle in the bronchi, biliary tract, gastrointestinal system, ureter, and uterus.
   E. Sublingual route is most often used to relieve an acute attack or immediately before exercise to prevent one.
   F. Oral and topical preparations may be used for prolonged prevention. Some preparations are available as sustained release capsules.
   G. Patients receiving long-acting preparations to prevent attacks may also use sublingual tablets to relieve acute attacks within 1–3 min.
II. Adverse responses.
   A. Central nervous system: headache, weakness, dizziness.
   B. Cardiovascular: postural hypotension.
   C. Skin: flushing, sweating.
   D. Drug interactions include:
      1. Severe hypotension leading to collapse when nitroglycerin or its relatives are combined with alcohol, tricyclic antidepressants (see Table 16–6).
      2. Bradycardia may result when adrenergic blocking agents (propranolol, nadolol) are combined with digitalis preparations.
      3. Adrenergic (see Table 17–2) and anticholinergic drugs (see Table 17–4) may reduce the effects of antianginal agents.
   E. Drug tolerance may develop with organic nitrates such as nitroglycerin. The drug must be stopped temporarily and restarted.
III. Nursing implications.
   A. Instruct the patient to stop activity, sit down, and rest at the first sign of angina. Medication for relief of acute pain should be taken in this position. If permitted by the physician, one additional tablet may be taken every 5 min if pain persists up to a maximum of three tablets.
   B. For oral administration, use the following guidelines:

1. Do not crush or chew sustained release capsules. Administer on an empty stomach with a full glass of water.

2. Instruct patient to chew chewable tablets slowly before swallowing.

3. Place sublingual tablet under the tongue and instruct the patient not to swallow until the tablet has completely dissolved naturally. Make sure mouth is moist before administering.

4. Check for and report an absence of burning under the tongue after sublingual administration. This symptom indicates either that the tablet has become inactive or that it is not dissolving properly.

5. Place transmucosal tablet in the space between the upper lip and gum.

6. Avoid handling tablets with hands since this practice reduces potency. Use good technique by pouring tablets into cap and then to a medicine cup.

C. For topical administration, use the following guidelines:

1. Take blood pressure and pulse before each dose and 1h after each dose. Report and record changes.

2. Remove previous dose of ointment if present and cleanse skin. Inspect the site for rash or irritation. Make sure previous patch is discarded out of reach of children. Old patches have caused symptoms in children who were found to be playing with them.

3. Choose a new site on the trunk. An acceptable site is relatively free of hair and several inches away from the previous site. Common sites include the chest, arms, abdomen, and upper back. Avoid distal parts of the body.

4. Squeeze the prescribed dose on the measured paper provided by the manufacturer.

5. Use the paper to spread the ointment over a 6×6-in. square. Do not use fingers or massage ointment into skin.

6. If protection of clothing is needed, cover the site with a piece of clean plastic wrap and tape.

7. If a transdermal patch is prescribed, apply at the same time daily according to the manufacturer's directions.

D. Report pain that lasts longer than 10 min and is not relieved by nitroglycerin. If at home, the patient should be driven by someone else to the nearest emergency room for immediate medical evaluation.

E. Store antianginal agents in tightly covered containers away from light.

F. For intravenous administration, follow manufacturer's directions carefully. Glass bottles or non-polyvinyl chloride (PVC) plastic administration sets must be used to avoid absorption of nitroglycerin by the tubing.

G. Encourage patients to wear identifying information about angina and specific drugs taken.

H. If nitroglycerin tablets are to be kept at the bedside of the hospitalized patient, use the following guidelines:

1. Place no more than five to ten tablets at the bedside and count them at the beginning and end of each shift.

2. Instruct the patient to report the onset of pain immediately, as soon as the first tablet has been taken.

I. Teach patients at home to keep a record of anginal attacks. A minimum record would include: The time of onset, the duration, activity that preceded the onset, and number of tablets taken to relieve the attack. Teach the patient to go to the nearest emergency room if anginal pain persists for longer than 10 min. Someone else should drive the patient.

J. Encourage the patient to undertake nondrug measures that relieve or prevent angina if these are permitted by the physician. Nondrug measures include: weight loss if appropriate, a graduated exercise program, avoidance of coffee, tea, and cola drinks, severe emotional stresses, sudden bursts of physical activity, avoidance of alcohol, smoking cessation if appropriate.

K. Instruct patients not to stop organic nitrates abruptly. This may trigger severe spasms in coronary arteries.

TABLE 18–5   Antiarrhythmics

Nonproprietary Name	Proprietary Name	Adult Dose Range	Notes
amiodarone	Cordarone	Dose individualized to patient	New drug used for patients with certain atrial and ventricular arrhythmias; may produce headaches, nausea, visual disturbances, blue-gray skin
bretylium	Bretylol	5–10 mg/kg IV infused over 10–20 min in dilute solution	Used only for emergency treatment of ventricular arrhythmias that do not respond to lidocaine, procainamide; severe hypotension may occur
disopyramide	Norpace	400–800 mg PO per day in four divided doses.	Used only for patients with ventricular arrhythmias; toxic to kidneys
flecainide	Tambocor	Dose individualized to patient	New drug recommended for patients with ventricular arrhythmias; may produce other arrhythmias, dizziness, blurred vision, nausea
lidocaine	Xylocaine	1–2 mg/kg IV single-dose bolus; 1–5 mg/min by continuous IV infusion 4–5 mg/kg IM	Used only for emergency treatment of ventricular arrhythmias; very short acting; solution without preservative should be used
mexiletine	Mexitil	Dose individualized to patient	New drug that suppresses ventricular arrhythmias; may produce nausea and vomiting, tremors, light-headedness, incoordination
phenytoin	Dilantin	1000 mg PO per day for first 1–4 days; then 400 mg PO per day as maintenance 100 mg IV every 15 min until arrhythmia is controlled or adverse responses occur	Anticonvulsant drug also used for premature ventricular contractions, ventricular or atrial tachycardia; see pp. 138–139 for additional information
procainamide	Procan-SR, Pronestyl	3–6 g PO per day in divided doses every 6 h	A broad-spectrum drug used mainly for patients who do not respond to quinidine; hypersensitive responses may be life-threatening
propranolol	Inderal	40–80 mg PO per day; up to 1,000 mg PO per day may be required for some patients 1 mg IV every 3–5 min	Adrenergic blocker used mainly for patients with atrial fibrillation, atrial flutter, supraventricular tachycardia; severe hypotension may develop; may increase anginal pain; see pp. 185–186 for additional information
quinidine sulfate or gluconate	Cin-Quin, Quinova, Quinidex, Cardioquin, Quinaglute	300–500 mg PO 4 ×/day, also available for IM, IV use; a loading dose of 600–1000 mg may be administered in emergencies	Broad-spectrum drug used to prevent or control a variety of atrial and ventricular arrhythmias
tocainide hydrochloride	Tonocard	400 mg PO every 8 h initially; gradually increased to 1200–1800 mg PO per day in three divided doses	New drug that suppresses ventricular arrhythmias; give with food to minimize gastrointestinal effects; monitor blood pressure and pulse; report symptoms of sore throat, chills, fever, coughing, dyspnea, bruising, bleeding
verapamil	Calan, Isoptin	40–120 mg PO every 8 h 0.1–5 mg/kg IV initial dose; 10 mg IV 30 min later	Slows conduction through the AV node; used for supraventricular tachycardias, atrial fibrillation, and flutter; DO NOT ADMINISTER WITH DISOPYRAMIDE OR PROPRANOLOL.

ANTIARRHYTHMIC AGENTS

Antiarrhythmic agents (Table 18–5) are drugs prescribed for the patient with an abnormal disturbance in heart rate, regularity, pathway of electrical conduction, or site of origin. The main cause of arrhythmias is heart disease. A number of other factors may cause an arrhythmia including fever or hypothermia, drugs, disease in the central nervous system, lung disease, disturbances in acid-base balance, electrolyte imbalance. Many types of arrhythmias have been identified. They are often named by the site of origin and type of rate or pattern. For example, a rhythm that is too fast and originates in the atria is called *atrial tachycardia*. A rate that originates in the SA node but is too slow is called *sinus bradycardia*. When impulses that originate in one place cannot be conducted through to the ventricles, the term *block* is used. When there is no rhythmic discharge of impulses but a wild disarray of uncoordinated electrical discharge, the term *fibrillation* is used. Table 18–6 defines common arrhythmias.

An arrhythmia may be minor, producing no symptoms, or major, resulting in complete collapse and death. The effect of the rhythm on the patient's cardiac output is a major influence on its severity. Arrhythmias may develop suddenly and unexpectedly or they may persist for years. For example atrial arrhythmias may be serious but are usually less urgent than ventricular arrhythmias. This is because ventricular arrhythmias produce an immediate reduction of cardiac output that affects vital organs.

The only way to know for certain that a person is experiencing an arrhythmia is to record it on an EKG or cardiac monitor attached to the patient. For this reason, hospitalized patients who develop an arrhythmia are often transferred to the coronary care unit for close observation and treatment by nurses and physicians with advanced training.

Arrhythmias produce several other harmful effects:

1. Tachycardias increase the workload of the heart and the consumption of oxygen.

TABLE 18–6   Common Arrhythmias

Atrial flutter	A rapid regular rhythm that originates outside the SA node; shortens filling time; increases workload of the heart; thrombi may form in atria
Atrial fibrillation	Chaotic uncoordinated discharge of impulses from atria; shortens filling time; thrombi may form in atria; reduces cardiac output
Premature atrial contraction (PAC)	Early discharge of one impulse that may originate in the SA node or in another atrial site
Atrial tachycardia	A rapid irregular rhythm that originates in the atria outside the SA node; increases workload of the heart; may lead to congestive heart failure or angina pectoris
Atrioventricular (AV) block	Slowed or impaired conduction through the AV node. In first-degree block, conduction is slowed. In second-degree block, some impulses do not get through to the ventricles. In third-degree block, no impulses reach the ventricles; severely reduces cardiac output; may increase workload of heart
Premature ventricular contraction (PVC, VPC)	Early discharge of impulse that originates in the ventricles instead of the SA node; not serious unless they occur frequently, in groups, or from multiple sites
Ventricular fibrillation	Chaotic uncoordinated discharge of impulses from the ventricles; no cardiac output; death results within 4–6 min unless the patient is successfully resuscitated
Ventricular tachycardia	Rapid discharge of impulses that originate in the ventricles; severely reduces cardiac output; emergency treatment needed to prevent death

2. Tachycardias also shorten diastole, the relaxation phase during which the atria and ventricles fill. This in turn may reduce cardiac output.
3. Bradycardias below the rate of 60 per minute reduce cardiac output and deprive vital organs of adequate blood supply.
4. Arrythmias that disrupt the resting phase of the cardiac cycle may further increase irritability of heart muscle and trigger more serious arrhythmias.

I. Actions and uses.
   A. Generally exert a depressant effect on the myocardium.
   B. Decrease electrical excitability of cells in heart muscle, especially pacemaker cells.
   C. Slow conduction of impulses through the myocardium.
   D. Prolong the resting period—the time in the electrical cycle when the heart cannot respond to a new stimulus.
   E. Some agents are specific to particular arrhythmias while others are broad-spectrum and may be prescribed for a variety of arrhythmias.
   F. Response to dose is highly individualized; patients under initial treatment are usually monitored continuously.
   G. Quinidine also affects the autonomic nervous system, producing dual effects including atropinelike (anticholinergic) and adrenergic blocking (vasodilatation) effects.

II. Adverse responses.
   A. Cardiovascular system: may produce other arrhythmias, bradycardia, syncope, hypotension, embolism.
   B. Gastrointestinal system: may produce dry mouth, nausea, vomiting, diarrhea, abdominal pain, anorexia.
   C. Central nervous system: quinidine may produce blurred vision, tinnitus, headache, photophobia, confusion, delirium, psychosis, hot flushed skin.
   D. Genitourinary system: urinary retention, urgency.
   E. Hypersensitive reactions—skin eruptions.
      1. Quinidine may produce drug fever, anaphylaxis, asthmalike respiratory symptoms, anemia.
      2. Procainamide may also produce agranulocytosis, systemic lupus erythematosus, Raynaud's phenomenon.
   F. Drug interactions include:
      • Shorter duration of action when quinidine is combined with phenobarbital, phenytoin.
      • A rise in plasma digoxin level when quinidine is combined with digoxin, bretylium.
      • A reduction in therapeutic effects of phenytoin when combined with disopyramide.
      • Excessive cardiac depression when lidocaine is combined with phenytoin.
      • Added hypotension when procainamide is combined with antihypertensives, methyldopa.
      • Severe postural hypotension when quinidine is combined with nitroglycerin.
      • A further increase in prothrombin time when quinidine is combined with oral anticoagulants.
      • See p. 138 for interactions of phenytoin. Potentially fatal bradycardia and hypotension when verapamil is combined with propranolol.
      • Increase in antiarrhythmic effects including adverse responses when they are combined with: other antiarrhythmics, anticholinergics, antihypertensives, diuretics, phenothiazines.
      • Decreased antiarrhythmic effects when combined with atropine.
      • Increased muscle relaxation when quinidine, procainamide are combined with skeletal muscle relaxants.
      • Decreased effects of cholinergics when they are combined with quinidine.
      • The following drugs inhibit the actions of propranolol: anticholinergics such as atropine, barbiturates, indomethacin.

III. Nursing implications.
   A. Collect a careful nursing history to identify patients more likely to develop an arrhythmia (those with fever, respiratory, or cardiovascular disease, hyperthyroidism, emotional dis-

tress, large consumers of coffee, tea, cola drinks, cigarette smokers, hyperventilators, and those taking certain drugs).

B. Take the apical pulse for a full minute on newly admitted patients. Record rate, rhythm, volume as a point of departure for changes.

C. Monitor the patient's blood pressure carefully because hypotension is a common adverse response to therapy.

D. Check the apical pulse for a full minute before each dose. Report bradycardia.

E. Know where emergency antiarrhythmic drugs and supplies are stored on your nursing unit. Double-check emergency supply of lidocaine to be certain it does not contain preservatives or epinephrine when used for an arrhythmia.

F. Monitor serum drug levels when ordered by the physician to adjust dosage.

G. Teach patients to change positions slowly to prevent symptoms associated with hypotension.

H. Teach patients how to take and record their pulses daily.

I. Teach patients to take antiarrhythmics like quinidine and procainamide on time. Late or missed doses cause serum blood levels to fall rapidly.

ANTICLOTTING AGENTS

Anticlotting agents are drugs that interfere with blood coagulation (Table 18–8). Normally, the process of coagulation or clotting provides protection from blood loss. The process begins when a blood vessel is impaired. The vessels contract immediately and platelets attach themselves both to the rough surfaces and to each other. This forms a plug which prevents further blood loss. The plug is later strengthened by fibrin that combines with it to form a clot or thrombus. Fibrin is a protein formed by a series of chemical interactions that involve over 15 different protein substances called *clotting factors*. Many of the clotting factors require vitamin K to be synthesized.

Some patients have abnormalities in blood flow, coagulation, or blood vessel walls that result in the formation of thrombi that do not protect but cause further damage. Table 18–7 contains a description of common conditions that may involve thrombi.

A thrombus may form in either an artery or a vein. A thrombus that occludes blood flow in an artery produces injury and potentially irreversible damage to the body part nourished by that artery. A thrombus that forms along a vein is more likely to detach from the wall and travel to the arterioles in vital organs such as the brain, heart, or lungs. This traveling thrombus, known as an *embolus,* moves through blood vessels until it lodges in an arteriole too small to pass it through. There it causes damage to the tissue nourished by that arteriole. The veins most likely to develop thrombi are deep

TABLE 18–7 Selected Conditions Involving Thrombi

Condition	Description
Cerebral embolism	A stroke caused by the movement of an embolus into a brain artery or arteriole
Cerebral thrombus	A stroke caused by the formation of a thrombus in a diseased cerebral artery
Peripheral vascular disease	A collection of diseases that affect arteries and/or veins in the extremities Thrombi develop more easily in diseased blood vessels
Phlebothrombosis	Thrombus formation along the wall of a vein
Pulmonary embolism	Emboli move through the right side of the heart and lodge in a pulmonary artery or arteriole
Thrombophlebitis	Thrombus formation and inflammation along the wall of a vein

TABLE 18–8 Anticlotting Agents

Nonproprietary Name	Proprietary Name	Adult Dose Range	Notes
Anticoagulants			
heparin sodium	Heparin Panheprin Liquemin	IV: intermittent injection, 10,000 U initially; 5,000–10,000 U every 4–6 h; SC dose same. IV: continuous infusion. 5,000–10,000 U injected into tubing as a loading dose. 1,000 U/h for a 70-kg patient	An indwelling rubber capped needle called a *heparin lock* is often used. An infusion pump is recommended. No more than 6 h of solution is hung at any time to prevent accidental overdosage. See Nursing Implications for SC administration
warfarin sodium	Coumadin Panwarfarin	10–15 mg PO per day initially; 2–15 mg PO for maintenance	Dosage may need adjustment according to the patient's prothrombin time
warfarin potassium	Athrombin K	Same as warfarin sodium	
dicumarol		300 mg PO initial dose; 200 mg second day; 25–150 mg PO per day for maintenance	Mild GI side effects are common. Antacids may impair drug absorption
acenocoumarol	Diatrom	16–28 mg PO initial dose; 8–16 mg PO second dose; 2–10 mg PO per day for maintenance	Mild GI side effects, dermatitis, urticaria, and alopecia (hair loss) have been reported
diphenadione	Dipaxin	20–30 mg PO initial dose; 10–15 mg PO second dose; 2.5–5 mg PO per day for maintenance	Mild GI side effects have been reported
phenprocoumon	Liquamar	21 mg PO initial dose; 9 mg PO second dose; 0.5–6 mg PO per day for maintenance	Nausea, diarrhea, dermatitis have been reported
anisindione	Miradon	Available in 50-mg tablets	Rarely used
Antithrombus Agents			
aspirin		0.325–1.3 g PO per day	
dipyridamole	Persantine	Dosage range not established. Available as 25-mg tablets	Used to prevent thrombi in patients with artificial heart valves; a vasodilator
dextran	Macrodex Gentran 75 10% Travert	500 ml IV	Used to prevent thrombus in surgical patients
Thrombolytic Agents			
streptokinase	Streptase	250,000 IU IV over 30 min initially; 100,000 IU/h by continuous IV infusion for 24–72 h	
urokinase	Abbokinase	4,400 IU/kg administered IV over 10 min initially; 4,400 IU/kg continuous IV for 12 h	This course of treatment is followed by heparin or oral anticoagulation

Abbreviations: GI, gastrointestinal.

veins in the pelvis and legs. Circulation to the body part distal to the venous thrombus becomes sluggish producing symptoms described below.

The patient with an arterial thrombus is most likely to experience symptoms of diminished blood flow: pain in the affected part that increases with activity, hypoxic changes in the affected part, disruption of function in the affected part.

The patient with a venous thrombus is likely to experience pain, tenderness, and warmth at the site of the thrombus, and swelling of the affected part. Erythema may also be present.

As soon as a thrombus is discovered, immediate steps are taken to remove it and to prevent it from getting larger or forming an embolus.

The patient with an arterial thrombus may be taken to the operating room for removal and restoration of blood flow. The patient with a venous thrombus is usually placed on bedrest to prevent the formation of an embolus.

Drug therapy may be prescribed to prevent or treat thrombi that form in blood vessels. *Anticoagulants* are drugs that interfere with clotting by suppressing the activity of clotting factors. This prevents existing clots from getting larger and/or prevents new clots from forming. *Antithrombotic* drugs suppress the activity of platelets. *Thrombolytic drugs* act to break up the fibrin in a thrombus.

I. Actions and uses.
   A. *Anticoagulants* act primarily by interfering with the activity of clotting factors. *Oral anticoagulants* act slowly and require 1–3 days before intended effects occur. Heparin acts immediately and its effects are short.
   B. Anticoagulants are prescribed primarily for the patient with a venous thrombus.
   C. *Antithrombus drugs* act primarily by suppressing the activities of platelets.
   D. Antithrombus drugs are prescribed primarily for the patient with arterial thrombus.
   E. *Thrombolytic drugs* promote the disintegration of a thrombus by enhancing the formation of an enzyme known as *plasmin*. Plasmin breaks up the fibrin in a clot.
   F. Thrombolytic drugs are prescribed mainly for the patient with severe pulmonary emboli or thrombophlebitis of the ileofemoral veins.
   G. Anticoagulant doses are adjusted using several laboratory tests as a guide.
      1. The *partial thromboplastin time* (PTT) is used to evaluate the effects of the anticoagulant heparin. The patient's pretreatment time is obtained as a baseline. A desirable therapeutic range is approximately twice the patient's baseline time.
      2. Oral anticoagulant doses are adjusted using a laboratory test called the *prothrombin time*. A desirable therapeutic range is twice the patient's baseline reading.
   H. Low-dose heparin may be used to prevent embolism in patients at risk for the formation of thrombi. For example, selected surgical patients and those with hemiplegia or quadriplegia following a complete stroke, may receive this therapy.
      1. Heparinized solutions may be used to flush cannulas, the heart-lung machine, a hemodialysis unit, or other similar equipment.
II. Adverse responses.
   A. Anticoagulants.
      1. Hypersensitive reactions to heparin include chills, fever, urticaria, anaphylactic shock.
      2. Transient hair loss.
      3. Osteoporosis and spontaneous fractures.
      4. Hemorrhage (ecchymosis, hematuria, uterine bleeding, melena, epistaxis, hematoma, gingival bleeding, hemoptysis, hematemesis).
      5. Thrombocytopenia.
      6. Drug interactions include:
         • An increase in anticoagulation effects when oral anticoagulants are combined with: aspirin and other salicylates, phenylbutazone, disulfiram, metronidazole, clofibrate, cimetidine, sulfinpyrazone.
         • A decrease in anticoagulation when oral anticoagulants are combined with barbiturates, glutethimide, rifampin, cholestyramine, large doses of vitamin C.
      7. Protamine sulfate is a specific antidote for heparin overdosage.
      8. Vitamine K_1 (phytonadione) is a specific treatment for bleeding from oral anticoagulants.
   B. Antithrombus agents.
      1. See p. 129 for adverse responses to aspirin.
      2. Dextran may produce wheezing, tightness in the chest, mild hypotension, occasional urticaria, anaphylaxis.

    C. Thrombolytic agents.
      1. Fever, bleeding, allergic reactions.
      2. Aminocaproic acid (Amicar) is a specific antidote for overdosage of thrombolytic drugs.

III. Nursing implications.

    A. Collect information about the patient's bleeding and bruising pattern before initiating drug therapy with anticlotting agents.

    B. Ask the patient about the use of prescribed and nonprescribed drugs that may enhance anticoagulation effects of drug therapy. For example, aspirin prolongs the bleeding time.

    C. Seek additional information when anticlotting agents are prescribed for a patient who has bleeding or a wound, blood disorders, a planned surgery on the brain, eye, spinal cord, severe hypertension, ulcers, tuberculosis, pregnancy, bacterial endocarditis. Most anticlotting agents are not recommended for patients with these conditions.

    D. Monitor the patient's PTT when administering heparin. Hold the dose and seek additional information if the PTT exceeds 120 s. Anticipate a reduction of dosage or an omitted dose.

    E. Monitor the patient's prothrombin activity when administering oral anticoagulants. Hold the dose and seek additional information if the prothrombin time is over 30 s. Anticipate a reduction of dosage that will not be visible in the laboratory test for 1–2 weeks. Vitamin K may be needed.

    F. Check the patient systematically and regularly for bleeding. A head to toe method is recommended.

    G. When administering heparin SC, use the following guidelines:
      1. Check the last PTT and get additional information if it is greater than 120 s.
      2. Select a small-gauge, short needle such as a ½-in. no. 26.
      3. Measure the dosage in a 1–ml tuberculin syringe for greater precision.
      4. After measuring the dosage, aspirate an additional 0.1 ml of air into the syringe. Position the air at the plunger end of the syringe.
      5. Select a SC site on the abdomen or iliac area well away from obvious muscle or deeper structures. Rotate injection sites.
      6. Cleanse the site using rotary motion and friction.
      7. Grasp 2.5–5 cm (1–2 in.) of SC tissue between the thumb and fingers of one hand.
      8. Inject the needle straight into the SC tissue perpendicular to the skin surface.
      9. Inject the heparin; then clear the needle with 0.1 ml of air that remains in the syringe.
      10. Withdraw the needle and apply firm pressure to the injection site for 1 min. Do not massage the site.

    H. Anticipate that patients with vitamin K deficiency due to inadequate intake or small bowel disease are more likely to have bleeding from oral anticoagulants.

    I. Teach patients to inspect themselves systematically and regularly for bruises and bleeding.

    J. Teach patients to use the same laboratory for every prothrombin time or PTT. Variations in laboratory methods may produce laboratory results that are difficult to interpret.

    K. Know where antidotes for anticlotting agents are. These include protamine sulfate for heparin, vitamin K_1 for oral anticoagulants, and aminocaproic acid for thrombolytic agents.

    L. Instruct the patient on long-term therapy to wear identifying drug information at all times.

    M. Use nondrug measures that prevent the formation of thrombi. Examples of nondrug measures include:
      • Ambulate the patient regularly.
      • Demonstrate leg exercises to hospitalized patients, encourage patients to perform these exercises regularly.
      • Provide passive exercises for patients unable to participate regularly.
      • Apply elastic stockings correctly.
      • Avoid constricting garments or pillows that impede blood flow to the lower extremities.
      • Encourage adequate fluid intake.

    N. Teach the patient to report the use of anticoagulants to other physicians, chiropractors, dentists, and other health professionals who provide care.

ANTIHYPERTENSIVES

Antihypertensives are drugs that reduce blood pressure in patients with *hypertension* (Table 18–9). The patient with hypertension has a persistently elevated blood pressure. When the average of two or more diastolic readings is greater than 90 mm Hg or the average of two or more systolic readings is greater than 140 mm Hg, a person may be diagnosed as having hypertension. A single elevated reading does not mean a person has hypertension. Elevation on two or more occasions, however, indicates hypertension.

Blood pressure is a measure of the force applied to arterial walls by the flow of blood. The measure is recorded in millimeters of mercury (mm Hg). A blood pressure reading contains two measurements: systolic and diastolic pressures. *Systolic pressure* reflects the pressure against arterial walls during systole when the heart is contracting. Normal systolic pressure is below 140 mm Hg. *Diastolic pressure* reflects pressure against the arterial walls during diastole when the heart is filling. Normal diastolic pressure is below 85 to 90 mm Hg.

Major factors affecting blood pressure are cardiac output and peripheral vascular resistance. *Cardiac output* is the amount of blood squeezed out of the ventricles each minute. *Peripheral vascular resistance* is a term that describes the amount of constriction or dilation present in arterioles.

Over 60 million people in the United States have been found to have elevations of blood pressure. Two types of hypertension have been identified. *Essential or primary hypertension,* the most common type, is a persistent elevation of blood pressure for which a primary cause cannot be found. *Secondary hypertension* occurs as a result of some other disease process. A person with persistent elevation of diastolic blood pressure in the 90- to 104-mm Hg range has *mild hypertension*. When diastolic readings persist in the 105- to 114-mm Hg range, a person has *moderate hypertension*. When diastolic readings persist above 115 mm Hg, a person has *severe hypertension*. When systolic blood pressure persists in the range of 140–159 mm Hg, without diastolic elevation, a person has *borderline isolated systolic hypertension*. When systolic blood pressure persists above 160 mm Hg without diastolic elevation, a person has *isolated systolic hypertension*. A *hypertensive emergency* is a clinical condition of high sustained blood pressure that must be reduced in minutes or hours to prevent death or disability.

Besides an elevation of blood pressure, there may be no other symptoms in a person with hypertension. The person may look and feel well. However, high blood pressure that persists for months and years causes damage in target organs such as the brain, heart, and kidneys. The result of damage includes stroke, heart attack, kidney failure, and declining vision that may lead to blindness. Factors that favor persistent elevations of blood pressure include obesity, high dietary intake of sodium and animal fat, heavy alcohol intake, cigarette smoking, and a sedentary life-style.

Antihypertensive drugs such as those described in Table 18–9 are an important part of the medical treatment plan. A second important feature is eliminating or modifying risk factors described earlier. When hypertension results from other diseases such as a tumor, thyroid disease, or coarctation of the aorta, medical treatment is directed at the underlying cause.

There are a variety of antihypertensive agents, and most of them carry risks of serious adverse responses. To reduce these risks, a specific regimen is recommended by the Joint National Committee on Detection, Evaluation, and Treatment of High Blood Pressure. This regimen, known as *stepped care,* is described in Table 18–10.

I. Actions and uses.
   A. Adrenergic blocking agents interfere with the effects of the sympathetic nervous system in one or more of the following ways:
      1. By interfering with the amount and activity of norepinephrine and dopamine in the central nervous system: methyldopa, clonidine.
      2. By blocking adrenergic receptor sites on the cell membrane: propranolol and its relatives, prazosin, phentolamine, phenoxybenzamine.
      3. By acting on postganglionic sympathetic nerves: guanethidine, reserpine.
   B. Calcium blocking agents relax smooth muscle of blood vessels by interfering with the movement of calcium ions through cell membranes.
   C. Diuretics lower blood pressure by depleting the body of sodium and water. A reduction of

TABLE 18–9   Antihypertensives

Nonproprietary Name	Proprietary Name	Adult Dose Range*	Notes
Adrenergic blocking agents			
acebutolol	Sectral	400 mg initially; may be increased to a maximum of 800 mg PO per day in divided doses	New drug similar to propranolol; has additional adverse responses of dysuria, nocturia; may also be used for arrhythmias; must be discontinued gradually over 2 weeks
atenolol	Tenormin	50 mg PO per day; up to 100 mg PO per day	
clonidine hydrochloride	Catapres	0.2 mg PO per day initially, gradually increased to a maximum of 1.2 mg PO per day in two divided doses	May not be discontinued abruptly; hypertensive crisis may result
guanabenz acetate	Wytensin	8 mg PO per day initially, gradually increased to a maximum of 32 mg PO per day in two divided doses	
guanadrel sulfate	Hylorel	5 mg PO 2×/day, gradually increased to 20–75 mg PO per day in two to four divided doses	New drug similar to guanethidine; shorter duration of action
guanethidine sulfate	Ismelin	10 mg PO per day initially, gradually increased to a maximum of 300 mg PO per day in two divided doses.	
labetalol hydrochloride	Normodyne, Trandate	200 mg PO per day initially, gradually increased to a maximum of 1,200 mg PO per day	
		20–80 mg IV single-dose bolus 2 mg/min Continuous IV infusions	IV doses are for hypertensive emergencies only
methyldopa	Aldomet	500 mg PO per day initially, gradually increased to a maximum of 2,000 mg PO per day in two divided doses	
		250–500 mg IV diluted in 100 ml and administered over 30–60 min	IV doses for hypertensive emergencies only
metoprolol	Lopressor	50 mg PO per day initially, gradually increased to a maximum of 300 mg PO per day	
nadolol	Corgard	40 mg PO per day initially, gradually increased to a maximum of 320 mg PO per day	
phenoxybenzamine	Dibenzyline	20–60 mg PO per day	Used when hypertension results from excess catecholamines
phentolamine mesylate	Regitine	50 mg PO; 5 mg IV	Used mainly to diagnose tumor of the adrenal gland (pheochromocytoma) as a cause of hypertension
pindolol	Visken	20 mg PO per day initially, gradually increased to a maximum of 60 mg PO per day in two divided doses	
prazosin	Minipress	1 mg PO 3×/day may be increased gradually to a maximum of 20 mg PO per day in two divided doses	First dose should be given at bedtime to reduce likelihood of postural hypotension
		5–15 mg IM 5–15 mg IV rapid-injection single-dose bolus; 200–400 mg/L continuous IV infusion	IM, IV doses for hypertensive emergencies only

TABLE 18–9   (cont.)

Nonproprietary Name	Proprietary Name	Adult Dose Range*	Notes
propranolol	Inderal	40 mg PO per day initially, gradually increased to a maximum of 160–480 mg PO per day in two divided doses	
timolol	Blocadren	20 mg PO per day initially, gradually increased to a maximum of 60 mg PO per day in two divided doses	Also used to prevent death or extension of infarction in patients with myocardial infarction
trimethaphan camsylate	Arfonad	0.3–3 mg per min continuous IV infusion	For hypertensive emergencies only
rauwolfia drugs			Rauwolfia drugs come from a climbing shrub; they have been used for centuries for hypertension but have been replaced by newer agents; not used when the hypertensive person also has depression
rauwolfia serpentina	Raudixin and others	50 mg PO initially, gradually increased to a maximum of 100 mg PO per day	
reserpine	Serpasil and others	0.05 mg PO per day initially, gradually increased to a maximum of 0.25 mg PO per day	
Calcium Blocking Agents			
diltiazem hydrochloride	Cardizem	120 mg PO per day initially, gradually increased to a maximum of 240 mg PO per day in three to four divided doses	Calcium channel blockers are currently used experimentally in the United States for hypertension
nifedipine	Procardia	30 mg PO per day initially, gradually increased to a maximum of 180 mg PO per day in three to four divided doses	
verapamil hydrochloride	Calan, Isoptin	240 mg PO per day initially, gradually increased to a maximum of 480 mg PO per day in three to four divided doses	
Diuretics			
See Tables 18–11 and 19–3			Diuretics may be used alone or in combination with other agents; thiazide diuretics are commonly used
Vasodilators			
diazoxide	Hyperstat	50–100 mg IV single-dose bolus every 5–10 min; 15–30 mg/min by continuous IV infusion over 20–30 min	For hypertensive emergencies only; continuous patient monitoring is essential
hydralazine	Apresoline	50 mg PO initially, gradually increased to a maximum of 300 mg PO per day in two divided doses	Lupuslike syndrome may develop even with normal doses
		10–50 mg IM every 20–30 min; 10–20 mg IV single-dose bolus diluted in at least 20 ml and administered at 0.5 ml/min; 200 mg/L by continuous IV infusion	IM, IV doses for hypertensive emergencies only
minoxidil	Loniten	5 mg PO initially, gradually increased to a maximum of 100 mg PO per day in two divided doses	
sodium nitroprusside	Nipride	0.5–10 μg 1 kg per min by continuous IV infusion	For hypertensive emergencies only; infusion must be covered and protected from light that decomposes drug

TABLE 18–9 (*cont.*)

Nonproprietary Name	Proprietary Name	Adult Dose Range*	Notes
Other Drugs			
captopril	Capoten	37.5 mg PO per day initially; gradually increased to a maximum of 150 mg PO per day in two divided doses	Affects the renin-angiotensin system in the kidney. This system promotes retention of salt and water; constriction of arterioles
enalapril	Vasotec	2.5–5 mg PO per day initially; gradually increased to 10–40 mg PO per day	New drug similar to captopril; angioedema is a rare but potentially fatal side effect; report swelling of face, lips, tongue or respiratory stridor immediately; report elevated serum potassium

*Maximum doses may be exceeded for some patients.

circulating fluid volume helps to bring blood pressure down. For complete information on diuretics see pp. 208–211 and Table 19–3.

   D. Vasodilators act on blood vessels to cause dilation. This, in turn, causes a decrease in peripheral vascular resistance. The combination of these two events reduces blood pressure. Some vasodilators act mainly on arterioles: diazoxide, hydralazine, and minoxidil. Other drugs act on both arterioles and venules: prazosin, nitroprusside.

   E. Captopril, and enalapril relatively new drugs, lower blood pressure by interfering with the renin-angiotensin system. This system regulates blood pressure by producing substances that promote salt and water retention and vasoconstriction.

   F. Combination therapy is common for patients with hypertension. The stepped care approach is recommended by the Joint National Committee on Detection, Evaluation, and Treatment of High Blood Pressure. The stepped care approach is described in Table 18-10. Some combinations come in one multi-ingredient form such as those listed in Table 18-11.

II. Adverse responses.
   A. Adrenergic blocking agents.
      1. Postural hypotension, reflex hypertensive crisis with abrupt withdrawal of clonidine.
      2. Increased gastrointestinal motility.
      3. Impaired ejaculation.
      4. Increased blood volume and sodium retention, edema.
      5. Nasal stuffiness.
      6. Extrapyramidal symptoms resembling Parkinson's disease.
      7. Reflex tachycardia or bradycardia.

TABLE 18–10   Stepped Care Drug Therapy for Hypertension

Step 1	The physician prescribes a *thiazide diuretic* (see Table 19–3). In some patients, a *beta-adrenergic blocking agent* may be used instead.
Step 2	The physician prescribes combination of two drugs: a diuretic and a beta-adrenergic blocking agent. In some patients, a *calcium blocking agent* may be prescribed instead.
Step 3	The physician prescribes a third drug to be added to those in step 2. Usually a *vasodilator* is prescribed.
Step 4	The physician prescribes another adrenergic blocking agent to be added or substituted. Guanethidine is frequently used.

TABLE 18–11   Selected Multi-ingredient Antihypertensives

Proprietary Name	Antihypertensive Ingredient*	Diuretic Ingredient*
Aldoril	methyldopa	hydrochlorothiazide
Diupres	reserpine	chlorothiazide
Hydropres	reserpine	hydrochlorothiazide
Inderide	propranolol	polythiazide
Regroton	reserpine	chlorthalidone
Salutensin	reserpine	hydroflumethiazide
Ser-Ap-Es	hydralazine, reserpine	hydrochlorothiazide
Timolide	timolol	hydrochlorothiazide

*Many preparation are available in several strengths of each ingredient.

8. Sensitivity to insulin and oral hypoglycemia.
9. Bronchoconstriction, bronchospasm, wheezing.
   B. Calcium blocking agents.
   1. Postural hypotension, palpitations, bradycardia (verapamil).
   2. Nausea, abdominal cramps, constipation or diarrhea, heartburn.
   3. Sexual difficulties, hyperglycemia.
   4. Joint stiffness and muscle cramps.
   5. Shakiness, nervousness, mood changes, headache, difficulty in balance.
   6. Urticaria, pruritus, fever, chills, sweating.
   C. Diuretics.
   1. Hypokalemia (low serum potassium) is a serious adverse response to all diuretics except spironolactone and triamterene. See p. 210 for further discussion.
   D. Vasodilators.
   1. Pericardial effusion (minoxidil only).
   2. Postural hypotension, angina, palpitations.
   3. Anorexia, nausea.
   4. Dizziness, tremors, paresthesias, drowsiness, syncope.
   5. Muscle cramps, peripheral neuropathy.
   6. Lupuslike syndrome, urticaria, skin rash, flushing.
   7. Anemias.
   8. Nasal stuffiness, increased tearing.
   9. Reflex sodium and water retention.
   10. Hyperglycemia.
   E. Drug interactions.
   1. Alcohol, antipsychotics, phenothiazines, peripheral vasodilators increase the likelihood of hypotension when combined with antihypertensives.
   2. Digitalis derivatives increase the likelihood of bradycardia when combined with propranolol.
   3. Amphetamines, monoamine oxidase inhibitors, oral contraceptives, tricyclic antidepressants decrease the effects of antihypertensives.

III. Nursing implications.
   A. Measure blood pressure using correct technique. Table 18–12 lists important points for obtaining a correct measurement.
   B. Anticipate orders for orthostatic blood pressures in patients with hypertension.
   C. Protect nifedipine capsules from light.
   D. Administer oral antihypertensives on a full stomach to reduce gastrointestinal side effects. An exception to this measure is captopril which should be administered on an empty stomach to ensure maximum absorption.
   E. Encourage nondrug measures that reduce blood pressure: weight loss, exercise, smoking cessation, salt restriction. Praise the patient's efforts and progress in these areas.

F. Monitor serum potassium when possible in patients receiving diuretics as drug therapy. Offer foods high in potassium such as bananas, carrots, celery, grapefruit, oranges, meats, potatoes, peanut butter, dried fruits, tomatoes.

G. Teach patients to change position slowly to avoid postural hypotension.

H. Anticipate and increase observations for adverse drug responses in patients who are elderly, receive multiple drug therapy, or have other illnesses requiring drug therapy (heart disease, respiratory disease, and so forth).

I. Assist the patient to develop a plan for taking antihypertensive drugs exactly as prescribed. A major issue for patients receiving drug therapy for hypertension is missed doses and/or stopping drug therapy. A minimum plan includes:
  1. What drugs are to be taken.
  2. When drugs are to be taken (in relation to the patient's daily schedule).
  3. How, when, and where refills may be obtained.
  4. What side effects may occur and how to report them.

J. Develop communication skills that enable patients to share problems they may be having with drug therapy. Economic difficulty, unfavorable changes in sexual performance, or other adverse drug responses may cause the patient to discontinue drug therapy. In some patients, drugs or dosages may need adjustment. In other cases, the patient may be assisted by the social worker, dietitian, or clinical nurse specialist.

K. Teach women patients with hypertension during childbearing years to:
  1. Consult the physician as a part of planning for pregnancy (the safety of many hypertensive drugs has not been established for use during pregnancy).
  2. Work closely with the physician to establish birth control measures that are safe and effective.

L. Give patients a telephone number to call before discontinuing drug therapy. Tell patients that abrupt withdrawal of some drugs may cause serious illness.

M. Request a stethoscope with dual earpieces and have the patient listen to the sounds of blood pressure as you measure it. For some patients, this helps to provide additional reinforcement of the need to continue therapy.

N. Develop a brief, simple explanation of what blood pressure is and offer it to patients regularly as you measure blood pressure. One example is: "Blood pressure is a measure of the force inside your heart and blood vessels. The top number represents the pressure during the beat—when your heart pushes blood out to your body. The bottom number represents the pressure between beats when your heart is filling with blood for the next beat."

TABLE 18–12   Checklist for Measuring Blood Pressure

1. Eliminate noise as much as possible.
2. Support the entire arm, elevated at the level of the heart in an extended position with the palm up.
3. Make sure that the legs are not crossed at the knees or ankles.
4. Select a cuff approximately 20% wider than the arm.
5. Apply the cuff snugly with the lower edge 1–2 in. above the elbow.
6. Check the tubings to be sure they are not twisted, kinked, or occluded.
7. Place the manometer directly in your line of vision as you would a book. Avoid looking down or up at a manometer.
8. Estimate systolic blood pressure by listening or feeling for the disappearance of sound or pulse as the cuff is inflated.
9. Inflate the cuff rapidly to approximately 30 mm Hg above the estimated systolic blood pressure.
10. Deflate the cuff more slowly—no more than 2–3 mm Hg/s.
11. Wait at least 30–60 s after the cuff is deflated before inflating it again if a second reading is needed.
12. Write the blood pressure down immediately after deflating the cuff.
13. Ask someone else to check the blood pressure if you are not sure of the reading.

TABLE 18–13   Antilipemics

Nonproprietary Name	Proprietary Name	Adult Dose Range	Notes
cholestryramine resin	Questran	12–16 g PO in two to four divided doses at mealtimes and bedtime	Mix powder with water, fluids, or pulpy fruit
clofibrate	Atromid-S	2 g PO per day in two to four divided doses	
colestipol hydrochloride	Colestid	15–30 g PO in two to four divided doses at mealtimes and bedtime	Mix powder with water, fluids, or pulpy fruit
dextrothyroxine sodium	Cholixin	1 mg PO per day for 1 month, gradually increased by 1 mg PO each month to a maximum of 8 mg if needed	
gemfibrozil	Lopid	600 mg PO bid 30 min before breakfast and dinner	
neomycin		0.5–2 g PO per day	An antibacterial also used to sterilize bowel for surgery; ototoxic, nephrotoxic
nicotinic acid	Niacin, Nicalex	2–9 g PO per day in three to four divided doses at mealtimes	Also used as a vasodilator in peripheral vascular disease
probucol	Lorelco	500 mg PO 2×/day with morning and evening meals	Not recommended during pregnancy; long-term effects not known; remains in body for up to 6 months after last dose
sitosterols	Cytellin	30 ml PO 30 min before meals and at bedtime	Mix with coffee, tea, fruit juice, or milk; occasionally produces nausea and vomiting, mild laxative; long-term effects not known.

ANTILIPEMICS

Antilipemics are drugs that reduce the concentration of lipoproteins in the bloodstream (Table 18–13). *Lipoproteins* are substances that carry cholesterol, triglycerides, and other lipids in the circulation. Elevations of certain lipoproteins are associated with atherosclerosis, the deposit of fatty plaques along arterial walls. Atherosclerosis is linked to heart disease, angina pectoris, strokes, and peripheral vascular disease.

A person with elevated lipoproteins may not know it unless special blood tests are done to measure the levels. Other symptoms may develop as the condition progresses to damage target organs.

Many different patterns of abnormal lipid elevations have been identified depending upon the specific lipids involved. Some antilipemics are more effective against one type than another.

Drug therapy is usually not as effective as diet therapy in lowering elevated lipoproteins. For this reason every effort is made to assist the patient to reduce intake of saturated fats such as meat and dairy products and sugar. Success in reducing elevated lipoproteins is often directly related to changes in life-style the patient is able to make.

I. Action and uses.
  A. Antilipemics may decrease the absorption and/or increase the breakdown of cholesterol. These are called bile-binding resins.
  B. Some antilipemics decrease the formation of triglycerides.
  C. Some antilipemics decrease low-density lipoproteins associated with hereditary factors.
  D. Drug therapy with antilipemics is generally prescribed only if 3 to 6 months of diet therapy has not been successful in reducing elevations.
  E. Drug therapy is generally indicated for patients with coronary heart disease, a strong family history of heart disease, or other risk factors.

II. Adverse responses.

A. Gastrointestinal system: nausea, vomiting, indigestion, abdominal distention, flatulence, constipation or diarrhea, steatorrhea, malabsorption of nutrients; cholelithiasis and cholecystitis (clofibrate only); hyperglycemia, impaired glucose tolerance, and abnormal liver function (nicotinic acid only).

B. Genitourinary: breast tenderness, decreased sexual interest, and impotence have all been reported with clofibrate.

C. Skin rash and hair loss, cardiac arrhythmias and flulike syndrome have all been reported with clofibrate; cutaneous flush and pruritus (nicotinic acid only).

D. Drug interactions include:
- Increased vasodilation and postural hypotension when nicotinic acid is combined with antihypertensives.
- Enhanced effects and toxicity of phenytoin, tolbutamide, oral anticoagulants when combined with clofibrate.
- Decreased effects of chlorothiazide, phenylbutazone, phenobarbital, anticoagulants, thyroxine, and digitalis preparations when combined with cholestyramine or colestipol hydrochloride.

III. Nursing implications.

A. Assess the patient for risk factors associated with atherosclerosis: high dietary intake of saturated fats and sugar, sedentary life-style, cigarette smoking, obesity, and positive family history, existing hypertension or diabetes mellitus.

B. Check to see if serum cholesterol is elevated (above 250 mg/ml) or serum triglycerides are elevated (above 150 mg/ml).

C. Provide referrals, direct teaching, and encouragement that assist the patient to reduce or eliminate risk factors, modify life-style.

D. Administer cholestyramine and colestipol hydrochloride mixed with water, fluid, or pulpy fruit before meals. Other drugs prescribed for the patient should be given either 1h earlier or 4 to 6 h after cholestyramine or colestipol hydrochloride.

E. Administer other antilipemics with or after meals to decrease gastrointestinal side effects.

F. Teach women patients during childbearing years to check with the physician as part of planning a pregnancy when taking antilipemic drugs.

BLOOD COMPONENTS AND VOLUME EXPANDERS

Blood components and *volume expanders* are products that change the volume or composition of blood (Table 18–14). They are always administered IV and may be prescribed for a variety of clinical conditions that affect either the volume of circulating blood or the substances circulating in it. Blood components and volume expanders are usually prescribed for one or more of the following reasons: to provide substances that are absent, to replace losses, and/or to restore balance.

I. Actions and uses.

A. Red blood cell components provide additional erythrocytes to carry oxygen. Thus they may be ordered to maintain or restore oxygen carrying capacity for a patient with hemorrhage, anemias not caused by nutritional deficiency, bone marrow failure, persistent blood loss.

B. Plasma components may be prescribed for a patient with a coagulation disorder, or to replace plasma lost during surgery or from burns.

C. Plasma derivatives provide plasma proteins such as albumin, immune globulins, and certain clotting factors. For these effects specific plasma derivates may be ordered for the patient with hypovolemic shock, decreased circulating proteins, deficient circulating immune substances, or hemophilia.

D. White blood cell transfusion provides granulocytes. For this effect they are occasionally ordered for the patient with malignancy and associated septicemia.

E. Volume expanders provide large molecules of substances that exert a pulling pressure to hold

TABLE 18–14   Selected Blood Components and Volume Expanders

Name	Description	Approximate Volume	Notes
Red Blood Cell Components			
Packed RBCs	Red blood cells are separated from most of the plasma and administered to the patient.	250–300 ml/U	May produce all of the adverse responses
Leukocyte-poor RBCs	All of the leukocytes are removed from packed RBCs which are then administered to the patient.	200 ml/U	May be ordered for patients who are immunosuppressed; who have developed specific antibodies from previous transfusions; or who have adverse responses limited to bacterial infection and hemolytic reactions
Deglycerolized RBCs	Plasma is removed from whole blood and glycerol is added; this enables blood to be stored for up to 3 years	200 ml/U	Same as above; also enables patients to be transfused with their own blood which has been previously collected and stored
Whole blood	An entire amount of unmodified blood collected from a donor	500 ml/U	Does not contain clotting factors after storage of several days; may produce all of the adverse responses; used mainly for acute massive blood loss
Fresh frozen plasma (FFP)	Plasma is separated from a unit of whole blood within 6 h after collection and frozen for up to 1 year	200–250 ml/U	Used primarily for the patient with coagulation disorders; may also be used for volume expansion; does not cause intravascular hemolytic reaction, hypothermia, or citrate toxicity
Platelets	Platelets are separated from whole blood from a single donor or from several donors within 6 h after collection	35–50 ml/U	Used for patients with thrombocytopenia, certain drug reactions, disseminated intravascular coagulation; adverse responses include bacterial and hepatitis infections, urticaria, anaphylaxis, febrile reaction, extravascular hemolysis
Cryoprecipitate	The insoluble part of plasma that remains after thawing; provides concentrated source of fibrinogen and factor VIII	10–15 ml/U	Used for hemophilia, other rare clotting disorders, adverse responses include anaphylaxis, hepatitis, urticaria
Plasma Derivatives			
Human serum albumin— 5%, 25% (Albuconn, Albumisol, Albutein, Buminate, and others)	Human albumin prepared from pooled plasma, serum, or placentas from human donors	5%—12.5 g/250 ml at 2–4 ml/min; 25%—12.5 g/50 ml at 1 ml/min	Used to expand plasma, replace protein; adverse responses include urticaria and circulatory overload
Plasma protein fraction (PPF) (Plamanate, Plasma-Plex, Plasmatein, and others)	Selected proteins are prepared from pooled blood, plasma, or serum from human donors	50 mg/ml at no more than 10 ml/min	Used to expand plasma; may produce circulatory overload, febrile reaction, urticaria
Granulocytes	Granulocytes are removed from whole blood from a compatible donor (usually a family member)	150 ml	Used mainly for the patient with advanced malignancy, septicemia

TABLE 18–14   (cont.)

Name	Description	Approximate Volume	Notes
Others			
Dextran (Gentran, Macrodex, Rheomacrodex, LMD, and others)	A commercially prepared solution that contains large glucose-related molecules	150 ml	Two forms are available in different molecular weights; check label carefully; used mainly to expand plasma volume; adverse response is urticaria
Hetastarch (Volex, Hespan)	Similar to dextran	500 ml	Used mainly to expand plasma volume

Abbreviations: RBC, red blood cell.

blood inside the circulatory system. For these effects, they may be ordered for the patient with blood or plasma loss in a variety of clinical conditions.

   F. The risks of adverse responses are decreased when a blood component or volume expander is selected to meet the patient's specific need.

II. Adverse responses.

   A. *Air embolism*—caused by air in the container or tubing that enters the patient's bloodstream, lodges in the right ventricle, and prevents blood from going into the pulmonary artery; the patient experiences a sudden onset of coughing, dyspnea, convulsions, and hypotension.

   B. *Anaphylaxis*—caused by hypersensitivity to the product; the patient experiences a sudden onset of coughing, respiratory distress, hypotension, abdominal cramps, shock loss of consciousness, vomiting, and diarrhea.

   C. *Circulatory overload*—caused by too-rapid administration; the patient experiences cyanosis, dyspnea, headache, elevated blood pressure and central venous pressure.

   D. *Citrate toxicity*—caused by the accumulation of citrate, an anticoagulant added to blood as a preservative; may develop from too-rapid administration; the patient experiences tingling about the mouth, nausea and vomiting, bradycardia and cardiac arrhythmias, hypotension, low serum potassium.

   E. *Delayed hemolytic reaction*—an incompatibility that develops 2 or more days after blood transfusion and involves red blood cells; the patient experiences fever, jaundice, continued anemia, presence of bilirubin and hemoglobin in the urine.

   F. *Extravascular hemolytic reaction*—an immediate incompatibility between the recipient's red blood cells and donor plasma; the patient experiences fever and chills several hours after the transfusion.

   G. *Febrile nonhemolytic reaction*—an immediate incompatibility of lymphocytes or platelets; the patient experiences fever, chills, hypotension, palpitations, headache, malaise.

   H. *Hypothermia*—an immediate response caused by too-rapid administration of cold blood components; the patient experiences shaking chills, cardiac arrhythmias, hypotension.

   I. *Infections*—caused by the presence of bacteria or viruses in donor blood that are transmitted to the recipient; acquired immune deficiency syndrome (AIDS), cytomegalovirus, hepatitis, and malaria have been reported.

   J. *Immediate hemolytic reaction*—caused by a major incompatibility of ABO or RH antigens that result in destruction of red blood cells; the patient experiences chills, fever, back pain, dyspnea, hypotension, shock, dwindling urine output that may lead to renal failure and death.

   K. *Urticarial reaction*—cause unknown; occurs with plasma infusions; the patient experiences local erythema, hives, itching, and fever.

III. Nursing implications.

   A. Use hospital policy and procedures to identify and verify blood or blood components with the written physician's order. In some cases, this procedure may be done only by registered nurses. A minimum identification procedure includes:

1. Matching the patient's name and identification number on a transfusion request with the receiver's chart.
2. A matching of the ABO/RH blood group on the donor bag to the ABO/RH blood group of the recipient as listed on the transfusion request.
3. Matching any identification numbers on donor bag with identification numbers on the transfusion request.
4. Checking the expiration date on the donor bag.
5. Verification of the physician's order for transfusion, specific product to be used, rate of administration.

B. Identify the patient correctly. A minimum identification procedure includes:

1. Matching the name and identification number on the patient's bracelet to that on the transfusion request or donor bag.
2. Asking the patient to pronounce and spell his or her full name if possible.

C. Collect, report, and record information about any previous transfusions and related problems.

D. Take and record vital signs before the transfusion is started.

E. Remain with the patient during the first 5 to 15 min of the initial transfusion to observe for an adverse response.

F. Use hospital policy and procedure if an adverse response develops. Anticipate some or all of the following guidelines:

1. Stop the transfusion immediately and notify the registered nurse. Do not remove the needle but prepare for a change of the entire administration set down to the hub of the IV catheter.
2. Remain with the patient and take vital signs until help arrives. Tell the patient that help is on the way.
3. Assist in changing the intravenous administration set. Experts do not recommend that a backup container of isotonic saline be infused with the old administration set. This is because additional blood remaining in the tubing will be infused. The severity of the patient's reaction may be directly affected by the amount of incompatible blood received.
4. Continue to observe the patient frequently and monitor vital signs. Assist other health professionals with activities needed to support the patient's vital functions.
5. Send the remaining blood component and the entire intravenous administration set to the blood bank as directed.
6. Collect the first urine specimen and others according to hospital policy and send it to the laboratory for hemoglobin analysis.

G. Monitor the flow rate as directed. Normally blood and its components should be infused within 4 h. Notify the registered nurse if the flow rate increases or decreases by more than five to ten drops per minute.

H. Report immediately any concerns expressed by the patient such as religious beliefs related to whether he or she can accept blood components, or concerns about contracting AIDS from blood transfusions.

I. Do not administer any other drugs through the IV administration set while blood is running.

J. Record the appropriate information according to hospital guidelines.

DIGITALIS GLYCOSIDES

Digitalis glycosides are drugs that strengthen myocardial contraction (Table 18–15). Originally these drugs were made from the dried leaf of the foxglove plant. Now they are made synthetically. Other terms used to describe these drugs include *cardiac glycosides*, *cardiotonics*, and *digitalis derivatives*.

Digitalis preparations are believed to act mainly by a complex process that affects the movement

TABLE 18–15   Digitalis Glycosides

Nonproprietary Name	Proprietary Name	Adult Dose Range	Notes
amrinone lactate	Inocor	0.75 mg/kg IV single-dose bolus administered over 2–3 min; may be repeated in 30 min 5–10 µg/kg/min by continuous IV infusion to follow after a single dose; total dose should not exceed 10mg/kg	New drug; not a digitalis derivative; does not affect heart rate or blood pressure; does not produce digitalis toxicity; used mainly for emergency treatment of the patient with congestive heart failure; may produce liver toxicity, thrombocytopenia. Do not dilute in IV solutions.
deslanoside	Cedilanid D	Available as 0.2 mg/ml for injection only	
digoxin	Lanoxin	0.125–0.5 mg PO per day or several times per week for maintenance; also available as PO elixir	Should never be administered IM because it causes severe pain and muscle necrosis; a shorter-acting preparation
		Available for IV administration as 0.25 mg/ml dose; IV doses should be diluted with 10 ml sterile sodium chloride	Dosage highly individualized to patient
digitoxin	Crystodigin Purodigin	0.05–0.2 mg PO per day or several times per week for maintenance; also available for IV administration	Dosage highly individualized to patient
ouabain		Available as 0.25 mg/ml ampules for IV administration only	Used only in an emergency when rapid onset of action is essential; short duration of action; high potential for toxicity

of calcium ions across the cell membrane during myocardial contraction. A second effect of digitalis derivatives that has important implications is a slowing of conduction through the heart.

The main use of digitalis derivatives is for the patient with congestive heart failure. The patient with congestive heart failure has a condition in which the heart is unable to pump enough blood to meet body requirements. In most patients, the cause is a weakened myocardium. The weakened pump is unable to squeeze all of the blood out of the heart's four chambers with each contraction. This, in turn, causes a backup of blood in the heart. Pulmonary embolism, infection, anemia, cardiac arrhythmias, hypertension, myocardial infarction, inflammation of the heart, and excessive exercise may cause a failure of the heart.

The patient experiences early symptoms of fatigue, weakness, and dyspnea on exertion. As congestive heart failure progresses, the patient is dyspneic at rest. Pillows may be needed to prop the patient in an upright position even to sleep (orthopnea). There may be cyanosis, more pronounced in the extremities. There may be edema which can be observed over the tibia, sacrum, and at the ankles.

The medical treatment plan contains three basic parts: digitalis to improve the strength of myocardial contractions: diuretics (see Table 19–3) to reduce circulating fluid volume; and rest to reduce the demands on the heart. There may be dietary restriction of sodium with small frequent meals. Elastic stockings may be applied to prevent thrombophlebitis. Oxygen may help to relieve the patient's dyspnea.

Digitalis derivatives are given to a high percentage of hospitalized adults. Almost every nurse practicing in a hospital will administer these drugs regularly. Thus it is important for nurses to have an excellent working knowledge of digitalis derivatives.

I. Actions and uses.
   A. Strengthens the force of myocardial contractions. For this effect, it is prescribed for the patient with congestive heart failure.
   B. A secondary action is to slow conduction through the heart. For this effect, it is occasionally

prescribed for the patient with an atrial arrhythmia such as atrial fibrillation or flutter.

    C. The actions of digitalis derivatives are cumulative. This means that there is a buildup of its effects.

    D. Improved myocardial contractions in turn increase blood flow to vital organs. This action usually results in *diuresis* (an increase in the formation and excretion of urine).

    E. Digitalis derivatives are prescribed using a special loading process called *digitalizing*. Initially there are several larger doses called *digitalizing doses*. This is followed by a prescription for a maintenance dose. The maintenance dose varies considerably. At first, maintenance doses are prescribed every day. This may be decreased to two to four times per week if possible. Because of the dangers of toxicity, an important goal is to arrive at the smallest dose possible that will be effective.

II. Adverse responses.

    A. The margin of safety for digitalis derivatives is small. This means that the dose required for therapeutic effectiveness is very close to the dose that produces toxicity.

    B. Digitalis toxicity occurs frequently and can be fatal. Symptoms of toxicity include:

        1. Cardiovascular: severe bradycardia, atrial arrhythmias, AV blocks, premature ventricular tachycardia, fibrillation.

        2. Gastrointestinal: anorexia, nausea, vomiting, abdominal pain, diarrhea.

        3. Nervous system: Early symptoms are headache, fatigue, malaise, neuralgia involving the lower part of the face and paresthesias, disorientation, confusion and delirium, visual disturbances (e.g., blurred vision, halos around objects, frosted objects, disturbances of color vision, especially yellow and green).

        4. Skin: rashes; gynecomastia in men.

        5. Drug interactions include:
- Increased plasma concentration when combined with quinidine.
- Signs of digitalis toxicity when combined with quinidine.
- Increased likelihood of arrhythmias when combined with adrenergics, succinylcholine, calcium, reserpine.
- Decreased effects of digitalis when combined with antacids, barbiturates, cholestyramine, penicillamine, phenylbutazone, phenytoin, rifampin.

    C. Digitalis toxicity cannot be reversed except by stopping the drug and allowing its effects to wear off slowly as the drug is eliminated over a period of days to weeks. Treatment is symptomatic.

    D. The likelihood of toxicity is greatly enhanced in patients who are elderly, have elevated serum calcium or magnesium, low serum potassium, have liver or kidney disease, take too large a dose, or take other drugs such as quinidine, diuretics, amphotericin B.

III. Nursing implications.

    A. Be sure to ask newly admitted patients when the last dose of a digitalis derivative was taken. Record the name, dose, and exact schedule.

    B. Monitor serum potassium, especially if the patient is also receiving a diuretic.

    C. Store digitalis preparations away from light.

    D. Take and record patient's apical pulse for a full minute before each dose. If the apical pulse is below 60 beats/min, temporarily withhold the dose and notify the physician. In some cases, the physician will direct that the dose be omitted. In other cases, the physician may want the drug administered. Unexpected changes in pulse rate or rhythm should also be reported. For example, if the patient's pulse has been regular and becomes irregular, the change should be reported before a dose is given.

    E. Before administering a digitalis derivative, ask the patient specifically about symptoms of toxicity. Report disturbances in vision and gastrointestinal upset that may be early warnings of digitalis toxicity.

    F. Teach patients to count the pulse and report abnormalities to the physician.

    G. Watch carefully for drug interactions. Anticipate multiple drug therapy for patient's receiving digitalis derivatives. Many digitalized patients are hospitalized for other reasons.

    H. Teach patients taking a digitalis drug the important relationship between it and other related drugs such as diuretics and potassium supplements. Missed doses or extra doses of any component of drug therapy may upset the delicate balance between therapeutic effects and toxicity.

I. Monitor serum digitalis levels when possible. Table 18–16 contains information about serum digitalis levels. However, a patient may develop toxicity when serum levels are below these points.

J. Help the patient to develop a method for recording drugs, doses, and pulse rate at home. This is especially important when the patient is elderly, lives alone, and when the patient takes maintenance doses at a frequency of one dose several time per week.

K. Anticipate the physician's orders for daily weighing of the patient as a way to assess changes in cardiac status. Weigh the patient at the same time on the same scale, and assure that the patient is wearing the same amount of clothing every day.

HEMOSTATICS

Hemostatics are drugs that stop bleeding by forming an artificial clot (Table 18–17). These drugs control only bleeding from small vessels and are not effective for bleeding from arteries or veins.

I. Actions and uses.
  A. Hemostatics act to control oozing from small vessels.
  B. Absorbable gelatin sponge may be moistened with sterile isotonic sodium chloride or thrombin solutions and placed inside a wound before it is sutured. The material is completely absorbed within 4 to 6 weeks.
  C. Oxidized cellulose promotes clotting by interacting with hemoglobin. Absorption of the active material usually takes place within 2 to 7 days. This hemostatic is supplied as specially treated surgical gauze which is not permanently implanted in fractures or used as a permanent dressing on skin surfaces.
  D. Thrombin is a powder applied topically to oozing surfaces during dental, nasal, or laryngeal surgery.
  E. Thromboplastin is a powder applied to bleeding surfaces during surgery. The powder contains the enzyme thrombokinase which converts prothrombin to thrombin.
  F. Human clotting factors are prepared from human plasma to replace clotting factors that are absent or deficient in patients with hemophilia. They may be used to prevent or treat bleeding.
  G. Aminocaproic acid is used to treat bleeding emergencies following surgery or administration of thrombolytic drugs. It acts by preventing disintegration of the clot.
II. Adverse responses.
  A. Oxidized cellulose interferes with bone regeneration and may cause the formation of cysts if implanted permanently in fractures.
  B. Oxidized cellulose slows the formation of new epithelium on wounded skin surfaces. For this reason, it is not used as a topical dressing except initially to control hemorrhage.
  C. Clotting factors contain human protein that may cause hypersensitivity reactions such as headaches, visual disturbances, flushing, tachycardia, chest tightness or wheezing, fever and chills, nausea and vomiting, muscle and joint pain, jaundice, viral hepatitis.
  D. Systemic hemostatics may cause intravascular clotting.

TABLE 18–16   Serum Digitalis Levels

Therapeutic Levels	Toxic Levels*
10–35 ng/ml digitoxin	Above 35 ng/ml
0.5–2.0 ng/ml digoxin	Above 2 ng/ml

*Patients may develop toxicity with serum levels well below these limits.

TABLE 18–17   Hemostatics

Nonproprietary Name	Proprietary Name	Adult Dose Range	Notes
Absorbable Agents			
Absorbable gelatin sponge	Gelfoam Gelfilm	Available as cones, packs, sponges, powders, films	Often moistened with isotonic saline or thrombin solution
Oxidized cellulose	Oxycel, Surgicel	Available as pledgets, gauze pads and strips	Cannot be used in fractures or as permanent topical dressings
Thrombin	Thrombinar Thrombostat	Available as a powder in vials containing 1,000, 5,000, or 10,000 units.	For topical use only; deteriorates in 48 h after reconstitution as a solution
Thromboplastin		Available as powder	
Systemic Agents			
Aminocaproic acid	Amicar	5 g initially; 1 g every hour PO, IV (no more than 30 g/24 h)	Used for overdose of fibrinolytic drugs such as streptokinase, urokinase; too-rapid intravenous administration may cause hypotension, bradycardia, cardiac arrhythmias; have vitamin K or protamine sulfate available
Antihemophilic factor	Actif VIII, Factor VIII, Hemofil, Kaoate	10–20 U/kg IV initially; subsequent doses adjusted to patient's response; maintenance doses 250–500 U/day	Used only to treat or prevent bleeding in patients with hemophilia A. Should not be administered faster than 10 ml/min
Anti-inhibitor coagulant complex	Autoplex	25–100 factor VII correctional units per kilogram IV	Used only to treat bleeding in certain patients with hemophilia; should not be administered faster than 10 ml/min
Carbazochrome salicylate	Adrenosem, Salicylate	5–10 mg PO, IM	Used to treat or prevent capillary oozing and bleeding; administer IM injection slowly to reduce pain and irritation at the site
Factor IX complex	Knoyne, Proplex	IV doses must be individualized to patient	Used to replace clotting factors II, VII, IX, or X, especially in patients with hemophilia

    E. Drug interactions include:
- Increased coagulation when aminocaproic acid is combined with oral contraceptives.
- Decreased coagulation when aminocaproic acid is combined with oral anticoagulants.
- Anti-inhibitor coagulant complex is not recommended with prothrombin products, aminocaproic acid, tranexamic acid.
- Antihistamines block effects of carbazochrome salicylate.

III. Nursing implications.
    A. Monitor vital signs in all patients with known or suspected bleeding.
    B. Obtain baseline blood pressure and pulse before the initial dose of any systemic hemostatic agent.
    C. Seek additional information when systemic hemostatic agents are ordered for patients with cardiac, renal, or hepatic conditions or pregnancy. Systemic agents are usually not recommended for patients with these conditions.
    D. Check for aspirin or salicylate allergy before administering carbazochrome salicylate.
    E. Store human clotting factors under refrigeration at 2–8°C. Do not freeze.
    F. Use the following guidelines to administer human clotting factors:
        1. Reconstitute the powder exactly as directed by the manufacturer.
        2. Agitate the reconstituted solution gently by rolling it between the palms of both hands. Do not shake.

TABLE 18–18   Peripheral Vascular Drugs

Nonproprietary Name	Proprietary Name	Adult Dose Range	Notes
Vasodilators			
cyclandelate	Cyclospasmol	100–200 mg PO 4×/day	
isoxsuprine hydrochloride	Vasodilan	10–20 mg PO 3–4×/day	
nylidrin	Arlidin, others	3–12 mg PO 3–4×/day	
papaverine	Pavabid, others	100–300 mg PO 3–5×/day	
Sclerosing Agents			
morrhuate sodium injection		1–5 ml	Skin above the injection site turns bronze in color and fades gradually
sodium tetradecyl sulfate	Sotradecol	0.5–2 ml per injection site; no more than 10 ml total volume should be injected	May cause pain at injection site; allergic and anaphylactic response have been reported; tissue sloughing may occur if drug is accidentally introduced outside the vein
Other			
pentoxifylline	Trental	800–1,200 mg PO per day with meals in three divided doses	New drug; not a vasodilator; improves blood flow by acting on red cell flexibility; may produce dyspnea, nausea, vomiting

3. Administer within the window of time directed by the manufacturer. Some drugs become inactive or contaminated shortly after reconstitution.
4. Administer at the rate ordered by the physician. Too-rapid administration may cause adverse responses.
5. Discard unused reconstituted solutions.
6. Slow the IV apparatus if the patient reports adverse responses. Report observations immediately and request further instructions.

G. Check the patient regularly for signs of abnormal clotting with systemic hemostatics.
H. Check bleeding surfaces for hemostasis when topical preparations are used.

PERIPHERAL VASCULAR DRUGS

Peripheral vascular drugs are agents that affect arteries or veins in the extremities, particularly the legs and feet (Table 18–18). One group of drugs, called *vasodilators*, is ordered to relieve ischemia in the patient's extremities. The patient with ischemia has diminished blood flow to a body part caused by obstruction, narrowing or spasm of arteries and arterioles. In peripheral vascular disease, ischemia is usually caused by atherosclerosis in the distal aorta, iliac, or femoral arteries or their branches. The patient with peripheral ischemia usually experiences *intermittent claudication*—leg pain related to exercise. Pulses in the legs or feet may be weak or absent; skin may be cool, pale, hairless, and/or shiny. There may be skin discoloration or ulcers in severe cases.

The effectiveness of peripheral vasodilators in ischemic conditions has not been proved. Some studies indicate that blood flow is primarily affected in nonischemic areas. In addition, the underlying atherosclerotic process is not affected by vasodilators.

Bypass surgical grafts are also used to create a detour around obstructed blood vessels. Nondrug nursing measures such as those listed below are also helpful.

Another group of drugs, called *sclerosing agents,* may be ordered to occlude diseased veins in the patient with peripheral vascular disease involving veins. The patient with varicose veins has a condition in which the valves inside veins do not close properly. This allows blood to flow backward, causing veins to become dilated and tortuous (twisted). The patient experiences a feeling of heaviness and fatigue in the affected legs. Dilated tortuous veins may be visible in the affected area and swelling may develop. In severe cases, the patient may develop varicose ulcers.

Drug therapy may be prescribed instead of surgery for the patient with varicose veins. A surgical procedure includes *ligation* (tying off the upper end of veins) and/or *stripping* (removing a portion of the vein). *Hemorrhoidectomy* is a surgical procedure in which varicose veins of the rectum are removed. All therapies are directed at closing off diseased veins so that venous blood flows into deeper veins.

I. Actions and uses.
   A. Most peripheral vasodilators relax smooth muscle of arteriole walls causing them to dilate.
   B. Peripheral vasodilators are prescribed orally to improve blood flow to ischemic areas when the patient has peripheral vascular disease involving arteries and arterioles.
   C. Sclerosing agents cause inflammation, scarring, and occlusion of veins.
   D. Sclerosing agents are injected by a specially trained physician at several segments along diseased veins. As occlusion of the diseased vein occurs, blood flows into deeper veins.
II. Adverse responses.
   A. Vasodilators.
      1. Gastrointestinal system: nausea, vomiting, abdominal distress, papaverine may produce liver toxicity.
      2. Cardiovascular system: hypotension, tachycardia, palpitations; papaverine may produce cardiac arrhythmias.
      3. Other: facial flushing, headache, weakness, dizziness.
   B. Sclerosing agents: local irritation, hypersensitivity, anaphylaxis, tissue sloughing; morrhuate sodium produces a bronze discoloration above the injection site.
III. Nursing implications.
   A. Assess peripheral blood flow in newly admitted patients. A minimum assessment includes observation of the extremities and palpation of pulses. If edema is present, the extremity circumference is measured as a baseline. Record and report findings.
   B. Teach the patient to improve blood flow by positioning the extremities correctly.
      1. Patients with arterial disease should place the extremities horizontally or in a dependent position when sitting or lying down.
      2. Patients with venous disease should elevate the legs to relieve edema and congestion when sitting or lying down.
   C. Encourage and assist the patient to participate in an exercise program that is designed to develop collateral circulation in affected areas.
   D. Teach the patient measures to protect the extremities from injury:
      1. wear well-fitted shoes and socks.
      2. cut toenails straight across.
      3. avoid constricting garments; avoid hot water bottles, heating pads applied to the feet.
      4. inspect the legs and feet daily for minor injuries and notify the physician if present.
   E. Encourage the overweight person to initiate and maintain a weight loss program.
   F. Encourage the patient with atherosclerosis to slow the disease process by reducing risk factors: reduce intake of sugars and saturated fats, stop smoking, exercise regularly.
   G. Check blood pressure when administering vasodilators known to cause hypotension. Caution the patient to change positions slowly to prevent postural hypotension.
   H. Administer vasodilators with or after meals to minimize gastrointestinal side effects.
   I. Know where emergency drugs and equipment are located when assisting the physician with injections of sclerosing agents.
   J. Apply elastic stockings correctly and teach patient to:
      1. Follow manufacturer's directions for measuring the legs so that the correct size is obtained. Apply stockings before getting out of bed.
      2. Elevate the legs above the heart for 10 min before the stockings are applied.
      3. Follow the manufacturer's directions for applying the stocking over the foot.
      4. Stand at the patient's head and pull the stocking up in one smooth movement.

5. Inspect the stocking to make sure the heel is well fitted; remove wrinkles and rolls.
6. Remove stockings at least once daily to bathe legs and feet, inspect the skin.
7. Wash stockings regularly and dry on a flat surface.

CASE STUDY 9

Mrs. Althea Cronin is a 35-year-old woman who is admitted to the hospital with thrombophlebitis following the birth of a healthy daughter 3 weeks ago. Mrs. Cronin tells the student nurse that she has had varicose veins ever since her first pregnancy 10 years ago. The physician's admitting orders include:

- Bedrest with legs elevated.
- Elastic stockings.
- Heparin 10,000 U IV q6h.

After 7 days of drug therapy, the physician writes an order for an additional drug: warfarin sodium (Coumadin) 10 mg PO daily × 3 days.
Answer the following questions:

1. How would you explain the term *thrombophlebitis* to Mrs. Cronin?
2. What observations might you find on initial admission assessment?
3. What is the intended effect of heparin?
4. What observation would lead you to suspect that Mrs. Cronin is having an adverse response to heparin?
5. What laboratory test will enable the physician to monitor Mrs. Cronin's response to heparin?
6. What laboratory test will enable the physician to monitor Mrs. Cronin's response to warfarin sodium?
7. How would you administer heparin SC if the physician had ordered that route?
8. In your own words, explain why drug therapy is sometimes used for the patient with varicose veins.
9. What drug should be available in case of heparin overdose?
10. What drug should be available in case of warfarin sodium (Coumadin) overdose?

CASE STUDY 10

Mr. Boris Madeira is a 45-year-old man admitted to the hospital with primary hypertension. On admission, Mr. Madeira's blood pressure is 162/106, height 5 ft 10 in., weight 200 lb. Mr. Madeira says that he smokes about one pack per day of filtered cigarettes and has two drinks every evening before dinner. For recreation Mr. Madeira likes to watch sports on television, especially football. Mr. Madeira has had an elevated blood pressure for over 6 months. He states he has been taking "water" pills twice a day but his blood pressure has come down only a little. He says that the doctor is going to try some "new pills." Then he makes the following statements: "Don't know why he's worrying about all this. I feel fine . . . work every day. In fact, I can only stay a couple of days . . . got a big presentation to make at the office next week." The physician's orders include:

- 1,800-cal, 2-g sodium diet.
- Serum cholesterol and triglycerides, serum electrolytes in AM.
- Orthostatic blood pressures qid.
- Hydrochlorothiazide (*Hydrodiuril*) 25 mg PO.
- Clonidine hydrochloride (*Catapres*) 0.1 mg PO bid.

Answer the following questions:

1. Underline the statements in the case study that describe risk factors for hypertension.
2. Respond in your own words to the statements made by Mr. Madeira about feeling fine and working every day.

3. Explain what is meant by *blood pressure* as you would describe it to Mr. Madeira.
4. What is hydrochlorothiazide and how does it affect blood pressure?
5. What is clonidine hydrochloride and how does it affect blood pressure?
6. What adverse drug responses should Mr. Madeira be instructed to report?
7. What actions should you take before administering antihypertensive drugs to Mr. Madeira?
8. What are orthostatic blood pressures and how should they be taken? Why have they been ordered for Mr. Madeira?
9. What statements in the case study should be reported to the professional nurse who is developing the nursing care plan?
10. What is the relationship between the physician's order for blood work, hypertension, and drug therapy?

CASE STUDY 11

Mr. Charles Scarlotti is an 82-year-old man who is admitted to the hospital with a diagnosis of mild congestive heart failure. The physician's orders include:

- Bedrest with bathroom privileges.
- Measure intake and output.
- Weigh daily.
- O_2 by nasal prongs at 3–4 L/min.
- Digoxin (Lanoxin) 0.25 mg PO q6h × four doses, then 0.25 mg PO qd.
- Serum Na, K stat.

Answer the following questions:

1. What is the intended effect of digoxin for Mr. Scarlotti?
2. Explain digitalis toxicity and identify statements in the case study that increase the risk of toxicity for Mr. Scarlotti.
3. What questions will you ask before administering digoxin to Mr. Scarlotti?
4. What action(s) should be taken if Mr. Scarlott's apical pulse is 55 beats/min before the next digoxin dose?
5. What is the term used to describe the following part of the physician's order: "0.25 mg PO q6h × four doses"?
6. What is the term used to describe the next part of the physician's order: "digoxin 0.25 mg PO qd"?
7. If digoxin is effective, what changes would you expect to see in Mr. Scarlotti?

EXERCISES

1. Make a list of instructions you would give to a patient who has nitroglycerin tablets at the bedside.

2. List the steps to be followed and taught to the patient when applying 1 in. of nitroglycerin ointment 1% transdermally.

3. Describe the effects of antiarrhythmic drugs on the four characteristics of the heart. A table has been provided to help you organize the information.

Name of Drug	Contractility	Automaticity	Rhythmicity	Conductivity

4. List five essential nursing actions to be taken when assisting with the administration of blood components or volume expanders.
   a. _____.
   b. _____.
   c. _____.
   d. _____.
   e. _____.

Chapter 19 | DRUG THERAPY AFFECTING THE PATIENT'S GENITOURINARY SYSTEM

EXPECTED BEHAVIORAL OUTCOMES

After completing this chapter, you should return to the expected behavioral outcomes and evaluate your ability to:

1. Relate the effects of a specific drug to the structure and/or function of the genitourinary system.
2. Compare the effects of male and female hormones from the perspective of the patient's condition, actions and uses, adverse responses, and nursing implications.
3. Relate the actions, uses, and adverse responses of diuretics to the implications for the nurse administering them.
4. Describe patient teaching appropriate for the patient receiving a urinary antiseptic.
5. Compare patient teaching appropriate for the woman using an oral contraceptive to that needed by the woman using a vaginal antiinfective.
6. List the kinds of hospitalized patients who are more likely to develop a vaginal infection, and prepare a plan for early detection.

STRUCTURE AND FUNCTION REVIEW

The genitourinary system contains organs for reproduction and urinary elimination. (See Figure 19-1.) Organs for reproduction are located very near to organs for the formation and excretion of urine. Thus, dysfunction in one location often affects the functions of nearby organs. Many drugs can cause damage to the kidneys. Such drugs are called *nephrotoxic*. Observing, reporting, and recording the patient's urinary output is an important nursing action during drug therapy.

I. Female reproductive system.
  A. *Ovaries*—produce ova, and sex hormones; estrogen and progesterone.
  B. *Fallopian tubes*—convey the ova from the ovaries to the uterus; aid in the upperward passage of the spermatozoa; the place where fertilization of the ovum takes place.
  C. *Uterus*—organ in which the embryo grows and develops.
  D. *Vagina*—(organ of copulation) place where semen is deposited; serves as exit for fetus at time of delivery and for the uterine excretions.
  E. *Vulva*—the external genitalia, which act as a protection and maintain secretions.
  F. *Breasts or mammary glands*—organs of lactation, which function after childbirth to provide sustenance for the offspring. Frequent site of cancer.

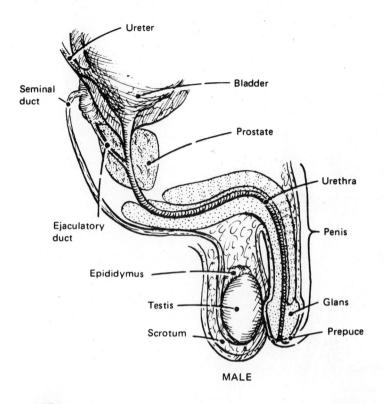

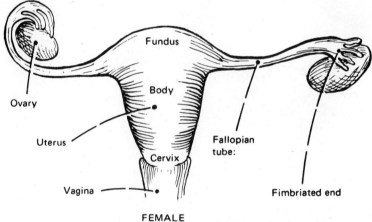

Reproductive organs

FIGURE 19–1   The female and male reproductive organs.

II. Male reproductive system.
   A. *Scrotum*—contains and supports the testes.
   B. *Testes*—produces spermatozoa and testosterone.
   C. *Prostate*—secretes a thin milky fluid that aids spermatic motility.
   D. *Penis*—conveyor of both semen and urine.
III. Urinary system. (See Figure 19-2.)
   A. *Kidneys*—two bean-shaped, compound, tubular glands located at the rear of the abdominal cavity. Their functions include:
      1. Regulating the acid-base ratio of the body.
      2. Regulating the electrolyte pattern.
      3. Excreting metabolic waste.

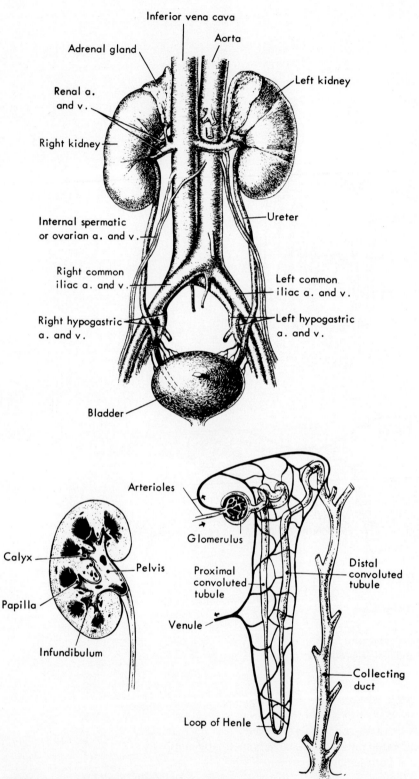

FIGURE 19–2 *A.* **Gross anatomy of the kidneys, ureters, and bladder.** *B.* **Gross structure of the kidneys and a nephron unit.** (From Keuhnelian, J. G., and Sanders, V. E.: *Urologic Nursing.* Macmillan, New York, 1970.)

4. Regulating the osmotic pressure of the extracellular fluids.
5. Influencing the blood pressure.
B. *Ureters*—tubes connecting the kidneys with the urinary bladder, allowing the passage of urine.
C. *Urinary bladder*—storage place for urine until it is voided.
D. *Renal arteries*—bring blood to the kidneys where it is circulated and filtered to remove waste products and water in the form of urine. Renal veins transport blood away from the kidneys; filtration in the kidney glomeruli separates waste products and water to form urine.
E. Factors that influence the secretion of urine include: amount of blood circulating through the kidneys; blood pressure; ability of kidney glomeruli to filter.

ANDROGENS

Androgens are male sex hormones normally manufactured by the testes in the male, the ovaries in the female, and the adrenal glands in both sexes (Table 19-1). In the male, androgens regulate the devel-

TABLE 19–1 Androgens

Nonproprietary Name	Proprietary Name	Adult Dose Range	Notes
calusterone	Methosarb	50 mg PO per day; 200 mg PO per day for breast cancer	Used mainly for anabolic effects
danazol	Danocrine	200–800 mg PO per day	Used mainly for endometriosis and breast disease; dosage for breast cancer may be two to three times larger
dromostanolone proprionate	Drolban	50 mg IM; 100 mg IM 3×/week for breast cancer	Solution is oily; used mainly for anabolic effects
ethylestrenol	Maxibolin	4–8 mg PO per day	Available as an elixir; used mainly for anabolic effects
fluoxymesterone	Halotestin, Oratestryl	2–30 mg PO per day	May be used for replacement, breast cancer, postpartum breast engorgement (rare)
methandrostenolone	Dianabol	5 mg PO per day	Anabolic steroid, used also for osteoporosis
methyltestosterone	Metandren, Oreton Methyl	5–25 mg buccal tablets per day; 10–50 mg PO per day (capsules)	Used for replacement therapy, breast cancer, postpartum breast engorgement (rare)
nandrolone decanoate	Deca-Durabolin	50–100 mg IM every 3–4 weeks	Anabolic steroid; used also for osteoporosis, anemia
nandrolone phenproprionate	Durabolin	25–50 mg IM every week	Anabolic steroid; used also for osteoporosis, anemia, breast cancer
oxandrolone	Anavar	5–10 mg PO per day	Anabolic steroid; used also for osteoporosis
oxymetholone	Anadrol-50	5–15 mg PO per day; up to 50–100 mg PO per day for anemia	Anabolic steroid; used also for osteoporosis, anemia
stanozolol	Winstrol	6 mg PO per day	Anabolic steroid
testolactone	Teslac	1 g PO per day in 4 divided doses	Anabolic steroid; IM dose for breast cancer
testosterone	Testoject Testaqua Oreton	Aqueous solution: 50 mg IM 3×/week; pellets 300 mg SC every 4–6 weeks	Dosage varies with patient's condition; used for replacement, osteoporosis, and decreased sperm production
testosterone enanthate	Delatestryl	100–400 mg IM every 2–4 weeks	Solution is oily; used for replacement, osteoporosis, decreased sperm production
testosterone proprionate	Testex	10–20 mg buccal tablets per day; 25 mg IM 2–4×/week	IM solution is oily; used for replacement, breast cancer

opment of sexual characteristics including sexual organs, body hair, oil gland secretion, skin thickening, musculoskeletal growth, and voice changes. In the female, androgens are transformed into estrogens through a complex series of chemical reactions in the body. In both sexes, androgens increase muscular development by regulating nitrogen and protein metabolism.

Testosterone is the androgen hormone of greatest importance in drug therapy. *Anabolic steroids* are synthetic drugs that resemble testosterone. Two key differences are stronger muscle-building activity and weaker masculinizing activity of anabolic steroids.

I. Actions and uses.
  A. Androgens may be used as replacement therapy when the patient's own production of testosterone is too low.
  B. Androgens may be used to increase muscle and bone growth for patients with chronic disabling conditions such as burns, trauma, and muscle-wasting diseases. Occasionally, androgens may be used to accelerate delayed growth in children.
  C. Androgens may be used for the female patient with postmenopausal osteoporosis because they improve calcium balance.
  D. Androgens may be used for women with *endometriosis* (growth of endometrial tissue outside the uterus).
  E. Androgens increase the formation of red blood cells. For this effect, they may be prescribed for patients with life-threatening anemias.
  F. Androgens suppress lactation in the female. For this effect, they may be used rarely postpartum for the woman who does not breastfeed.
  G. Androgens may be used for women with breast cancer.
II. Adverse responses.
  A. Women: increased masculinization such as appearance of facial and/or body hair, deepening of voice, menstrual irregularities, prominent musculature and veins, acne.
  B. Men: priapism (painful erection), urinary obstruction caused by prostate enlargement; impotence and decline in sperm production with long-term use contraindicated in men with prostate cancer.
  C. Children: disturbances in growth, bone development and sexual development, acne.

TABLE 19–2   Antidiuretic Drugs

Nonproprietary Name	Proprietary Name	Adult Dose Range	Notes
Replacement Drugs			
desmopressin acetate	DDAVP	2.5–20 µg intranasally twice daily	Dosage adjusted to control nocturia first, then daytime polyuria
lypressin	Diapid	0.1–0.4 ml via nasal spray up to every 4 h	Very short-acting
posterior pituitary injection	Pituitrin-S	Capsules for inhalation	
vasopressin injection	Pitressin	0.25–0.5 ml SC, IM, intranasally, IV	Used primarily for short-term replacement following brain surgery or trauma
vasopressin tannate oil suspension	Pitressin tannate	2–5 U IM every 2–3 days	May produce sterile abscess at injection site
Diuretics			Thiazide diuretics such as those listed in Table 19–3 may be prescribed to reduce polyuria.
Other Drugs			
chlorpropamide	Diabenese	Dose individualized to reduce urine output	An oral hypoglycemic drug that may occasionally be prescribed for the patient with diabetes insipidus; appears to enhance the effects of whatever ADH is present in the circulation

    D. Other: edema caused by salt and water retention, jaundice and gallbladder disease; liver cancer, stomatitis, fever, gastrointestinal disturbances.

    E. Anabolic steroids have been abused, particularly by athletes who take them to develop strength.

    F. Drug interactions include:
- A reduction of therapeutic effects of androgen when combined with aminopyrine, antihistamines, barbiturates, calcitonin, chlorocyclizine, estrogens, phenylbutazone.

III. Nursing implications.

    A. Collect a careful nursing history. Androgens are usually not used for patients with heart disease, cirrhosis, kidney disease, prostate cancer, during pregnancy or lactation.

    B. Monitor laboratory tests prescribed to identify adverse responses: liver function studies, serum electrolytes; report abnormalities.

    C. Weigh and measure the patient before administering the first dose and regularly during long-term therapy.

    D. Administer oral preparations before or with meals to reduce gastrointestinal upset.

    E. Encourage good oral hygiene to prevent local irritation when the buccal route is prescribed.

    F. Administer IM injections deeply into a large muscle mass.

    G. Encourage careful skin care to control acne.

    H. Encourage a balanced diet.

ANTIDIURETICS AND DIURETICS

Antidiuretics

Antidiuretics are drugs that act on the kidney to conserve water (Table 19–2). The hypothalamus normally secretes antidiuretic hormone (ADH) when the blood becomes too concentrated, when blood volume falls, and when there is fever, pain, and severe emotional stress.

The primary use of antidiuretic drugs is for the patient with *diabetes insipidus*. The patient with diabetes insipidus has a deficiency of antidiuretic hormone. The kidneys do not absorb water and the patient excretes large amounts of dilute urine. Up to 5 to 40 L of urine per day may be excreted. This enormous water loss causes the patient to become very thirsty (*polydipsia*) and the patient may drink up to 5 to 40 L/day. If the patient is not treated, hypotension develops from severe volume depletion.

Several factors are known to cause a deficiency of antidiuretic hormone. Disease or injury in the hypothalamus or pituitary glands in the brain may destroy cells that manufacture ADH. In some patients, there may be a defect in the renal tubules that prevents them from reabsorbing water.

    I. Actions and uses.

    A. Antidiuretic drugs may replace deficiencies in antidiuretic hormone when disease has affected the hypothalamus or pituitary glands.

    B. Thiazide diuretics (see Table 19–3) may be used when the kidney tubules are unable to reabsorb water.

  II. Adverse responses.

    A. Cardiovascular system: arrhythmias, decreased cardiac output; peripheral vasoconstriction that may lead to gangrene, elevated blood pressure.

    B. Skin and mucous membranes: marked facial pallor, local irritation of nasal mucosa when snuff is used.

    C. Gastrointestinal system: nausea, eructation, abdominal cramps, urge to defecate.

    D. Genitourinary system: women may experience uterine cramps that resemble menstrual cramps.

    E. Respiratory system: pulmonary fibrosis has been reported.

    F. Other: headache, sterile abscess with IM route; hypersensitivity reactions that may range from urticaria to anaphylaxis; water intoxication may develop when vasopressin drugs are used (headache, nausea, vomiting, confusion, lethargy, coma, convulsions).

    G. Drug interactions include: increased effects of vasopressin when combined with general anesthetics, chlorpropamide, trimethaphan; decreased effects of vasopressin when combined with lithium carbonate.

III. Nursing implications.

    A. Observe the patient receiving antidiuretic drugs for decreased urine specific gravity, and decreased thirst.

    B. Measure and record intake and output.

    C. Seek additional information when antidiuretics are prescribed for the patient with asthma, epilepsy, or heart disease. These patients are more likely to experience serious adverse responses.

    D. Anticipate the physician's order to restrict fluids when starting the patient on an antidiuretic drug.

    E. Use the following guidelines to administer vasopressin tannate in oil suspension IM:

        • Rotate the ampule between the palms of both hands to warm the solution and distribute the hormone evenly throughout the suspension.

        • Inject deeply into a large muscle mass.

        • Follow manufacturer's directions located in package insert.

Diuretics

Diuretics are drugs that increase the rate of urine formation and excretion (Table 19–3). Most diuretics act directly on the tubules of the kidney. Diuretics are prescribed primarily to prevent or treat edema. The patient with edema has an accumulation of too much body fluid in the tissues. This may be caused by an abnormally high intake of fluids or abnormally low excretion. Many underlying diseases cause edema, including heart and blood vessel disease, liver or kidney disease, cancer. Edema may develop in one or more of the following ways:

• Damage to wall of blood vessels and capillaries allows fluid to leak out into tissues.
• Interference with venous blood flow by constricting garments, venous disease, or sedentary life-style.
• A reduction of plasma proteins causes an abnormally low oncotic pressure in the bloodstream; fluid leaks out through capillary routes.
• Excess fluid in the bloodstream causes an abnormally high pressure in the bloodstream; fluid is squeezed out into the tissues.
• Obstruction of the lymph system causes edema from accumulation of lymph.

The most common sites where edema can be directly observed are the eyelids, wrists, fingers, buttocks, ankles, tibia, and sacral area. When excess fluids collect in the patient's abdominal cavity, the term *ascites* is used. When the accumulation of fluids is generalized and massive edema is present, the patient is said to have *anasarca*. When an indentation from finger pressure remains visible in the tissue, the patient is said to have *pitting edema*.

Edema causes the patient to feel weak and tired. Tachycardia and increased respiratory rate may develop as the patient's heart and lungs work harder to provide oxygenated blood to body tissues and remove waste products. As edema progresses, other symptoms may develop from pressure on body organs by excess fluid. For example, the patient may experience nausea or indigestion from pressure on gastrointestinal organs. Fluids may collect inside the lungs or compress the lungs from the thoracic cavity.

In addition to observing the patient, the two most common methods for estimating edema are weighing the patient daily and measuring intake and output. Ascites may be estimated by measuring the patient's abdominal girth daily.

I. Actions and uses.

    A. *Osmotic diuretics* increase osmotic pressure in the bloodstream by adding particles in solution. Increased osmotic pressure pulls fluid from tissue spaces into the bloodstream. For these effects, osmotic diuretics are prescribed for the patient with edema from acute renal

TABLE 19–3   Diuretics

Nonproprietary Name	Proprietary Name	Adult Dose Range	Notes
Osmotic Diuretics			
glycerin	Glyrol, Osmoglyn	1–5 g/kg PO available as 50% or 75% solution	Used to reduce intraocular pressure before ophthalmic surgery
isosorbide	Ismotic	1.5 g/kg PO	Used to reduce intraocular pressure before ophthalmic surgery
mannitol	Osmitrol	50–200 g IV over a 24-h period; available in concentrations of 5–25% solutions, and volumes of 50–1,000 ml	A test dose may be prescribed to evaluate the patient's response; dosage adjusted to maintain urine output from 30–50 ml/h; used to increase urine output; may also be used to reduce intraocular pressure before ophthalmic surgery or during acute glaucoma
urea	Ureaphil Urevert	1–1.5 g/kg IV	Available as a powder that must be reconstituted according to directions
Thiazide Diuretics			
bendroflumethiazide	Naturetin	2.5–15 mg PO per day	Teach the patient taking thiazide diuretics to avoid alcohol and eating licorice.
benzthiazide	Exna	50–200 mg PO per day	
chlorothiazide	Diuril	50–2,000 mg PO per day	
chlorthalidone	Hygroton	25–200 mg PO per day	
cyclothiazide	Anhydron	1–6 mg PO per day	
hydrochlorothiazide	Esidrex Hydrodiuril Oretic	25–100 mg PO per day	
hydroflumethiazide	Saluron	25–50 mg PO per day	
indapamide	Lozol	2.5–5 mg PO per day	Not recommended for patients taking lithium; actions are similar to thiazide diuretics
methychlothiazide	Enduron	2.5–10 mg PO per day	
metolazone	Diulo Zaroxolyn	2.5–20 mg PO per day	
polythiazide	Renese	1–4 mg PO per day	
quinethazone	Hydromox	50–200 mg PO per day	
trichlormethiazide	Metahydrin Naqua	2–8 mg PO per day	
High-Ceiling diuretics			
bumetanide	Bumex	0.5–2 mg PO per day up to a maximum of 10 mg per day; may also be given IM, IV	
ethacrynic acid	Edecrin Edecrin Sodium	50–200 mg PO per day; 50 mg IV	Gastrointestinal disturbances are more common.
furosemide	Lasix	40–200 mg PO per day; 20 or 40 mg IM, IV per dose	IV dose often exceeds 40 mg
Potassium-Sparing Diuretics			
amiloride hydrochloride	Midamor	5–10 mg PO per day	
spironolactone	Aldactone	100 mg PO per day in divided doses	Often combined with other agents (see Table 18–11); side effects include gastrointestinal upset, gynecomastia; watch for *hyperkalemia* (abnormal elevation of serum potassium)
triamterene	Dyrenium	100–300 mg PO per day in divided doses	Often combined with other agents (see Table 18–11); side effects include nausea, vomiting, leg cramps, dizziness; watch for *hyperkalemia* (abnormal elevation of serum potassium)

TABLE 19–3   *(cont.)*

Nonproprietary Name	Proprietary Name	Adult Dose Range	Notes
Other Diuretics			
acetazolamide*	Diamox	250–500 mg PO per day	
dichlorphenamide*	Daranide	200 mg PO per day	
ethoxyzolamide*	Cardrase	125–1000 mg PO per	
	Ethamide	day in divided doses	
methazolamide*	Neptazane	100–300 mg PO per day	

*These drugs inhibit the action of an enzyme, carbonic anhydrase, to increase excretion of urine, sodium, potassium; they are rarely used except to reduce intraocular pressure in patients with glaucoma, and to reduce certain seizures.

failure, cardiovascular surgery, brain or spinal cord injury or surgery, severe jaundice, hemolytic transfusion reaction.

B. Osmotic diuretics reduce intraocular pressure. For this effect, they may be prescribed for the patient with acute glaucoma or ophthalmic surgery.

C. *Thiazide diuretics* increase the excretion of sodium, chloride, and water. For this effect they may be prescribed for the patient with hypertension, edema associated with congestive heart failure or mild liver or kidney disease.

D. *High-ceiling diuretics* promote greater diuresis than other agents, increasing the excretion of sodium, chloride, and water. These diuretics act more rapidly than others and are eliminated more quickly. For these effects they may be prescribed for the patient with acute pulmonary edema, nephrosis, chronic liver and kidney failure, or edema originating from heart, liver, or kidney disease.

E. *Potassium-sparing diuretics* produce increases in the formation and excretion of urine without accompanying potassium depletion that is typical of other agents. For these effects, they may be prescribed in combination with other diuretic agents for patients requiring long-term diuretic therapy.

II. Adverse responses.

A. Osmotic diuretics: fluid overload from rapid expansion of blood volume before urine output increases; headache, nausea, vomiting, hypersensitivity; thrombosis or pain if accidentally introduced outside the vein.

B. Thiazide diuretics: hypokalemia, elevated serum levels of uric acid, calcium; reduced serum phosphatase, hyperglycemia, deterioration of mental function leading to coma in patients with cirrhosis of the liver; hepatitis, acute pancreatitis, hypersensitive reactions.

C. High-ceiling diuretics: hypokalemia; other fluid and electrolyte imbalances; temporary or permanent deafness; gastrointestinal disturbances, hypersensitivity, disturbances in blood pressure; liver dysfunction; skin rash, paresthesia, hypoglycemia; not recommended during pregnancy.

D. Potassium-sparing diuretics: hyperkalemia, nausea, vomiting, leg cramps, dizziness (triamterene only); breast enlargement, minor gastrointestinal symptoms (spironolactone only).

E. Long-term diuretic therapy may deplete the patient of sodium and/or water. In addition, the patient may develop magnesium deficiency.

F. Drug interactions include:

- Interference of therapeutic effects when high-ceiling diuretics are combined with warfarin sodium (Coumadin) and clofibrate (Atromid-S).
- Increased potential for lithium toxicity when high-ceiling diuretics are combined with lithium.
- Increased potential for kidney toxicity when high-ceiling diuretics are combined with cephalosporins.
- Increased potential for ototoxicity when aminoglycoside antibiotics (see Table 24–2) are combined with ethacrynic acid.
- Antihypertensive and diuretic combinations increase the likelihood of hypotension.

- Increased potential for hypokalemia when corticosteroids (see Table 22–2) are combined with diuretics.
- Decreased diuretic effects when combined with epinephrine and norepinephrine.

III. Nursing implications.

A. Observe the patient on admission and regularly for edema in the eyelids, wrists, buttocks, sacrum, thighs, tibia, and ankles. Ask if rings have become tighter lately.

B. Anticipate the physician's order for daily weights (on the same scale, at the same time of day, wearing similar clothing).

C. Monitor intake and output carefully and report changes in urine output.

D. Place the bedpan or urinal close at hand for the patient on bedrest; empty and measure contents frequently.

E. Provide excellent skin care to edematous areas and perineum. Change the patient's position frequently.

F. Monitor blood pressure and report orthostatic hypotension; teach the patient to change positions slowly.

G. Observe, report, and record changes in the patient's underlying condition.

H. Check serum potassium before each dose and report hypokalemia or hyperkalemia (potassium-sparing diuretics).

I. Adminster oral diuretics in the early morning and afternoon, if permitted, to prevent sleep interruptions from nighttime voiding.

J. Observe and report developing fluid overload when administering an osmotic diuretic: increasing edema, tachycardia, dyspnea, blood pressure, falling urine output.

K. Explain to the patient how drugs and diet work together when multiple therapies are prescribed.

L. Provide a list of food and fluids to be encouraged and avoided when a low-sodium diet or potassium-rich foods are prescribed.

M. Ask the physician if a salt substitute can be used by the patient on a low-sodium diet.

N. Ask the female patient about possible pregnancy before administering a diuretic initially. Many diuretics are not recommended during pregnancy and lactation. Many diuretics are excreted in breast milk.

O. Observe and report hyperglycemia that develops during diuretic therapy. This condition occurs more often when the patient with diabetes is taking a diuretic.

P. Review the signs and symptoms of digitalis toxicity. This condition occurs more often when diuretic therapy is combined with a digitalis drug (see Table 18–15).

Q. Instruct the patient to report sexual difficulties that develop during diuretic therapy. This condition occurs more frequently when diuretics are prescribed for hypertension (see pp. 182–188).

DRUGS AFFECTING URINE ACIDITY OR ALKALINITY

Drugs may be used to make the patient's urine either more acid or more alkaline (Table 19–4). The usual reasons for changing the *pH* (measure of acidity, alkalinity) of urine are either to promote or slow down elimination of body chemicals or drugs.

I. Actions and uses.

A. Urine acidifiers may be used to increase the effectiveness of certain anti-infective drugs such as methenamine, nitrofurantoin.

B. Urine alkalinizers may be used to reduce excessive excretion of acids following drug therapy with certain cancer drugs, uricosuric agents (see Table 22–3), or sulfonamides (see Table 24–11).

C. Urine alkalinizers may also be used for the patient with a overdose of salicylates or phenobarbital.

II. Adverse responses.

TABLE 19–4　Drugs Affecting Urine Acidity or Alkalinity

Nonproprietary Name	Proprietary Name	Adult Dose Range	Notes
acetohydroxamic acid	Lithostat	10–15 mg/kg PO per day up to a maximum of 1.5 g/day; usually prescribed every 6–8 h	New drug that causes urine to become more acid; used with antibiotics for the patient with recurrent urinary tract infection associated with renal calculi; may prevent formation of staghorn renal calculi; adverse responses include headache, depression, and anxiety; anorexia, nausea, and vomiting; anemia; administer on an empty stomach
ammonium chloride		500 mg–1 g PO every 2–3 h	Causes the urine to become more acid
citrates (citric acid, potassium citrate, sodium citrate)		1–2 packets diluted in one glass of water	Causes the urine to become more alkaline; follow manufacturer's directions for correct administration
sodium bicarbonate		10–15 g PO per day	Causes the urine to become more alkaline
tromethamine	Tham, Tham-E		Available as powder to be dissolved in IL sterile water or as solution; causes urine to become more alkaline; not recommended during pregnancy or for patients with uremia or chronic respiratory acidosis; not to be administered for longer than 1 day

TABLE 19–5　Estrogens, Progestins, and Oral Contraceptives

Nonproprietary Name	Proprietary Name	Adult Dose Range	Notes
Estrogens			
chlorotrianisene	Tace	12–25 mg PO per day	Used for menopause, delayed sexual development, postpartum breast engorgement, prostate cancer
conjugated estrogens	Ovest, Premarin	0.3–10 mg PO per day; 2–4 g vaginal cream per day; 25 mg IV for emergency control of dysfunctional uterine bleeding	Dosage varies greatly according to patient's condition; used for delayed sexual development, menopause, uterine bleeding, postpartum breast engorgement, prostate cancer; may be given in cycles
dienestrol	DV	Topical vaginal cream: 1–3×/day initially, then 1–3×/week	Used for senile atrophic vaginitis
diethylstilbestrol (DES)	Stilbestrol	0.2–15 mg PO per day	Dosage varies greatly according to patient's condition; used for dysfunctional uterine bleeding, delayed sexual development, postpartum breast engorgement, prostate cancer, breast cancer; higher incidence of side effects; cannot be used during pregnancy
diethylstilbestrol diphosphate	Stilphostrol	50–200 mg PO 3×/day; 500 mg–1 g IV per day initially; dosage and frequency reduced to 250–500 mg 1–2×/week for maintenance	Used primarily for prostate cancer
esterified estrogens	Amnestrogen Menest		Dosage and uses similar to conjugated estrogens

TABLE 19–5 *(cont.)*

Nonproprietary Name	Proprietary Name	Adult Dose Range	Notes
estradiol	Estrace	1–2 mg PO per day	Prescribed in 3-week cycles to relieve menopausal symptoms
estradiol cypionate	Depo-Estradiol, Depogen	1–5 mg IM per month	Dosage varies with patient's condition; used for menopausal symptoms, delayed sexual development
estradiol valerate	Delestrogen	10–30 mg IM; 1–2×/month	Dosage varies with patient's condition; used for menopausal symptoms, delayed sexual development, postpartum breast engorgement, prostate cancer.
estrone (in various combinations)	Ogen, Theelin and others	0.1–4 mg IM per day or week; also available as vaginal suppositories	Dosage varies greatly with patient's condition; used for dysfunctional uterine bleeding, menopausal symptoms, delayed sexual development, postpartum breast engorgement, prostate cancer, senile atrophic vaginitis
ethinylestradiol quinestrol	Estinyl; Feminone Estrovis	0.02–1 mg PO 1–3×/day 0.1–0.2 mg PO once/week	Dosage varies greatly with patient's condition; used for dysfunctional uterine bleeding, menopausal symptoms, delayed sexual development, postpartum breast engorgement, prostate and breast cancer
Progestins			
hydroxyprogesterone caproate	Delalutin	375 mg IM per menstrual cycle	Used for menstrual disorders; may also be used for adenocarcinoma of the uterus
medroxyprogesterone acetate (MPA)	Depo-Provera Provera	5–10 mg PO per day; 150 mg IM every 3 months for endometriosis	Used for menstrual disorders, endometriosis; may also be used for endometrial cancer
megestrol acetate	Megace	40–320 mg PO per day in divided doses	Used for advanced cancers of breast or endometrium
norethindrone, norethindrone acetate	Norlutin; Norlutate	5–30 mg PO per day	Dosage and frequency varies with patient's condition; used for menstrual disorders, endometriosis; may be prescribed in cycles
progesterone	Gesterol, Lipolutin	5–10 mg IM/day	No more than 50 mg per dose should be injected into one IM site; used for menstrual disorders; dosage varies with patient's specific condition

    A. Urine acidifiers may produce acidosis, nausea, vomiting, gastric irritation.
    B. Urine alkalinizers may produce metabolic alkalosis.
III. Nursing implications.
    A. Observe and record characteristics of urine output.
    B. Monitor the patient for acidosis.
    C. Monitor the patient for alkalosis.
    D. Follow manufacturer's directions for oral administration of citrate acidifiers. Administer drugs after meals to prevent or reduce cathartic effects.
    E. Provide excellent perineal care and teach the patient how it is done.

OBSTETRIC AND GYNECOLOGIC AGENTS

Estrogens, Progestins, Oral Contraceptives.

Estrogen and *progestin* are female sex hormones manufactured in the ovaries in females, in the testes in males, and in the adrenal glands in both sexes (Table 19–5), pp. 212–213. In the female, estrogens and progestins regulate the development of sexual characteristics including sexual organs, breast development, menstrual cycle. Progestins resemble the actions of the hormone progesterone. During pregnancy, progesterone is secreted first by the corpus luteum and later by the placenta to maintain the endometrial lining and promote milk-producing cells in the breast.

Oral contraceptives are hormones that prevent pregnancy (see Table 19–6). Most oral contraceptive preparations currently in use contain a combination that includes an estrogen and a progestin. Most oral contraceptives work by inhibiting female ovulation. A postcoital hormone is available that prevents fertilization and implantation. Currently, researchers are investigating androgens (see pp. 205–206) as a contraceptive for men.

  I. Actions and uses.

    A. Estrogens may be used as replacement therapy for women who experience unpleasant menopausal symptoms such as "hot flashes," chilly sensations, muscle cramps, dizziness, palpitations, hyperventilation. When prescribed for this condition, estrogens are usually taken in 28- to 30-day cycles that resemble the menstrual cycle.

TABLE 19–6 Selected Oral Contraceptives

Proprietary Name	Estrogen Dose	Progestin Dose	Notes*
Brevicon, Modicon	ethinyl estradiol 0.035 mg	norethindrone 0.5 mg	Several preparations available; one contains seven inert tablets so the patient takes a tablet every day
Demulen	ethinyl estradiol 0.05 mg	ethynodiol diacetate 1 mg	Same as above
Enovid E	mestranol 0.10 mg	norethynodrel 2.5 mg	Three preparations are available
5 mg	mestranol 0.075 mg	norethynodrel 5 mg	
10 mg	mestranol 0.15 mg	norethynodrel 9.85 mg	
Loestrin			
1/20	ethinylestradiol 0.02 mg	norethindrone 1 mg	Each preparation includes seven additional tablets that contain iron; also know by the trade name Zorane
1.5/30	ethinylestradiol 0.03 mg	norethindrone 1.5 mg	
Lo/Ovral	ethinyl estradiol 0.03 mg	norgestrel 0.3 mg	
Micronor	none	norethindrone 0.35 mg	Must be taken every day
Nor-QD			
Norinyl			Also known by the trade name Ortho-Novum 1/50
1 + 50	mestranol 0.05 mg	norethindrone 1 mg	
1 + 80	mestranol 0.08 mg	same as above	
2 mg	mestranol 0.10 mg	norethindrone 2 mg	
Norlestrin			
1/50	ethinyl estradiol 0.05 mg	norethindrone acetate 1 mg	
2.5/50	same as above	norethindrone acetate 2.5 mg	
Ortho-Novum 10 mg	mestranol 0.06 mg	norethindrone 10 mg	See other Ortho-Novum preparations
Ovcon			Also known by the trade name Zorane 1/50
35	ethinyl estradiol 0.035 mg	norethindrone 0.4 mg	
50	ethinyl estradiol 0.05 mg	norethindrone 1 mg	
Ovral	ethinyl estradiol 0.05	norgestrel 0.5 mg	
Ovrette	none	norgestrel 0.075 mg	Must be taken daily
Ovulen	mestranol 0.10 mg	ethynodiol diacetate	
Stilbesterol	diethylstilbestrol 25 mg PO bid	none	Must be taken bid for 5 days within 72 h after sexual intercourse; nausea and vomiting are common; vaginal carcinoma may develop in female children if taken during pregnancy

*Except where noted, oral contraceptives are taken daily for 21 days; none for 7 days; then cycle is repeated.

    B. Women with senile atrophic vaginitis or postmenopausal osteoporosis may also be helped by estrogen therapy.

    C. Estrogen may also be used when a woman has delayed or failure of ovarian or other sexual development, hirsutism, or acne during puberty.

    D. Estrogen may be prescribed for males with prostate cancer or females with certain types of breast cancer that are estrogen sensitive.

    E. Progestins may be used for the patient with symptoms of premenstrual tension such as headaches, increased irritability, breast tenderness, weight gain.

    F. Progestins may be used for the patient with endometriosis.

    G. Progestins may be used for the patient with recurrent or metastatic cancer of the endometrium.

    H. Estrogens and progestins alone or combined may be used as oral contraceptives; to suppress postpartum lactation; for dysmenorrhea (painful menstruation); or for dysfunctional uterine bleeding.

  II. Adverse responses.

    A. Estrogens and progestins.

      1. Anorexia, nausea, vomiting, diarrhea.

      2. Edema and weight gain.

      3. Altered glucose lipoproteins and triglycerides.

      4. Increased incidence of benign and malignant tumors.

      5. Gynecomastia (breast enlargement), feminization, impotence, thrombosis, or embolism may develop in men.

      6. When taken during pregnancy, estrogens are associated with increased incidence of vaginal cancer in daughters and increased incidence of genital abnormalities in sons.

      7. When taken during lactation, estrogens may lead to a decreased milk supply and lowered levels of vitamins, proteins, and fat content in breast milk.

    B. Oral contraceptives.

      1. Increased frequency of cardiovascular disorders including thrombophlebitis, thromboembolism, cerebral and coronary thrombosis, hypertension, myocardial infarction.

      2. Estrogenlike side effects such as nausea, vomiting, dizziness, breast discomfort, weight gain may occur.

      3. Irregular menstrual bleeding is common.

      4. Ocular disturbances such as corneal sensitivity.

      5. Skin changes including chloasma, rashes, photosensitivity, jaundice have been reported.

      6. Birth defects have been reported when oral contraceptives are taken during pregnancy.

      7. Same effects as estrogens and progestins on lactation.

    C. Drug interactions include:

      • Reduction of therapeutic effects of estrogens, progestins, or oral contraceptives when combined with barbiturates.

      • Estrogen and progestin may decrease effect of oral anticoagulants, hypoglycemic drugs.

      • Oral contraceptives may decrease effectiveness of anticonvulsants, antihypertensives, tricyclic antidepressants.

      • The following drugs may decrease the effectiveness of oral contraceptives: ampicillin, anticonvulsants, antimigraine agents, barbiturates, chloramphenicol, isoniazid, neomycin, nitrofurantoin, penicillin, phenylbutazone, rifampin, sulfonamides, tetracyclines, tranquilizers.

 III. Nursing implications.

    A. Collect a careful nursing history. Female hormones or oral contraceptives may not be recommended for the patient with pregnancy, cardiovascular disease, diabetes, migraine headaches, underlying conditions associated with edema, or for lactating women.

    B. Administer oral preparations after meals or at bedtime to reduce nausea.

    C. Administer IM preparations deeply into a large muscle such as the gluteus.

    D. Encourage women taking oral contraceptives to stop smoking, eat a balanced diet, and have medical checkups including Pap smears every 6 to 12 months.

    E. Create opportunities to explain the menstrual cycle and develop a simple explanation that lay people can understand.

    F. Teach patients to take hormones exactly as prescribed.

    G. Teach patients what side effects to expect and when to report them.

    H. Weigh and measure the patient before administering the initial dose and weekly during therapy.

    I. Report the patient's questions and concerns to the registered nurse or physician.

Fertility Drugs

Fertility drugs are hormones that produce ovulation in women who are unable to become pregnant because they do not ovulate (Table 19–7). Most fertility drugs cause the release of one or more hormones that stimulate ovulation: gonadotrophic luteinizing hormone (LH) or follicle-stimulating hormone (FSH).

  I. Actions and uses.

    A. Fertility drugs are useful primarily for infertile women who do not ovulate.

    B. Several fertility drugs may be used occasionally for infertile men to stimulate the formation of more sperm.

 II. Adverse responses.

    A. The incidence of multiple births is greatly increased.

    B. Hot flashes, headache, nausea, breast enlargement, and abdominal bleeding, fluid retention, abnormal ovarian enlargement, and liver dysfunction may occur.

III. Nursing implications.

    A. Show the wife and husband how to take and record the wife's basal body temperature to detect ovulation.

    B. Weigh and measure the patient before the first dose is administered and regularly during therapy.

    C. Observe and report blurring, visual disturbances, edema that develop during drug therapy.

    D. Be sensitive to the high anxiety and mood swings that couples often experience during therapy, especially after several unsuccessful attempts at pregnancy.

    E. Report the couple's concerns and/or questions to the registered nurse or physician.

Oxytocics and Tocolytics

Oxytocics are drugs that stimulate uterine contraction (Table 19–8). One group of drugs resembles oxytocin, a natural hormone produced by the hypothalamus and released during the later stages of pregnancy and during labor. Another group of drugs are selected *prostaglandins*. These drugs also resemble naturally occurring hormones that increase in the body during late pregnancy and labor. A

TABLE 19–7 Fertility Drugs

Nonproprietary Name	Proprietary Name	Adult Dose Range	Notes
chorionic gonadotropin for injection	Antituitrin-S, APL Secules, Follutein, Libigen, Pregnyl	8000–10,000 IU IM for ovulation	Dosage highly individualized; menotropins must be administered first; also used to increase sperm production in men
clomiphene citrate	Clomid	25–200 mg PO per day	Dosage and frequency highly individualized; course of therapy varies from a few days to a few weeks; also used to increase sperm production in men
menotropins for injection	Pergonal	75 IU IM per day for 9–12 days	Dosage highly individualized and followed by chorionic gonadotropin injection

third group of oxytocics are called *ergots* and/or *ergot alkaloids*. Ergots produced by a fungus have been known and used for over 400 years. *Tocolytics* are drugs that inhibit uterine contractions during premature labor.

I. Actions and uses.

    A. Oxytocin acts on the myometrium to produce uterine contractions during late pregnancy. For this effect it is used to initiate labor, or improve the force of uterine contraction when labor is dysfunctional.

    B. Oxytocics are often used to augment uterine contractions following the delivery of the placenta and for several hours during the fourth stage of labor.

TABLE 19–8 Oxytocics amd Tocolytics

Nonproprietary Name	Proprietary Name	Adult Dose Range	Notes
Oxytocics			
oxytocin citrate buccal tablets	Pitocin Citrate		
oxytocin injection	Pitocin Syntocinon	10 U/L IV fluid at 0.2 ml/min initially; gradually increased to a maximum of 2 ml/min; total dose usually ranges from 600 to 12,000 U	Infusion pump should be used; patient should be monitored continuously by trained nursing staff; physician should be in attendance
oxytocin nasal solution		Single burst of nasal spray in each nostril 2–3 min before nursing	Used occasionally to stimulate milk ejection before breast-feeding
Prostaglandins			
carboprost tromethamine	Prostin 15M	250 mg IM every 1.5–3.5 h until abortion occurs; total dose not to exceed 1,200 mg (12 mg)	
dinoprost tromethamine	Prostin F2 alpha	40 mg × one dose 20 mg 6 h later	Instilled into amniotic fluid to produce abortion in the second trimester
dinoprostone	Prostin E2	Each vaginal suppository contains 20 mg	
Ergots (Selected)			
ergonovine	Ergotrate	0.2 0.4 mg PO 3×/day×7 days; 0.2–0.3 mg IM; 0.2 mg IV	
methylergonovine	Methergine	0.2–0.4 mg PO 3× per 7 days; 0.2–0.3 mg IM; 0.2 mg IV	
chorionic gonadotropin for injection	Antuitrin-S APL Seciles, Follutein, Libigen, Pregnyl	8,000–10,000 IU IM for ovulation	Dosage highly individualized; menotropins must be administered first; also used for men
Tocolytics			
alcohol		10% solution IV at 7.5 mg 1 kg per h initially; then 1.5 mg 1 kg per h for 10 h	
magnesium sulfate		6 g IV for 20 min initially, gradually reduced over 24–72 h	
ritodrine hydrochloride	Yutopar	0.1 mg/min initially; gradually increased until labor controlled; 10–20 mg PO every 4–6 h for maintenance	adrenergic drug
terbutaline	Brethine, Brethaire, Bricanyl		

    C. Oxytocin also forces milk from milk channels to large sinuses for the nursing infant. For this effect, known as *milk ejection,* oxytocin may occasionally be used in nursing mothers.

    D. Selected prostaglandins produce uterine contractions at any time during pregnancy. For this effect, they may be used to produce intended abortion in the second trimester of pregnancy.

    E. Ergots are used primarily to stimulate uterine contractions after delivery to control postpartum bleeding. Ergots are also used for the patient with migraine.

    F. Prostaglandins may also be used for incomplete abortion, elective abortion, intrauterine fetal death, and similar abnormal conditions of pregnancy and labor.

    G. Tocolytics inhibit uterine motility. For this effect, they are used to delay premature labor. Another use of tocolytics is to delay delivery in order to use other therapeutic measures.

  II. Adverse responses.

    A. Ergots.

      1. Hypertension, nausea, vomiting, allergic reactions.

      2. Ergot poisoning may develop from long-term use: extremities become cool, pale, numb; anginal pain, changes in heart rate and blood pressure may develop; headache, nausea, vomiting, diarrhea, dizziness are common; confusion, depression, drowsiness may be present.

      3. May produce long sustained uterine contractions without rest periods if accidentally administered during labor.

    B. Oxytocics.

      1. Tachycardia, initial fall in blood pressure followed by sustained elevation, cardiac arrhythmias in mother or fetus, increased bleeding.

      2. Pelvic hematoma, uterine spasm, tetany, or rupture.

      3. Fetal distress, fetal death.

      4. Nausea and vomiting.

      5. Hypersensitivity including anaphylaxis.

    C. Prostaglandins.

      1. Nausea, vomiting, diarrhea.

      2. Hypersensitivity, including anaphylaxis.

      3. Hypotension, cardiac arrthythmias.

      4. Breast engorgement, lactation.

      5. Headache, grand mal seizures.

      6. For midtrimester abortion: cervical or uterine laceration, rupture of placenta; delivery of live fetus.

      7. Fever and bronchospasm.

    D. Tocolytics.

      1. Tachycardia, circulatory overload, myocardial ischemia, cardiac arrest.

      2. Respiratory depression.

      3. Hyperglycemia, hypokalemia.

III. Nursing implications.

    A. Monitor vital signs, progression of labor, and fetal condition frequently; report changes to the registered nurse or physician.

    B. Report immediately uterine contractions lasting longer than 60 s or occurring faster than every 2 min without intermittent uterine relaxation.

    C. Seek additional information from the registered nurse or physician about any orders to administer ergot preparations during labor; accidental administration may cause dangerously abnormal uterine contractions.

    D. Know where emergency drugs and supplies are located whenever oxytocics and tocolytics are administered.

    E. Administer antiemetics if nausea and vomiting occur.

    F. Check the patient's uterine fundus and vaginal blood flow (lochia) frequently after delivery.

    G. Observe and assist the new mother while nursing and report difficulties to the registered nurse.

    H. Report the patient's questions and concerns to the registered nurse or physician.

URINARY ANTISEPTICS, ANALGESICS, ANTISPASMODICS

Urinary antiseptics are drugs that inhibit the growth of bacteria in the urinary tract (Table 19–9). A unique feature of these drugs is their limited action on the urinary tract. Doses high enough to produce systemic effects also cause toxicity. Anti-infectives used for systemic effects are discussed in Chapter 24, Tables 24–2 and 24–11.

Normally urine is sterile. That patient with a urinary tract infection has an inflammation caused by the growth of bacteria in the urethra, bladder, or kidneys. Bacteria most likely to cause urinary tract infection are normally found in the intestines: *Escherichia coli,* Klebsiella, Enterobacter, Pro-

TABLE 19–9   Urinary Antiseptics, Analgesics, and Antispasmodics

Nonproprietary Name	Proprietary Name	Adult Dose Range	Notes
Urinary Antiseptics			
amdinocillin	Coactin		New penicillin, antibioticlike drug (not an antiseptic) specifically for urinary tract infections caused by *E. coli*, Klebsiella, Enterobacter species; adverse responses reported include rashes, phlebitis
cinoxacin	Cinobac	1 g PO per day in four divided doses for 7–14 days	
methenamine		0.5–2 g PO per day	
methenamine hippurate	Hiprex Urex	1 g PO bid	
methenamine mandelate	Mandelamine	0.5–2 g PO per day	
methylene blue	Lurolene	65–130 mg PO tid	Tell patient that this drug turns urine blue-green color
nalidixic acid	NegGram	4 g PO per day in four divided doses for 1–2 weeks; then 2 g PO per day	Instruct patient to avoid bright sunlight
nitrofurantoin	Furadantin Macrodantin	50 mg PO qid × 14 days	Not recommended during pregnancy
oxlinic acid	Utibid	750 PO bid	CNS toxicity more common
Urine Analgesics			
ethoxazene hydrochloride	Serenium	300 mg PO per day in divided doses	Tell patient that this drug turns the urine an orange-red color; administer before meals
phenazopyridine hydrochloride	Pyridium	200 mg PO tid	Tell patient that this drug turns the urine an orange-red color
phenazopyridine hydrochloride and sulfisoxazole	Azogantrisin	Each tablet contains 50 mg phenazopyridine and 500 mg sulfasoxazole	Combines a urinary antiseptic with a sulfa drug (see Table 24–11); turns urine an orange-red color
phenazopyridine hydrochloride and sulfamethoxazole	Azogantanol	Each tablet contains 100 mg phenazopyridine and 500 mg sulfamethoxazole	Combines a urinary antiseptic with a sulfa drug (see Table 24–11); turns urine an orange-red color
Urinary Antispasmodics			
flavoxate hydrochloride	Urispas	300–800 mg per day in three to four divided doses	May cause drowsiness and blurred vision; caution patient not to drive car or operate heavy machinery; has anticholinergic side effects (see p. 159)
oxybutynin chloride	Ditropan	5 mg PO tid; maximum dosage not to exceed 20 mg PO per day	Used for the patient with spasms of bladder associated with neurogenic bladder, urinary retention overflow, incontinence

Abbreviations: CNS, central nervous system.

teus, Pseudomonas. The physician diagnoses the patient's condition from a urine culture that shows greater than 100,000 colonies of bacteria per milliliter, and from symptoms reported by the patient.

The patient with an infection of the urethra (*urethritis*) and/or bladder (*cystitis*), usually reports frequent, urgent and painful, burning urination that may be accompanied by hematuria, spasms in the suprapubic area, and low back pain. If infection is located in the kidney (pyelonephritis), the patient may report fever, chills, and flank pain. The urine of a patient with a urinary tract infection may be cloudy, reddish brown, and/or foul smelling.

Women develop urinary tract infection more often then men because the female urethra is shorter and closer to the rectum. Other factors known to increase the occurrence of urinary tract infection are pregnancy; poor perineal hygiene, especially after urinating, defecating, and sexual intercourse; catheterization and retention catheters; surgical or diagnostic procedures on the urinary tract; stasis of urine caused by retention or obstruction.

It is very important to cure a urinary tract infection as quickly as possible. An acute infection may develop into a chronic one that causes permanent scarring and damage to the urinary system. In addition to urinary antiseptics to inhibit bacterial growth, the physician may also prescribe a urinary analgesic or antispasmodic to relieve pain or spasm. In addition to administering drug therapy, the nurse uses and teaches nondrug measures that discourage bacterial growth, promote patient comfort, and prevent recurrence.

I. Actions and uses.
  A. Urinary antiseptics inhibit the growth of bacteria in the urinary tract.
  B. Urinary analgesics and antispasmodics relieve symptoms of frequency, urgency, burning, dysuria.
II. Adverse responses.
  A. Gastrointestinal system: nausea, vomiting, indigestion, abdominal pain, diarrhea, liver damage.
  B. Urinary system: painful, frequent urination, crystals in urine (methenamine); kidney damage.
  C. Skin: allergic rashes, pruritus, urticaria, photosensitivity.
  D. Central nervous system: headache, drowsiness, vertigo, visual disturbances, chills, fever.
  E. Blood: various anemias, bone marrow depression.
  F. Respiratory system: acute pneumonitis in persons with hypersensitivity to nitrofurantoin.
  G. Drug interactions include:
    • Decreased effects of methenamine drugs when combined with acetazolamide, sodium bicarbonate, or thiazide diuretics.
    • Increased potential for crystals in the urine when methenamine is combined with sulfonamides.
    • Decreased effects of nalidixic acid when combined with oral antacids, nitrofurantoin.
    • Increased anticoagulent effect when nalidixic acid combined with oral anticoagulants.
    • Decreased effect of nitrofurantoin when combined with acetazolamide (Diamox), oral antacids, anticholinergics (see Table 17–4), sodium bicarbonate.
III. Nursing implications.
  A. Collect information on usual voiding practices of newly admitted patients as a basis for planning patient teaching.
  B. Use good technique to obtain urine for the urine culture.
  C. Unless otherwise instructed, collect a urine culture before administering the first dose of a urinary antiseptic.
  D. Administer oral agents during or after meals with a full glass of water to prevent gastrointestinal side effects.
  E. Identify patients with liver or kidney disease, marked decreases in urine output. Urinary antiseptics are generally not recommended for these patients. Anticipate the physician's order for an antibiotic instead.
  F. Encourage and assist the patient to force fluids. Bacteria cannot reproduce as quickly in dilute urine. Three to 4 L/day of fluid intake is desirable.

G. Offer cranberry juice to the patient receiving methenamine agents. These fluids increase urine acidity and enhance effectiveness.

H. Teach and use perineal hygiene practices that prevent recurrence of infection in the urinary tract:
- Cleanse and dry the perineal area from front to back after urinating and defecating.
- Urinate when the voiding sensation is first noted. Avoid delaying urination which may lead to urinary stasis and more concentrated urine, factors that increase the likelihood of infection.
- Maintain sufficient fluid intake. Limit intake of xanthine beverages such as coffee, tea, colas.

I. Be alert for patients with other conditions that limit mobility and ability to cleanse the perineum adequately. For example, patients with rheumatoid arthritis or stroke may need the nurse's help for perineal care.

J. Use excellent technique during catheterization and when caring for the patient with a retention catheter.

K. Flag the chart according to hospital policy for patients receiving urinary antiseptics. Many drugs affect laboratory tests.

L. Teach the patient to take the complete course of therapy even if symptoms subside and return for a follow-up urine culture if ordered by the physician. The only way to know for certain that a urinary tract infection has been cured is by urine culture that is sterile.

M. Observe and record the characteristics of urine in all hospitalized patients. Early detection and treatment of minor infection may prevent its spread and/or recurrence.

VAGINAL ANTI-INFECTIVES

Vaginal anti-infectives are drugs that kill or inhibit growth of common pathogens that cause vaginitis (Table 19–10). The woman with vaginitis has an inflammation of the vagina that is often caused by microorganisms. The organisms that most often cause vaginitis are *Candida albicans* (a yeast), *Hemophilis vaginalis* (a bacteria), and *Trichomonas vaginalis* (a fungus). Factors that favor the development of vaginitis include pregnancy, destruction of normal flora from antibiotic therapy, frequent douching, use of feminine hygiene sprays, diabetes mellitus, oral contraceptives, continuous irritation from tight clothing, nylon clothing, menopause, stress.

The patient with vaginitis often notices a change in vaginal drainage. The appearance varies according to the causative organism. The patient may also experience local pruritus, burning, dyspareunia. The sexual partner may experience the same symptoms.

A diagnosis is made during a pelvic examination. A smear of vaginal secretions is examined under a microscope. The physician identifies the causative organism and prescribes a specific anti-infective for it.

I. Actions and uses.
- A. Anti-infectives are often administered as vaginal suppositories, tablets, or creams to kill or inhibit the growth of microorganisms causing vaginitis.
- B. Additional jelly or douches may be used to restore normal pH to the vagina which is normally slightly acid.

II. Adverse responses.*
- A. Local irritation may occur including stinging, burning, swelling, blistering.
- B. Metronidazole may produce nausea, diarrhea, headache, urticaria, metallic taste, leukopenia.
- C. Hypersensitivity to iodine may cause serious allergic responses if povidone-iodine is administered.

*Adverse responses are limited to those encountered when drugs are used for vaginitis. For other routes of administration and conditions, refer to appropriate section elsewhere in the text.

TABLE 19–10   Vaginal Anti-infectives

Nonproprietary Name	Proprietary Name	Adult Dose Range	Notes
candicidin	Candeptin Vanobid	1 capsule, tablet, or ap- plicatorful inserted into vagina in AM and PM for 14 days	Used for vaginitis caused by yeast infection
clotrimazole	Gyne-Lotrimin Lotrimin Mycelex	1 tablet inserted into the va- gina every night for 7 days	Used for vaginitis caused by yeast infection
metronizadole	Flagyl Metryl	250 mg PO 3 ×/day for 7 days	Used for vaginitis caused by Trichomonas; male partner may also need treatment; al- cohol should be avoided because of alco- hol-metronizadole interaction
miconazole nitrate	Monistat 2%	1 applicatorful inserted into the vagina every night for 2 weeks	Used for vaginitis caused by fungus
nystatin	Mycostatin	Vaginal tablets 100,000–200,000 U in- serted into vagina every day for at least 2 weeks	Used for vaginitis caused by fungus
povidone-iodine	Betadine Anti- septic Gel 10%	1 applicatorful inserted into vagina every night for 7 days	Used for vaginitis caused by Trichomonas or mixed organism; check for iodine sen- sitivity before administering

    D. Drug interactions include:
- A reduction of anticoagulant affects when warfarin is combined with metronidazole.
- A serious interaction that produces nausea, vomiting, headaches, abdominal cramps, flushing when alcohol is consumed during metronidazole therapy.

III. Nursing implications.
    A. Check for allergies before administering vaginal anti-infectives. Report iodine or seafood allergy and anticipate change of drug if povidone-iodine has been prescribed.
    B. Administer vaginal creams, suppositories high into vagina.
    C. Observe and report vaginal drainage in hospitalized patients. Patients who are diabetic, or who are receiving antibiotics or steroids are more likely to develop vaginitis.
    D. Review the physician's prescription with the patient in the clinic or office; report questions or concerns to the registered nurse or physician.
    E. Teach the patient to continue therapy as directed even if symptoms disappear or menses occurs. Severe local reaction should be reported to the registered nurse or physician.
    F. Protect the patient's clothing from medication stain by providing sanitary pad.
    G. Teach the patient nondrug measures to prevent recurrence of infection: perineal cleansing; avoid nonprescribed douches and sprays; avoid constricting clothing, nylon underwear and wet bathing suits; ensure use of condoms by the male partner during therapy; report early signs of reinfection (change in vaginal drainage); encourage patient to get appropriate rest and nutrition.
    H. Teach patient that sexual partner may need to be treated simultaneously.
    I. Assist the patient with comfort measures such as rinsing the vulva after each urination using a plastic squeeze bottle (peri-bottle) and warm tap water.

EXERCISE

The list below contains examples of common drugs affecting the patient's genitourinary system. In the space provided next to each drug, describe its effects on the structures or functions of the patient's genitourinary system. One example is provided to help you.

Drug	Effects on Structures and/or Functions
1. ammonium chloride	
2. chlorothiazide	
3. clomiphene citrate	
4. clotrimazole	
5. furosemide	Acts on the kidney tubules to increase the rate of urine formation and excretion
6. nitrofurantoin	
7. Ovulen (proprietary name)	
8. oxytocin injections	
9. testosterone	

CASE STUDY 12

Mrs. Yvonne Lovey is a 58-year-old woman who has been experiencing unpleasant menopausal symptoms including hot flashes, chilly sensations, muscle cramps, dizziness, and hyperventilation. The physician prescribed conjugated estrogens (Premarin) 1.25 mg PO every day for 21 days; then no drug for 7 days; then repeat cycle.

Answer the following questions about drug therapy for Mrs. Lovey.

1. What is the purpose of estrogen therapy for Mrs. Lovey?
2. For what other reasons are estrogens prescribed?
3. What is the relationship between the uses of estrogen therapy and various conditions for which a physician might prescribe androgen therapy?
4. What observations would indicate that Mrs. Lovey is having an adverse response to estrogens? Compare these observations to those you would look for in a patient receiving androgen therapy.
5. List the nursing implications related to estrogen therapy for Mrs. Lovey. Compare these implications to those you would consider for a patient receiving androgen therapy.

CASE STUDY 13

Martha Lopez is a 25-year-old woman who reports to the clinic and tells you that she has been having frequent burning, painful urination since yesterday. In gathering information for the nursing history, you learn that Mrs. Lopez is using an oral contraceptive listed in Table 19–6. Mrs. Lopez also reports that she has had a vaginal discharge ever since her last menstrual period.

Answer the following questions about drug therapy for Mrs. Lopez.

1. What additional information do you need to plan appropriate nursing care for Mrs. Lopez?
2. What procedures can you anticipate during Mrs. Lopez's office visit? Explain the purpose and rationale for each selection.
3. The physician prescribes methenamine mandelate 1 g PO qid. What patient teaching will Mrs. Lopez need?
4. The physician also prescribes clotrimazole vaginal tablets every night for 7 days. What additional patient teaching will Mrs. Lopez need?
5. What are the nursing implications associated with Mrs. Lopez's use of oral contraceptives? Explain your rationale where appropriate.
6. Mrs. Lopez asks you if it is okay to continue the oral contraceptives with the new drugs. How should you respond?
7. Mrs. Lopez tells you that her sister got a bladder infection in the hospital recently. Mrs. Lopez adds, "I thought hospitals were supposed to be so clean." What explanation would add to Mrs. Lopez's understanding?

Chapter 20 | DRUG THERAPY AFFECTING THE PATIENT'S RESPIRATORY SYSTEM

EXPECTED BEHAVIORAL OUTCOMES

After completing this chapter you should return to the expected behavioral outcomes and evaluate your ability to:

1. Relate the effects of a specific drug to the structure and function of the respiratory system.
2. Compare nondrug nursing actions that enhance the effectiveness of antitussives, expectorants, bronchodilators, and nasal decongestants.
3. Describe nursing actions to prevent and/or detect adverse responses for each group of drugs affecting the patient's respiratory system.

STRUCTURE AND FUNCTION REVIEW

The respiratory system contains organs for exchanging gases, regulating body temperature and acid-alkaline balance, and communicating sounds. (See Figure 20-1.) *Ventilation* is the process of taking air into the lungs (inspiration) and expelling air from the lungs (expiration). *Respiration* is the exchange of oxygen and carbon dioxide across the cell membrane.

1. *Nose*—the organ of smell; serves as a passageway that warms and filters air going to the lungs; transports air from the lungs; contains a membrane lining that is continuous with the sinuses.
2. *Sinuses*—four pairs of hollow cavities located in head; drain mucus directly into nose; give reasonance to voice.
3. *Larynx*—the organ of voice located between the base of the tongue and the trachea; air passing over vocal cords during expiration causes them to vibrate and produce sounds that are formed into words by the lips, teeth, and tongue.
4. *Trachea*—extends from larynx to the mainstream bronchus; serves as a passageway for air from the upper respiratory system to the lower airway system.
5. *Bronchi and bronchioles*—a branching treelike structure that begins with the right and left

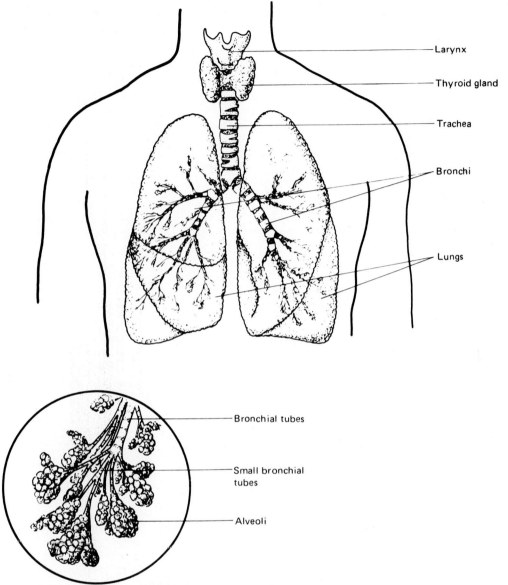

Larynx

Thyroid gland

Trachea

Bronchi

Lungs

Bronchial tubes

Small bronchial tubes

Alveoli

FIGURE 20–1   The lower respiratory tract.

bronchi and leads to progressively smaller tubes known as bronchi and bronchioles; serve as passageways directly to lungs.

6. *Lungs*—two cone-shaped organs located on the right and left sides of the thoracic cavity; left lung contains two lobes and right lung contains three; covered by a two-layered membrane known as the *pleura* that also covers the diaphragm and lines the thoracic cavity.

7. *Alveoli*—highly elastic sacs that are the working units of the lung; oxygen and carbon dioxide are exchanged between each alveolus and a capillary that surrounds it.

8. *Respiratory muscles*—diaphragm, intercostal muscles, other thoracic and abdominal muscles change the shape of the thoracic cavity during inspiration and expiration.

9. *Circulation*—bronchial arteries and veins supply the airways and lung tissue; pulmonary veins carry oxygenated blood from the lungs to the heart; pulmonary arteries carry carbon-dioxide-rich blood from the heart to the lungs; lymphatic vessels regulate immune responses in the lung and are believed to affect the amount of fluid in the lungs.

10. *Respiratory controls*—a respiratory center is located in the medulla oblongata and pons in

TABLE 20–1   Antitussives, Expectorants, and Mucolytics

Nonproprietary Name	Proprietary Name	Adult Dose Range	Notes
Antitussives			
benzonatate	Tessalon	100 mg PO 3–6×/day to maximum of 600 mg/day	Higher doses may be prescribed; do not chew
codeine phosphate, sulfate		5 ml PO of elixir; 15 mg PO	Narcotic; elixir may also contain terpin hydrate
dextromethorphan hydrobromide	Pertussin 8-hour Romilar Sucrets and others	15–30 mg PO 3–4×/day	Available as syrup; should not be administered to patients taking monoamine oxidase inhibitors
diphenhydramine hydrochloride	Benylin and others	25 mg PO every 4 h to a maximum of 100 mg/24 h	Also acts as an antihistamine; may produce drowsiness and drying of secretions
hydrocodone bitartrate	Hycodan	5–10 mg PO in a multi-ingredient syrup	Narcotic; multi-ingredient syrup also contains analgesic antipyretic
levopropoxyphene napsylate	Novrad	5–100 mg PO every 4 h up to a maximum of 600 mg/day	Available in capsules and syrup
noscapine	Tusscapine	15–30 mg PO 3–4×/day 60 mg PO single dose	
Expectorants			
guaifenesin (glyceryl guaiacolate)	Robitussin and many others	200–400 mg PO every 4 h to a maximum of 2.4 g/day	Elixir
potassium iodide	SSKI and others	Highly individualized	Older drug rarely used; see manufacturer's directions; administer with juice and have patient sip through a straw
terpin hydrate		5–10 ml PO every 3–4 h as needed	Elixir contains alcohol
Mucolytics			
acetylcysteine	Mucomyst	2–20 ml of 10% solution; 1–10 ml of 20% solution; by nebulizer every 2–6 h	May also be used experimentally for treatment of acute acetaminophen poisoning
tyloxapol	Alevaire	500 ml/12–24 h via nebulizer	Not used for patients with asthma because it increases incidence of bronchospasm

the brain; chemoreceptor bodies in the aorta and carotid arteries respond to changes in oxygen, carbon dioxide, and hydrogen ion levels in the bloodstream and cerebrospinal fluid; phrenic nerves and branches of the vagus nerve provide local control by the nervous system.

11. *Bony protection*—the thorax, ribs, and vertebrae provide bony protection for respiratory organs.

ANTITUSSIVES, EXPECTORANTS, MUCOLYTICS

Antitussives are drugs that suppress coughs. *Expectorants* are drugs that thin respiratory secretions making it easier for the patient to clear them by coughing. Mucolytics are drugs that break up and thin mucus so that it may be expectorated. (See Table 20–1.)

A *cough* is a normal physiological mechanism that helps a person expel foreign bodies and clear the respiratory system of secretions. Cough generally indicates irritation in the respiratory system. In some cases, irritation is produced by substances such as smoke, dust, or chemicals. In other cases, cough develops because excessive amounts of mucus are being secreted. Asthma, bronchitis, common cold, emphysema, lung tumor, pneumonia, and tuberculosis are respiratory diseases that may cause a person to cough. A cough that persists for longer than 2 weeks is one of the danger signals of cancer.

Usually a cough is desirable because it clears the patient's respiratory system. The physician prescribes expectorants and mucolytics for the patient with excessive or thickened secretions. Occasionally a cough is unproductive, annoying, or undesirable: when the cough center in the brain is irritated by disease, or when the patient has *hemoptysis*. For these patients, the physician may prescribe an antitussive to suppress cough.

I. Actions and uses.
   A. *Narcotic antitussives* depress the cough center in the brain to suppress the cough reflex.
   B. *Nonnarcotic antitussives* act centrally to suppress cough but the exact mechanism is not known.
   C. *Expectorants* are drugs given orally to thin respiratory secretions and make them easier for the patient to cough up.
   D. *Mucolytics* act as detergents to liquefy thick mucus by breaking up mucoproteins that hold thick mucus together. Most mucolytics are administered by inhalation via a nebulizer.
   E. Antitussives and expectorants are often administered as elixirs.

II. Adverse responses.
   A. Antitussives.
      1. May suppress the cough reflex excessively and may contribute to retained secretions in the tracheobronchial tree. Atelectasis, hypoxia, elevated carbon dioxide levels, and respiratory failure may result from retained secretions.
      2. Narcotic antitussives may produce nausea, vomiting, constipation, drug dependence. See p. 127 for additional information.
      3. Self-medication with nonprescribed antitussives and expectorants is common. This practice may prevent a person from seeking medical attention for a cough.
      4. Adverse effects may develop from individual ingredients present in multi-ingredient preparations.
   B. Mucolytics—nausea and vomiting, bronchospasm, stomatitis, hypersensitivity.
   C. Infection may result when solutions and equipment used for the inhalation route are contaminated.

III. Nursing implications.
   A. Collect a careful nursing history. A minimum of information includes: length, duration, and description of cough, prescribed and nonprescribed drugs being taken, allergies, and information about the patient's respirations.
   B. Administer elixirs last if several oral drugs are to be administered at the same time. Do not administer water with elixirs.
   C. Seek additional information before administering elixirs to patients with alcoholism taking disulfiram as treatments. Some elixirs contain alcohol that may produce a drug interaction.
   D. Record changes in the amount, color, odor, consistency of sputum.
   E. Provide additional tissues, bag for disposal, and receptacle for sputum collection.
   F. Encourage increased fluid intake and provide warm liquids to reduce irritation of mucous membrane linings in respiratory system.
   G. Teach the patient how to cough effectively when expectorants or mucolytics are prescribed.
   H. Seek additional information before administering to women during pregnancy. Antitussives are generally not recommended during pregnancy.
   I. Teach patients not to eat or drink for 15 min after taking expectorant, antitussive syrups.
   J. Assist the patient to wash face and hands, rinse mouth after drugs are administered by inhalation.
   K. Follow hospital procedures for aftercare of equipment used to administer drugs by inhalation.
   L. Teach patients to avoid other nonprescribed drugs and alcohol while taking antitussives, expectorants, mucolytics.
   M. Teach patients to read labels on all nonprescribed drugs for cough, expectoration.
   N. Teach family, friends, and neighbors to seek medical attention for any cough that persists for more than a week.
   O. Encourage patients, family members, friends, and neighbors not to smoke. Suggest a stop smoking program to smokers who want to quit.

TABLE 20–2   Bronchodilators

Nonproprietary Name	Proprietary Name	Adult Dose Range	Notes
Adrenergic Agents (See also Table 17–2)			
albuterol	Proventil Ventolin	2–4 mg PO 3–4/day; 1–2 in- halations every 4–6 h	
bitolerol	Tornalate	One inhalation every 5–8 h	New adrenergic drug; longer acting; may be used with corticosteroid or theophylline preparation
ephedrine sulfate		15–50 mg PO, SC; 20 mg IV	Longer acting
epinephrine bitartrate	Medihaler-Epi	0.3 mg per oral inhalation	
epinephrine inhala- tion 1:100		1:100 solution is placed in a nebulizer or positive-pres- sure breathing machine	Dosage highly individualized; must never be injected; read label care- fully and do not confuse with epi- nephrine for injection
epinephrine injec- tion 1:1,000	Adrenalin, Epinephrine	1:1,000 aqueous solution 0.1–0.5 ml SC, may be re- peated in 20 min if neces- sary; 0.25 mg IV	Used mainly to relieve acute bron- chospasm
epinephrine suspen- sion 1:200	Asmolin Sus-Phrine	0.1–0.3 ml SC, may be re- peated after 4 h if neces- sary	Longer acting; must never be injected IV; check label carefully
ethylnorepinephrine hydrochloride	Bronkephrine	1–2 mg SC, IM	
isoetharine	Bronkosol Bronkometer	1–2 inhalations 4 ×/day; also available as a solution for a nebulizer or positive-pres- sure breathing machine	
isoproterenol hydro- chloride inhalation	Isuprel Mistometer Norisodrine Aerotrol	0.5 of a 0.5% solution di- luted in water or saline and inhaled as mist over 10–20 min	
metaproterenol sulfate	Alupent Metaprel	0.2 mg PO 3–4 ×/day; 2–3 inhalations every 4 h; daily dose should not ex- ceed 12 inhalations	
methoxyphenamine hydroxide	Orthoxine	50–100 mg PO every 3–4 h if needed	
protokylol hydro- chloride	Ventaire	2–4 mg PO 2–4 ×/day	
terbutaline sulfate	Brethine Bricanyl	2.5–5 mg PO 3 ×/day at 6-h intervals; 0.25 mg SC, may be repeated in 30 min	May be used as tocolytic (see p. 217)

BRONCHODILATORS

Bronchodilators are drugs that widen bronchial airways to relax smooth muscle (Tables 20–2 and 20–3). The patient with narrowing of bronchial airways has spasm of smooth muscle in bronchioles. Spasms prevent sufficient air from entering the lungs; they lead to excess mucus production, swelling, and inflammation of bronchiole tissue. The patient experiences dyspnea, wheezing, tachycardia, fatigue, cough, and fear.

Common causes of bronchospasm include allergy, asthma, bronchitis, drug hypersensitivity, emphysema, infection, nasal polyps. Status asthmaticus is a medical emergency in which the patient has continuous bronchospasm that does not respond to treatment. Respiratory failure and death may follow.

Air pollution, cold air, exercise, emotional stress, and smoke are factors known to induce bronchospasm in individuals with underlying disease of the respiratory system.

TABLE 20–2 (*cont.*)

Nonproprietary Name	Proprietary Name	Adult Dose Range	Notes
Theophylline Derivatives			
aminophylline	Lixaminol, Somophyllin	500–1,000 mg for acute asthma attack; IV rate should not exceed 25 mg/min; also available as rectal suppositories	Dosage highly individualized; used mainly for acute attacks. For IV administration, see manufacturer's directions; too-rapid IV administration may cause cardiac arrhythmias, hypotension, cardiac arrest
dyphylline	Airet Lufyllin Neothyllin and others	15 mg/kg PO every 6 h. 250–500 mg IM every 6 h	Dosage highly individualized
oxtriphylline	Choledyl	200 mg PO 4×/day	
theophylline	Aerolate Brondokyl Liquophyllin SloPhyllin Theolair and others	160 mg/kg PO per day in three to four divided doses	Serum concentrations of 8–10 μg/ml are considered therapeutic; sustained release preparation available—these should not be crushed
theophylline sodium glycinate	Synophylate	330–660 mg PO every 6–8 h after meals	
Other Antiasthmatics			
beclomethasone diproprionate	Beclovent Vanceril	2–4 inhalations 3–4×/day; total dose should not exceed 20 inhalations per day	Not a bronchodilator but a corticosteroid that acts directly on mucous membranes; may be prescribed for the patient with severe chronic lung disease; systemic side effects may develop from long-term use; oral candidiasis is a frequent side effect; see p. 260 for additional information.
cromolyn sodium	Intal	20 mg capsule puctured and inhaled via inhaler 4×/day	Used only as prevention; not effective once bronchospasm has developed.
triamcinolone acetonide	Azmacort	2–4 inhalations 3–4×/day; total dose should not exceed 16 inhalations per day	Not a bronchodilator; a glucocorticoid that acts directly on mucous membranes; may be prescribed for patients with severe chronic lung disease; systemic side effects may develop from long-term use; see p. 260 for additional information.

Abbreviations: CNS, central nervous system.

I. Actions and uses.
  A. *Adrenergic bronchodilators* are drugs that mimic sympathetic nerves. This group of drugs acts directly on adrenergic receptors in smooth muscle to produce relaxation.
  B. *Theophylline bronchodilators* are central nervous system stimulants that relax smooth muscle in bronchioles and also stimulate respiratory centers in the medulla. These drugs may be used to prevent asthma attacks and/or relieve them. Serum theophylline levels of 5-8 mg/ml indicate a therapeutic range.
  C. *Corticosteroids* are adrenal hormones administered orally, IV, or by inhalation to relieve bronchospasm. These drugs relieve bronchospasm by suppressing associated inflammation, influencing the immune responses, and increasing the effects of epinephrine and morepinephrine during stressful situations. Additional information can be located on p. 260.
  D. Cromolyn sodium is a drug that prevents an asthma attack by suppressing the release in his-

TABLE 20–3   Selected Combination Bronchodilator Preparations

Proprietary Name	Ingredients	Adult Dosage
Asminyl	aminophylline 130 mg, ephedrine sulfate 26 mg, phenobarbital 8 mg	1–2 tablets PO
Bronkotabs	theophylline 100 mg, ephedrine sulfate 24 mg, guaifenesin 100 mg, phenobarbital 8 mg	1 tablet PO
Marax	theophylline 130 mg, ephedrine sulfate 25 mg, hydroxyzine hydrochloride 10 mg	1 tablet PO 4×/day
Quadrinal	theophylline 65 mg, ephedrine sulfate 24 mg, potassium iodide 320 mg, phenobarbital 24 mg	1 tablet PO
Quibron	theophylline 150 mg, guaifenesin 90 mg	1–2 capsules PO every 6–8 h, 15–30 PO elixir
Tedral, Theofedral	theophylline 130 mg, ephedrine hydrochloride 24 mg, phenobarbital 8 mg	1–2 tablets PO every 4 h

   tamine and other chemical substances by mast cells during an allergic response. The drug is
   not a bronchodilator and is used only to prevent asthma attacks.
   E. Many drugs contain multiple ingredients. A typical combination includes theophylline bronchodilator and an expectorant or an adrenergic bronchodilator (see Table 20–3).
II. Adverse responses.
   A. Adrenergic bronchodilator.
      1. Headache, restlessness, tremors, weakness, fear, and anxiety.
      2. Cerebral hemorrhage, cardiac arrhythmias, increased anginal pain, palpitations.
      3. See also p. 155.
   B. Theophylline bronchodilators.
      1. Central nervous system—nervousness, restlessness, tremors, insomnia; toxicity may produce fatal convulsions.
      2. Cardiovascular system—tachycardia, cardiac arrhythmias, hypotension, cardiac arrest.
      3. Diuresis.
      4. Respiratory system: respiratory rate increases.
      5. Gastrointestinal system: nausea, vomiting.
      6. Serum theophylline levels greater than 15 mg/ml indicate toxicity.
   C. Cromolyn sodium—cough, bronchospasm, nasal congestion, hoarseness, urticaria, rash, myositis, gastroenteritis.
   D. Inhalers may produce dryness and irritation of mucous membranes, infection.
   E. Drug interactions include:
      • An increase of plasma levels that can produce toxicity and death when bronchodilators are combined with monoamine oxidase inhibitors, cimetidine, clindamycin, erthromycin, lincomycin, phenytoin, troleandomycin.
      • A decrease in therapeutic effects of bronchodilators when combined with lithium, phenobarbital, propranolol and its relatives (see Table 18–5).
      • A reduction of antihypertensive effects of guanethidine, reserpine when combined with adrenergic bronchodilators.
III. Nursing implications.
   A. Collect a careful nursing history because bronchodilators must be used with great caution in patients with cardiovascular or liver disease.
   B. Gather information about nonprescription drugs the patient uses at home. Most nonprescription drugs for breathing problems contain an adrenergic brochodilator. Cumulative effects may produce toxicity when combined with the physician's prescription.
   C. Observe and record information about the patient's respiratory state. Minimum information

includes: respiratory rate and characteristics, presence or absence of cough, description of mucus if productive cough is present, wheezing, tachycardia, skin color, and behavior.

    D. Use nondrug measures that improve breathing: position the patient in semi-Fowler's, force fluids to 3 L/day to keep mucus thin; encourage and demonstrate effective coughing techniques.

    E. Anticipate the patient's need for frequent rest periods, assistance with hygiene, eating and ambulation because of fatigue associated with increased work of breathing.

    F. Use nonverbal touch to convey caring and reassurance. Excessive conversation increases the patient's fatigue and dyspnea.

    G. Provide additional tissues, a paper bag for tissue disposal, and a receptacle for sputum.

    H. Administer oral preparations with at least 1 full glass of water to reduce gastrointestinal side effects and encourage fluid intake. Follow with antitussive syrup if both are ordered for the same hour.

    I. Administer SC preparations to rotated sites when repeated injections are needed. The deltoid area is often used.

    J. Follow manufacturer's direction for IV administration of aminophylline. Do not administer too rapidly. Use a volume control pump or administration set when large volumes are ordered.

    K. Review the procedure for administering bronchodilators by inhalation and cleaning equipment (see p. 106). Teach these procedures to the patient.

    L. Teach patients taking theophylline preparations to avoid excessive intake of coffee, tea, colas and other caffeinated beverages. Caffeine increases central nervous system side effects.

    M. Monitor serum theophylline levels when available.

    N. Teach patient to avoid substances that irritate bronchial airways and stimulate brochospasm: known allergens, smoking, noxious fumes, aerosol cosmetics, and household cleaning products.

    O. Never increase the liter flow of prescribed oxygen when the patient is known to have asthma or chronic lung disease. High doses of oxygen may remove the hypoxic stimulus to breathe and produce respiratory arrest.

NASAL DECONGESTANTS

Nasal decongestants are drugs that reduce swelling and discharge of secretions from the nose (Table 20–4). The patient with an allergy or the common cold usually has swollen mucous membranes, rhinitis (inflammation), and rhinorrhea (runny nose).

   I. Action and uses:

    A. Most nasal decongestants are adrenergic drugs that relieve or prevent congestion by producing vasoconstriction of arterioles in the nose.

    B. Nasal decongestants may be used to relieve symptoms of allergy, common cold.

    C. Nasal decongestants may also be used to reduce bleeding during surgery on the nose and to improve visualization of the nose during physical examination, reduce congestion around the eustachian tubes during ear infections of air travel.

    D. Local applications via nose drops or nasal spray may be ordered for short-term use of nasal decongestants. The oral route is generally preferred for long-term use.

  II. Adverse responses.

    A. Adverse responses for adrenergic drugs can be located on p. 155.

    B. Even local application may produce systemic side effects either by absorption through nasal mucosa or swallowing of excess drug and absorption via the gastrointestinal system.

    C. Stinging, dryness, burning may occur after local applications.

    D. Rebound nasal congestion and damage to nasal muscosa may occur with long-term local applications.

    E. Adrenergic agents increase intraocular pressure in patients with glaucoma.

TABLE 20–4   Nasal Decongestants

Nonproprietary Name	Proprietary Name	Adult Dose Range	Notes
ephedrine hydro-chloride sulfate	Efedron Nasal, Vantronol	2–4 drops in each nostril every 3–4 h	Also available as a jelly in various strengths
epinephrine hydro-chloride	Adrenalin Chlo-ride	1–2 drops in each nostril every 4–6 h	
naphazoline hydro-chloride	Privine and others	2 drops or spray in each nostril every 4–6 h	Available as 0.05% nebulizer, 0.1% ophthalmic solution; causes stinging and irritation to mucous membranes
oxymetazoline hydro-chloride	Afrin and others	2–3 drops or spray in each nostril twice per day	Available as 0.25% and 0.05% solutions. Should not be used longer than 3–5 days
phenylephrine hydro-chloride	Neo-Synephrine, others	2–3 drops or spray in each nostril every 3–4 h; 10 mg PO 3×/day	Available as 0.25–1% solutions
phenylpropanolamine hydrochloride	Propradrine	25–50 mg PO every 3–8 h depending upon dose	Also available as elixir (4 mg/ml)
propylhexadrine	Benzedrex	Inhale once or twice through each nostril while blocking the other nostril	
pseudophedrine hydrochloride	Sudafed	60 mg PO 3–4×/day; 120 mg PO 2×/day for sustained release capsules	
terfenadine	Seldane	60 mg PO twice a day	New antihistamine prescribed for the patient with allergic rhinitis
tetrahydrozoline hydrochloride	Tyzine	2–4 drops in each nostril no more often than every 3 h	Available as 0.05 and 1% nasal solutions, also available as ophthalmic solutions
tuaminoheptane sul-fate	Tuamine	4–5 drops in each nostril no more often than 4–5×/day	Should not be used for longer than 4–5 days
xylometazoline hydro-chloride	Otrivin, others	2–3 drops or spray in each nostril every 8–10 h	Available as 0.05 and 0.1% nasal solutions

 F. Drug interactions include:
  • Potentially fatal interaction when combined with MAOIs (Table 16–6).
  • See p. 155 for interactions associated with adrenergic drugs.
III. Nursing implications.
 A. Collect and record the nursing history. A minimum of information includes: allergies, respiratory status, characteristics of nasal discharge if present, use of prescribed and nonprescribed drugs.
 B. Anticipate the patient's need for additional tissues, disposal bag.
 C. Administer local application using correct procedure (for review see p. 105).
 D. Use hospital procedure for aftercare of equipment following local application.
 E. Teach patients to blow the nose gently to help relieve congestion.
 F. Teach patients not to loan or borrow nasal decongestants.
 G. Teach patients to dispose of nasal sprays after 10–12 days of use.
 H. Teach patients to read labels on nonprescribed drugs.

CASE STUDY 14

Mr. Stanley Ludgate is a 72-year-old man with emphysema who is admitted to your nursing unit in respiratory distress. During the initial nursing assessment, you observe that Mr. Ludgate is dyspneic and wheezing with an occasional dry cough. The physician's orders include:

 • aminophylline 500 mg in 1,000 ml 5% dextrose in 0.45% normal saline by IV infusion over 6 hours.

A registered nurse prepares the infusion and asks you to get Mr. Ludgate ready for it. You will also be monitoring Mr. Ludgate during the infusion.

Answer the following questions about drug therapy for Mr. Ludgate.

1. What kind of drug is aminophylline and what are its intended effects for Mr. Ludgate?
2. What additional information needs to be obtained before the IV infusion of aminophylline is started?
3. What will you do to get Mr. Ludgate ready for the infusion?
4. What adverse responses will you look for while monitoring Mr. Ludgate during the IV infusion of aminophylline?
5. If the drop factor on the IV administration set reads 12 drops/ml, how fast should the intravenous administration unit run?
6. What nursing interventions are indicated for Mr. Ludgate in addition to those related to drug therapy?
7. After the infusion is completed, a serum theophylline level is drawn. The laboratory report indicates that Mr. Ludgate's drug level is within the therapeutic range. What clinical observations can you anticipate in view of this report?

EXERCISES

Circle the best answer for each of the following multiple-choice questions.

1. Antitussives are drugs that:
   a. Thin mucus.
   b. Stimulate respiration.
   c. Suppress cough.
   d. Dilate bronchi.
2. An adverse response to antitussive drugs that might occur includes:
   a. Retained secretions in the tracheobronchial tree.
   b. A respiratory infection from a contaminated inhaler.
   c. Swelling of mucous membrane lining the respiratory tract.
   d. Excessive coughing from irritation of mucous membranes.
3. Epinephrine may be prescribed subcutaneously in order to:
   a. Suppress cough and reduce associated fatigue.
   b. Dilate bronchioles and reduce bronchospasm.
   c. Liquefy sputum and reduce wheezing.
   d. Dilate blood vessels and raise blood pressure.
4. A nursing implication associated with administering elixirs is:
   a. Administer with a large glass of water to increase fluid intake.
   b. Use sterile equipment for each dose to prevent respiratory infection.
   c. Administer with meals to reduce gastrointestinal effects.
   d. Administer without food, water, and after oral drugs.
5. Decongestant nasal sprays and drops act primarily by:
   a. Dilating blood vessels in the nose.
   b. Stimulating breathing centers.
   c. Constricting blood vessels in the nose.
   d. Increasing nasal secretions.
6. If used too often as nose drops or nasal spray, ephedrine sulfate may cause:
   a. Rebound gastric distress.
   b. Hemoptysis.
   c. Rebound nasal congestion.
   d. Essential hypotension.

7. A nursing implication associated with decongestant nasal sprays or nose drops is:
   a. Administer daily to prevent adverse responses.
   b. Refrigerate drops and sprays to prevent contamination.
   c. Do not administer to a patient with respiratory infection.
   d. Teach patients to blow the nose gently to relieve congestion.

8. A nursing intervention that reduces adverse effects of nasal decongestant sprays or drops is:
   a. Use the correct method for instilling drops or sprays.
   b. Culture the nasal secretions before the first dose.
   c. Position the patient in the lateral Sims position.
   d. Discard all sprays and drops after 5 days.

9. A nursing intervention that enhances the effects of an expectorant is:
   a. Provide frequent rest periods.
   b. Place the patient in the supine position.
   c. Administer oxygen at the lowest possible dose.
   d. Assist the patient to use effective coughing techniques.

10. A nursing intervention that prevents theophylline toxicity is:
    a. Administer the theophylline drug before meals.
    b. Do not administer theophylline drugs with expectorants.
    c. Provide decaffeinated beverages when administering theophylline drugs.
    d. Do not administer theophylline drugs with antibiotics.

Chapter 21 | DRUG THERAPY AFFECTING THE PATIENT'S GASTROINTESTINAL SYSTEM

EXPECTED BEHAVIORAL OUTCOMES

After completing the chapter you should return to the expected behavioral outcomes and evaluate your ability to:

1. Relate the effects of a specific drug to the structure and function of the gastrointestinal system.
2. Compare antidiarrhea agents and laxatives with respect to their actions and uses; characteristics of bowel movements, adverse responses, and nursing implications.
3. List nursing implications to be considered when administering an antiemetic drug.
4. Identify the essential elements of patient teaching when administering mineral and vitamin supplements.
5. Explain the use of appetite suppressants, using terms appropriate for a teenager interested in losing weight.

STRUCTURE AND FUNCTION REVIEW

The gastrointestinal system contains organs for *digestion,* a process that transforms food into substances that can be used by the cell. (See Figure 21-1.) The entire digestive process includes at least three interrelated phases: ingestion, propulsion, storage, absorption, and elimination.

Included in the gastrointestinal system are the alimentary tract and accessory organs of digestion. Table 21-1 describes the structures and functions of the alimentary tract. Table 21-2 describes the structures and functions of accessory organs of digestion.

Digestion occurs as both a mechanical and chemical process. *Physical or mechanical digestion* is the breaking up of food into smaller parts and substances. *Chemical digestion* is primarily a process of hydrolysis brought about by the actions of enzymes. Carbohydrates are converted to simple sugars.

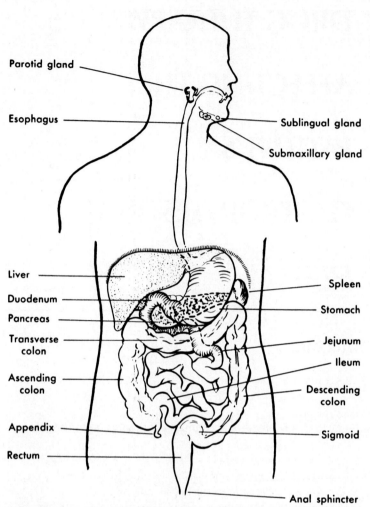

FIGURE 21–1   The digestive tract. (From Robinson, C. H.: *Basic Nutrition and Diet Therapy*, 3rd ed. Macmillan, New York, 1975.)

TABLE 21–1   The Alimentary Tract

Structure	Functions
Mouth	Receives food and contains some accessory organs for moistening and mastication, deglutition
Pharynx	Receives food and transports it to esophagus
Esophagus	Receives food and propels it to the stomach
Stomach	Receives food and stores it; processess food through mechanical and chemical activities; propels food in small portions into small intestines
Small intestines	Receives bile from the gall bladder; receives pancreatic secretions; digests and absorbs foods and drugs
Large intestines	Digests and absorbs food; propels waste products of digestion to rectum; forms feces; eliminates waste products via feces

TABLE 21–2   Accessory Organs of Digestion

Structure	Functions
Tongue	Assists in mastication, deglutition, digestion; organ of taste
Teeth	Assists in mastication
Salivary glands	Form saliva containing enzymes and secrete it to moisten food
Pancreas	Manufactures and secretes pancreatic fluid for digestion; manufactures and secretes insulin and glucagon for glucose metabolism
Liver	Manufactures bile, glycogen, fibrinogen, heparin, immune substances, plasma proteins, prothrombin; stores blood, vitamins, iron, copper; detoxifies alcohol, drugs, metals, and other harmful substances
Gallbladder	Stores bile and secretes it into the duodenum for fat digestion

Fats are transformed into fatty acids and glycerols. Proteins are transformed into amino acids. These simpler substances are then absorbed into the bloodstream and carried to the cells for nourishment.

Gastrointestinal functions strongly influence the fate of drugs administered by the oral route. The effects of drugs may be profoundly increased or decreased by changes in gastrointestinal activity.

ANTACIDS

Antacids are drugs that neutralize or remove acid from the stomach (Table 21–3). They are prescribed primarily for the patient with reflux esophagitis, peptic ulcer disease, or other conditions involving gastric hyperacidity. The patient with reflux esophagitis has an inflammation of the esophagus caused by a backup of gastric contents from the stomach into the esophagus. The patient with peptic ulcer disease has an erosion of the mucous membrane lining the duodenum or stomach. This erosion is associated with an increase in gastric acid.

Antacids have become abused by laypeople who are persuaded by advertising that normal gastrointestinal activities or occasional discomfort ought to be controlled by taking a particular brand of antacid. Thus, a particular role for the nurse is to explain how the gastrointestinal system works and how to maintain normal function. This helps the nonmedical person make choices about nonprescribed drugs that are based upon facts.

I. Actions and uses.
   A. Most antacids are chemical bases that neutralize acid content in the stomach. As the acid content of the stomach becomes more alkaline, gastric emptying time speeds up.
   B. Antacids relieve pain and burning associated with reflux esophagitis and peptic ulcer.
   C. Antacids help to shorten the healing time in patients with peptic ulcer disease.
   D. Antacids may be prescribed for prevention or treatment of stress ulcers.
   E. Antacids may be prescribed just prior to anesthesia, endoscopy, or caesarian section or for the patient in coma. The intention is to prevent aspiration pneumonia or pneumonitis if the patient accidentally aspirates gastric contents.
   F. Antacids may be administered by nasogastric drip for the patient with gastrointestinal bleeding.
   G. Antacids containing aluminum may be prescribed for the patient with diarrhea.
   H. Antacids containing magnesium may be prescribed as a laxative for the patient with constipation.
   I. Antacids may be prescribed occasionally to prevent some patients from developing kidney stones.

TABLE 21–3　Selected Antacid Combinations

Proprietary Name	Ingredients	Adult Dose Range	Notes
Alka Seltzer	citric acid, potassium bicarbonate, sodium bicarbonate	1–2 tablets dissolved in water	Not recommended for persons on a sodium-restricted diet
Amphogel	aluminum hydroxide, sodium	2 tablets or 10 ml PO as directed by physician	See text for dose regimens; may cause constipation
Basaljel	aluminum carbonate, sodium	1–2 capsules or tablets, 5–10 mg as directed by the physician	Same as above
Camalox	aluminum hydroxide, calcium carbonate, magnesium hydroxide, sodium	10–20 ml or 2–3 tablets PO per day as directed by physician	
Creamalin	aluminum hydroxide, magnesium hydroxide, sodium	See Amphogel	
Delcid	aluminum hydroxide, magnesium hydroxide, sodium	5 ml PO as directed by the physician	Maximum dose should not exceed 30 ml/24 h
Di-Gel	aluminum hydroxide, magnesium hydroxide, simethicone, sodium	2 chewable tablets or 10 ml PO as directed by physician	Maximum dose should not exceed 20 tablets or 100 ml/24 h
Gaviscon	aluminum hydroxide, magnesium trisilicate, sodium hydroxide	See package insert	
Gelusil	aluminum hydroxide, magnesium hydroxide, simethicone, sodium	10 ml or 2 tablets PO as directed by physician	Maximum dose should not exceed 60 ml or 12 tablets/24 h; Gelusil II contains the same ingredients in larger doses
Kolantyl Gel	aluminum hydroxide, magnesium hydroxide, sodium	5–20 ml or 1–4 wafers PO as directed by physician	Maximum dose should not exceed 60 ml or 12 wafers per 24 h
Maalox	aluminum hydroxide, magnesium hydroxide, sodium	10–30 ml or 1–4 tablets PO as directed by physician	Maalox Plus contains the additional ingredient of simethicone; check labels of specific preparations for maximum doses
Marblen	calcium carbonate, magnesium carbonate, magnesium phosphate, magnesium trisilicate	See package insert	May produce diarrhea
Mylanta	aluminum hydroxide, magnesium hydroxide, simethicone, sodium	5–10 ml or 1–2 tablets PO as directed by physician	Mylanta II contains the same ingredients in larger doses
Riopan	magaldrate, sodium	400–800 mg (5–10 ml) PO as directed by the physician	Riopan Plus contains additional ingredient of simethicone; available as tablets for chewing or swallowing
Silain Gel	aluminum hydroxide, magnesium hydroxide, simethicone, sodium	See package insert	
Titralac	calcium carbonate, glycine, sodium	5–10 ml PO as directed by physician	Maximum dose should not exceed 40 ml (8 g)/day; available as chewable tablets
Trisogel	aluminum hydroxide, magnesium trisilicate, sodium	See package insert	
Win-Gel	aluminum hydroxide, magnesium hydroxide, sodium	5–10 ml or 1–2 tablets PO up to 4×/day as directed by physician	
Other Drugs			
Carafate	sucralfate	4 g PO per day in four divided doses before meals and at bedtime	Acts locally to form a protective coating over ulcerated gastrointestinal area; short-term use only; check with patient daily about constipation, do not administer antacids for 30 min before or after each dose

TABLE 21–3 *(cont.)*

Proprietary Name	Ingredients	Adult Dose Range	Notes
Tagamet	cimetidine	300 mg PO 4 ×/day with meals and at bedtime; 800 mg PO daily 300 mg IM every 6 h 300 mg IV every 6 h; must be diluted and infused according to package insert	Suppresses secretion of gastric acid by blocking effects of histamine; used for prevention and treatment; caution patient not to stop taking drug abruptly to prevent rebound symptoms from occurring
Zantac	ranitidine	150 mg PO 2 ×/day 50 mg IM, IV every 6–8 h	Same as for cimetidine above
500		1 tablet PO daily	

J. The dosage and frequency for antacids depends upon the patient's condition. For example, when antacids are prescribed for pain, the patient is usually instructed to take them as needed when the pain occurs. When antacids are prescribed to speed ulcer healing, the physician usually prescribes large doses 1 and 3 h after eating, at bedtime, and as needed. Thus, the minimum number of doses per day is seven.

K. A combination antacid preparation is most likely to be prescribed. The combination includes aluminum hydroxide and magnesium hydroxide. Combination preparations combine faster- and slower-acting ingredients for a more sustained action, reduce the side effects of constipation or diarrhea that may develop with a single-ingredient drug, and enable a lower dose to be administered. Selected combination preparations are described in Table 21–3.

L. Cimetidine and ranitidine are termed *histamine blockers*. These drugs suppress the secretion of gastric acid by blocking the effects of histamine.

M. Sucralfate is a drug ingested orally that promotes ulcer healing by forming a protective coat over the eroded area. Treatment with this agent is not prevention but short-term healing of an existing ulcer.

II. Adverse responses.

  A. Antacids.

    1. May cause metabolic acidosis in patients with renal failure.

    2. Persistent alkaline urine resulting from antacid use may predispose the patient to urinary tract infection and kidney stones.

    3. Prolonged use of aluminum hydroxide may cause nausea, vomiting, constipation; accompanying diet low in phosphorous may cause osteomalacia, low serum phosphorus; intestinal obstruction.

    4. Prolonged use of magnesium hydroxide may cause diarrhea.

    5. Neutralization of gastric acid may cause rebound hypersecretion and increased acidity in the stomach.

    6. The patient may develop elevated levels of aluminum, calcium, magnesium, sodium depending upon the specific antacid taken.

    7. The patient taking an antacid containing carbonates may develop belching, abdominal distention, nausea, flatulence

    8. Drug interactions include:
- Antacids interfere with absorption of other oral agents.
- Antacids decrease the effects of anticoagulants, benzodiazepines, digoxin, iron preparations, phenothiazines, phenytoin, propranolol, sulfadiazine, tetracyclines.
- Increased nausea, vomiting, gastric irritation when antacids cause enteric coating on tablets to break down too soon.

  B. Histamine blockers.

    1. Central nervous system side effects include headache, dizziness, fatigue, confusion, slurred speech, delirium, hallucinations, coma. Alterations in consciousness more likely in the elderly.

2. Constipation or diarrhea.
3. Bradycardia or other cardiac effects may occur with rapid IV injection.
4. Gynecomastia, reduction of sperm count and sexual interest, impotence in men, galactorrhea in women.
5. Liver or kidney damage has been reported with cimetidine.
6. Malaise, muscle pains, skin rash, fever.
7. Relapse of symptoms progressing to ulcer perforation have been reported with abrupt withdrawal of cimetidine.
8. Drug interactions include:
   - Potentially toxic effects of oral anticoagulants, benzodiazepines, theophylline may develop when combined with cimetidine.
   - Cimetidine may affect the absorption of other oral agents.

C. Sucralfate.
   1. Nausea, vomiting, indigestion, dry mouth, constipation may develop.
   2. Miscellaneous symptoms include rash, dizziness, drowsiness, back pain.
   3. Drug interactions include:
      - Reduction of effects of tetracyclines when combined with sucralfate.
      - Reduced absorption of sucralfate when combined with an antacid.
D. Anticholinergics increase the effects of antacids and cholinergics tend to decrease the effects of antacids.

III. Nursing implications.
   A. Gather and record a careful nursing history. Antacids must be selected carefully on the basis of sodium content for the patient on a sodium-restricted diet, with liver or kidney disease.
   B. Shake suspensions well before administering. Offer the patient only a sip of water after he or she has taken suspensions.
   C. Instruct patients to moisten chewable tablets thoroughly before swallowing. Offer ½ glass of water or milk.
   D. Administer antacids at least 1 h before or 2 h after other medications to prevent drug interactions. Request help from the registered nurse to schedule medication times.
   E. Check manufacturer's instructions before IM, IV administration of cimetidine, ranitidine. Avoid rapid IV infusion which may trigger cardiovascular side effects.
   F. Assess, report, and record characteristics of the patient's pain. Dosage adjustments may be made according to the patient's pain. A minimum of information includes: location and description of pain, onset related to last meal, intensity, factors that increase or decrease pain intensity.
   G. Monitor and record the patient's food intake.
   H. Record the number and characteristics of the patient's stools. Constipation, fecal impactions, and intestinal obstruction have been reported with aluminum and calcium antacids. Diarrhea may develop with magnesium compounds.
   I. Teach the patient nondrug measures that reduce gastrointestinal symptoms: eat small- or medium-sized meals at regular intervals; eat a balanced diet; eat sitting up in a comfortable chair; avoid reclining after meals; avoid substances that increase gastric secretions (caffeine beverages, alcohol, cigarette smoking).
   J. Teach patients to avoid nonprescribed drugs, especially aspirin.
   K. Teach family, friends, neighbors, patients to seek medical attention when indigestion persists or when it is accompanied by chest pain, diaphoresis, dyspnea, a feeling of doom, or tarry stools.

ANTIDIARRHEA AGENTS

Antidiarrhea agents are drugs that relieve diarrhea (Table 21–4). The patient with diarrhea has an increased number of stools related to increased peristalsis that speeds the movement of food and fluids through the large intestine. Stools may be semiliquid, liquid, or watery and the number may vary

TABLE 21–4 Antidiarrhea Agents

Nonproprietary Name	Proprietary Name	Adult Dose Range	Notes
Adsorbent and Protective Agents			
activated charcoal		Dose varies according to patient's condition	Adsorbing agent; check package insert or with pharmacist for recommended doses
aluminum hydroxide	Amphojel and others	5–10 ml PO as directed by the physician	Protective agent
aluminum trisilicate		1 g PO 4×/day as directed by physician	Protective agent
bismuth salts	Pepto-Bismol and others	1 tablet or 5 ml PO 4×/day as directed	Protective and adsorbent; used more often in peptic ulcer disease
kaolin, pectin	Kaopectate and others	60–120 ml PO after each loose bowel movement	Adsorbing agent; pectin alone may used by administering one ground apple
simethicone	Mylicon	40–80 mg PO after each meal and at bedtime, available as chewable tablets	Adsorbing agent especially helpful for flatulence; often used in combination with antacids
Opiate Derivatives			
diphenoxylate hydro-chloride and atro-pine sulfate	Lomotil and others	20 mg PO per day in di-vided doses	May produce atropinelike side effects
loperamide hydro-chloride	Imodium	4–8 mg PO per day up to a maximum of 16 mg PO per day	May produce fatigue, drowsiness, nau-sea, vomiting; overdose produces usual central nervous system depres-sion
opium tincture		0.5–1 ml PO mixed with water	Contains morphine; mixing with water causes milky-white appearance; read label carefully to avoid interchanging accidentally with paregoric
paregoric		5–10 ml PO	Contains morphine; read label carefully to avoid accidental interchange with opium tincture
Other Agents			
antibiotics	See Chapter 24	See Chapter 24	Antibiotics may be used when diarrhea is caused by infection from micro-organisms
anticholinergic agents	See Table 17–4	See Table 17–4	Anticholinergics may be used to relieve cramping pain or spasms associated with diarrhea
bulk-forming laxatives	See Table 21–7	See Table 21–7	Bulk-forming laxatives absorb water and increase stool mass but may increase sodium and potassium losses when used for diarrhea
cholestyramine resin	Questran	12–16 g PO per day in two to four divided doses be-fore meals and at bed-time; mix with a full glass of water as directed	A resin that binds bile acids; may be used for the patient with diarrhea caused by Crohn's disease, surgical procedures on the intestines, used primarily to lower lipoproteins; review pp. 188–189 for adverse responses and nursing implications
pancreatin	Viokase	300–1,000 mg PO with meals or snacks	Used for replacement when diarrhea re-sults from deficiency of natural pan-creatic enzymes

from 1 to 40 or more stools per day. The patient may also have abdominal cramps, nausea, vomiting, weakness, and/or fever.

Diarrhea is not a disease but a symptom of irritation in the bowel. Some of the causes of diarrhea include infection, regional enteritis, ulcerative colitis, and partial bowel obstruction. Laxative abuse, vitamin deficiences, and side effects of drug therapy may also produce diarrhea. Systemic diseases associated with diarrhea include accidental or intentional poisoning, cardiac decompensation, electrolyte imbalance, uremia, endocrine disorders, or neurologic disease. An important part of the treatment for diarrhea is locating the cause and correcting it if possible.

Diarrhea may lead to dehydration and metabolic acidosis by depleting body stores of water, sodium, chloride, and bicarbonates. Bloody diarrhea may lead to anemia from blood loss. Diarrhea in infants is very serious and may be fatal if medical treatment is delayed.

In addition to the antidiarrhea agents list in Table 21–4, the physician may also prescribe an anticholinergic drug from among those listed in Table 17–4 to reduce peristalsis and relieve abdominal cramps. The nurse assists the patient with diarrhea by: observing, recording, and reporting information about the stools, administering drug therapy, observing the patient for complications, and selecting nondrug measures that prevent complications and promote comfort.

I. Actions and uses.
  A. *Adsorbents* are powders that attract and retain bacteria, gases, toxins, and other substances associated with diarrhea. *Protectives* are drugs that cover the mucous membrane lining of the colon to prevent further irritation. These agents are ingested orally but act locally in the colon.
  B. *Opiate derivatives* are narcotic drugs that tend to act selectively on opiate receptors in the brain and intestinal muscles (see Chapter 16).
  C. *Antibiotics* are drugs that kill or inhibit the growth of microorganisms that cause diarrhea. See Chapter 24 for additional information.
  D. *Anticholinergics* are drugs that block the effects of acetylcholine on parasympathetic nerves. They may be prescribed for the patient with cramps and abdominal pain associated with diarrhea. See pp. 157–160 for additional information.
  E. *Bile-binding resins* are drugs that react with bile acids. The main use of these agents is to lower cholesterol levels in patients at risk for atherosclerosis. However, they may also be prescribed for the patient with diarrhea caused by Crohn's disease or surgical procedures on the intestines (ileostomy, colostomy, and similar procedures). See pp. 188–189 for additional information.
  F. *Bulk-forming laxatives* such as those listed in Table 21–7 may be prescribed occasionally for the patient with acute diarrhea associated with irritable colon, colostomy, diverticulosis, or ileostomy. These agents increase the mass of stool.
II. Adverse responses—see also adverse responses associated with anticholingerics, bile-binding resins, bulk-forming laxatives, and narcotics.
  A. Adsorbents and protectives may interfere with absorption of other drugs, particularly anticholinergics and tetracyclines. Antacid protectives may produce adverse responses similar to those described on p. 239.
  B. Opiate derivatives produce few side effects at recommended doses. At higher doses, euphoria and physical dependence may develop. In very high doses, typical central nervous system depression and other adverse responses may occur similar to those described on p. 127. Preparations combined with atropine may produce dry mouth, rash, dizziness, drowsiness, urinary retention. Abdominal cramps have been reported with loperamide.
  C. Opiate derivatives may interact with barbiturates to increase central nervous system depression. When combined with monoamine oxidase inhibitors, opiate antidiarrhea agents may produce hypertensive crisis. Antidiarrhea opiates also enhance the effects of other narcotics the patient may be receiving.
  D. Bulk-forming laxatives may increase the loss of sodium, potassium, and water.
III. Nursing implications.
  A. Measure and record, and report the volume, consistency, color, and other relevant informa-

tion about each of the patient's stools. Record the presence of blood, mucus, pus, as well as related symptoms such as cramping, weakness, nausea.

B. Anticipate the patient's need for easy access to the bathroom or bedpan. Provide additional toilet tissues and extra bedpan if diarrhea is especially severe.

C. In severe cases, watch the patient for dizziness, and weakness that may lead to accidents and falls. Place a commode chair next to the bedside and place the call bell in the patient's hand.

D. Prevent irritation to the skin in the anal area by cleansing gently with soap and water after each stool and drying the skin thoroughly. A protective coating of emollient may be applied to prevent acid fecal contents from coming in contact with the patient's skin.

E. Wash hands carefully after handling fecal material or clothing and linens soiled with fecal material. Offer the patient a washcloth after each diarrhea stool if handwashing at the sink is not possible.

F. Encourage an increased fluid intake orally if permitted. Extremely hot or cold beverages are generally avoided because they may stimulate peristalsis. The physician may prescribe warm clear liquids such as weak tea, jello, and broth. In some cases, the patient may be NPO and IV fluids may be ordered.

G. Measure intake and output carefully and record accurately; weigh the patient carefully and record. These measurements help the physician to estimate fluid loss.

H. Monitor laboratory studies when available. Electrolyte loss may be observed in a serum electrolyte report. Protein loss may be observed in the reports of total serum protein and albumin and globulin levels. Blood loss may be monitored through the hematocrit and hemoglobin reports.

I. Prevent diarrhea in the hospital, clinic, nursing home, doctor's office and at home by: washing hands thoroughly at appropriate times during the day; storing and preparing food safely; avoiding laxatives; keeping refrigerators clean.

J. Consult the registered nurse to schedule drug therapy at times least likely to cause diarrhea as a side effect.

K. Administer paregoric in 30 ml of water and anticipate the milky-white appearance of the mixture. Read label carefully to avoid confusing paregoric with tincture of opium.

L. Administer antidiarrhea agents in solution with the calibrated dropper provided by the manufacturer.

M. Teach patients to use caution when participating in activities that require judgment and coordination after taking opiate derivatives.

N. Advise family members, friends, neighbors, and patients that a change in bowel habits is one of the warning signals of cancer that should stimulate a trip to the doctor for medical evaluation.

O. Advise parents of infants with diarrhea not to delay seeking medical attention. Infants are extremely susceptible to complications of diarrhea.

P. Report to the physician or registered nurse immediately the sudden development of abdominal distention in a patient with diarrhea. This may indicate toxic megacolon, a potentially fatal complication.

ANTIEMETICS, EMETICS

Antiemetics are drugs that prevent, relieve, or control nausea, vomiting, or motion sickness. *Emetics* are drugs that induce vomiting. (See Table 21–5.) Vomiting is the forceful evacuation of stomach contents through rhythmic abdominal and gastrointestinal muscle contractions. *Emesis or vomitus* are terms that describe stomach contents that have been vomited. *Nausea* is a sensation often felt in the throat or epigastric area, indicating a desire to vomit. *Motion sickness* is a sensation of nausea and vomiting brought about by certain kinds of motion, particularly in a boat or airplane.

There are two control centers located in the medulla that affect nausea and vomiting. One con-

TABLE 21–5 Antiemetics, Emetics

Nonproprietary Name	Proprietary Name	Adult Dose Range	Notes
Antiemetic Phenothiazines			
chlorpromazine	Thorazine	10–25 mg PO every 6–8 h, 25–50 mg IM every 3–4 h, one 25 to 100-mg suppository every 6–8 h	Also available as liquid, sustained release capsules; may also be used as antipsychotic or to control hiccoughs; see pp. 139–142 for additional information
perphenazine	Trilafon	8–16 mg PO per day, 5 mg IM	Also available as liquid, sustained release capsule; also used as antipsychotic
prochlorperazine	Compazine	5–10 mg PO, IM 3–4 ×/day; one 25-mg suppository 2 ×/day	IM dose should not exceed 40 mg/day; also available as sustained release capsule
promethazine	Phenergan	12.5–25 mg PO, IM, 1 suppository every 4–6 h	Also available as liquid
thiethylperazine	Torecan	10–30 mg PO, suppository/day, 10 mg IM 1–3 ×/day	
triflupromazine	Vesprin	20–30 mg PO/day, 5–15 mg IM every 4–6 h	PO dose is a liquid; IM dose should not exceed 60 mg per day
Antiemetic Antihistamines			
cyclizine hydrochloride	Marezine	50 mg PO, IM every 4–6 h	Also used for motion sickness
dimenhydrate	Dramamine and others	50 mg PO, IM every 4–6 h	
diphenhydramine	Benadryl	25–50 mg PO, IM every 4–6 h	Also used as antipruritic
hydroxyzine hydrochloride	Atarax, Vistaril	25 mg PO, IM every 6–24 h	Also used as antipruritic for allergies; use Z-tract technique for IM injections
meclizine hydrochloride	Antivert	25–50 mg PO every 12–24 h	Also used as antipruritic and for motion sickness

trol center, known as the *vomiting center*, receives impulses from the gastrointestinal tract, other body parts, the cerebral cortex, the labyrinth of the ear, and the chemoreceptor trigger zone (CRTZ, CTZ). The other control center, known as the *chemoreceptor trigger zone*, is activated by various drugs and other chemical stimuli. When the vomiting center is sufficiently stimulated, it sends impulses to the phrenic nerves in the diaphragm, spinal nerves located in abdominal muscles, and visceral nerves present in the stomach and esophagus. This results in a sequence of involuntary muscle contractions that ends in emesis or vomiting.

Occasionally, emesis is helpful to the patient. For example, vomiting enables a person to expel poisons that have been accidentally or intentionally ingested. Nausea and vomiting may warn a person of serious illness and the need for medical attention. For example, repeated vomiting is associated with infections, gastrointestinal disease, central nervous system disorders, hormone imbalances, certain heart diseases, emotional disorders, and radiation or chemotherapy.

Vomiting may deplete the patient of vital substances including water, electrolytes. Aspiration of stomach contents during vomiting may cause the patient to develop serious or even fatal pneumonitis or pneumonia. Aspiration is more likely when a patient's level of consciousness is decreased. The major responsibilities of the nurse when a patient is vomiting include: positioning the patient's head to the side so that emesis can be expelled and aspiration prevented; observing and recording characteristics of the emesis, administering an antiemetic if prescribed; assisting with hygiene measures such as washing the patient's face and hands, oral hygiene, and providing clean clothing or linens as needs.

I. Actions and uses.

A. Antiemetic phenothiazines act by depressing neurons in the CRTZ.

TABLE 21–5 (*cont.*)

Nonproprietary Name	Proprietary Name	Adult Dose Range	Notes
Other Antiemetics			
benzquinamide	Emete-Con	0.5–1 mg/kg IM, 0.2–0.4 mg/kg IV	Used for nausea and vomiting associated with anesthesia; inject IM into a large muscle mass; do not reconstitute with sodium chloride
dronabinol	Marinol		New cannabinoid drug specifically for patients with nausea and vomiting associated with antineoplastic chemotherapy; adverse responses include drowsiness, incoordination, visual blurring, anxiety, hallucinations
droperidol	Inapsine	2.5–10 mg IM	Used preoperatively to prevent emesis
nabilone	Cesamet	2 mg PO	See dronabinol
scopolamine hydrobromide		0.6 mg PO, IM	Anticholinergic; most effective agent for motion sickness; also available as transdermal patch
trimethobenzamide	Tigan	250 mg PO, one 200-mg IM suppository every 6h	
Emetics			
apomorphine		5 mg SC	Morphine derivative; vomiting can be expected in 2–5 min after injection; cannot be used for patients with respiratory depression
syrup of ipecac		15 ml PO; may be repeated in 20–30 minutes if vomiting has not occurred	Administer with a full glass of tepid water

B. Antiemetic antihistamines act by blocking the receptors on the cell membrane from responding to histamine, a neurotransmitter.

C. Certain antiemetics may also exert a direct influence to relax smooth muscle in the gastrointestinal system.

D. Antiemetics may be specific to nausea and vomiting or may be specific to motion sickness.

E. Antiemetics may be prescribed for nausea and vomiting associated with disease, anesthesia and surgery, diagnostic procedures, radiotherapy and chemotherapy of cancer, and motion sickness that occurs during travel. Antiemetics may be prescribed as prevention, relief, or control.

F. Emetics work by stimulating vomiting centers. The primary use of emetics is for the patient who has accidentally or intentionally ingested an overdose of drugs or a poison.

II. Adverse responses.

    A. Antiemetic phenothiazines—see also p. 141.

        1. Central nervous system—tremors, dry mouth, blurred vision, oversedation, parkinsonian symptoms.

        2. Cardiovascular system—orthostatic hypotension, palpitations.

        3. Gastrointestinal system—constipation, jaundice.

        4. Blood dyscrasias.

        5. Skin reactions—rashes, petechiae, edema, urticaria, photosensitivity.

        6. Phenothiazine tolerance may develop.

        7. Drug interactions include:

- Increased sedation and depression when combined with other central nervous system depressants such as alcohol, analgesics, sedatives.
- Increased hypotension when combined with antihypertensives.
- Increased likelihood of dry mouth, urinary retention when combined with anticholinergics.

  B. Antiemetic antihistamines, other antiemetics.
  1. Central nervous system: headache, dizziness, drowsiness, fatigue, tinnitus, blurred vision, tremors.
  2. Cardiovascular system: chest tightness, hypotension, palpitations.
  3. Gastrointestinal system: loss of appetite, nausea and vomiting, epigastric distress, dry mouth and throat, constipation or diarrhea.
  4. Urinary system: urinary frequency or retention, dysuria.
  5. Hypersensitivity: skin rashes, urticaria, drug fever, blood dyscrasias.
  6. Drug interactions are the same as for phenothiazines.

  C. Emetics
  1. Ipecac occasionally produces hypotension, tachycardia, dyspnea, chest pain when very large doses are administered.
  2. Apomorphine is an opiate derivative that produces respiratory depression and therefore cannot be used for the patient with respiratory depression or other drugs that depress respirations.

III. Nursing implications.

  A. Assess the patient's report of nausea and vomiting. A minimum of information needed would include: characteristics of nausea, vomiting; other gastrointestinal symptoms such as belching, indigestion, heartburn, flatulence; pattern and characteristics of bowel movements; other prescribed and nonprescribed drugs being taken, usual eating practices; current height and weight together with recent gains or losses.

  B. Prevent nausea and vomiting when possible by administering antiemetics early and by minimizing the patient's exposure to unpleasant sights, sounds, odors.

  C. Seek help from the registered nurse to schedule drug therapy with other agents in a way that minimizes nausea and vomiting as a side effect.

  D. Administer pain medication appropriately to prevent nausea and vomiting associated with incomplete pain relief.

  E. Observe and record characteristics of the patient's emesis: time, amount, color, odor, presence of unusual substances like blood clots, undigested food, foreign bodies.

  F. Position the patient at risk for vomiting on the side to prevent aspiration of gastric contents into the lungs.

  G. Assist the patient with hygiene measures after an episode of vomiting: offer a washcloth and towel for the face and hands, assist with oral hygiene, change clothing and linens as needed.

  H. Administer IM injections into a large muscle mass and rotate injection sites as needed.

  I. Administer antiemetic injections without mixing them with other drugs in the same syringe. An exception to this is promethazine which may be mixed with meperidine as a preanesthetic agent.

  J. Use safety precautions after administering an antiemetic: raise siderails; place the call bell in the patient's hand; place an emesis basin and tissues within easy reach; instruct the patient not to get out of bed unassisted.

  K. Seek additional information before administering antiemetics to women who may be pregnant. Most preparations are not recommended during pregnancy because they may affect the fetus.

  L. Increase observation efforts related to hypotension and oversedation when the patient is also receiving analgesics or antihypertensives.

  M. Teach the patient not to combine antiemetics with other drugs such as alcohol and nonprescribed allergy or cold remedies. This is especially important when the drug is to be used as prevention for motion sickness.

  N. Anticipate vomiting when an emetic has been administered and provide several large emesis basins, tissues. If the patient must be left alone during the interim, return frequently to observe and instruct the patient to call as soon as vomiting begins.

O. Stay with the patient who is vomiting. Do not leave a vomiting patient unattended.

P. Teach the patient not to drive or operate heavy equipment or machinery involving coordination and judgment after taking an antiemetic at home.

APPETITE SUPPRESSANTS

Appetite suppressants are drugs that stimulate the central nervous system to elevate mood, reduce feelings of hunger, and increase feelings of concentration and self-confidence (Table 21–6). These drugs may be prescribed occasionally for short-term adjunct to a weight reduction diet. However, they are widely available as nonprescribed diet aids. Most experts believe that the risks from using these drugs outweigh the benefits.

Most appetite suppressants are amphetamine stimulants. The actions and uses, adverse responses, and nursing implications associated with this group of drugs can be located in Chapter 16, pp. 146–147. Table 21–6 lists those particular preparations used to suppress appetite.

The best-known methods for permanent weight loss at this time include a combination of calorie-restricted diet, exercise programs, retraining related to eating habits, and emotional support. The nurse assists the patient best by suggesting and encouraging participation in a program that includes these basic components.

TABLE 21–6   Appetite Suppressants and Digestants

Nonproprietary Name	Proprietary Name*	Adult Dose Range	Notes
Appetite Suppressants			
amphetamine sulfate	Benzedrine	5–10 mg PO 3×/day 30–60 min before meals	Not recommended for persons with hypertension, hyperthyroidism, history of alcohol or drug abuse; high potential for drug tolerance and dependence; for short-term use only; read labels on nonprescribed agents; see also p. 147
benzphetamine hydrochloride	Didrex	25–50 mg PO 1–3×/day 60 min before meals	
chlorphentermine hydrochloride	Pre-Sate	65 mg PO per day after breakfast	
chlortermine hydrochloride	Voranil	50 mg PO per day at midmorning	See above.
dextroamphetamine sulfate	Dexedrine	Same as amphetamine sulfate	See above.
diethylpropion hydrochloride	Tenuate	25 mg PO 3×/day 60 min before meals	See above.
fenfluramine hydrochloride	Pondimin	20–40 mg PO 3×/day before meals	Sustained-release tablet for daily use also available; see above.
mazindol	Sanorex	1 mg PO 3×/day or 2 mg/day	
methamphetamine	Desoxyn, Stimdex	2.5–5 mg PO 3×/day	Long-acting form 10–15 mg PO per day in AM.
phendimetrazine tartrate	Anorex	35 mg PO 2–3×/day or 1 timed release capsule per day	Administer in AM
phenmetrazine hydrochloride	Preludin	25 mg PO 2–3×/day or 50–75 mg sustained release capsule PO per day	
phentermine hydrochloride	Phentrol	15–30 mg PO per day before breakfast	

TABLE 21–6   (cont.)

Nonproprietary Name	Proprietary Name*	Adult Dose Range	Notes
Digestants			
bile salts	Bilron	150–600 mg PO with or after meals	Bile salts may produce diarrhea as a side effect; effectiveness not well established; prolonged use may cause liver damage and damage to mucous membrane lining of the gastrointestinal system. Also used to treat the patient with gallstones that can be seen on x-ray film but who are not good candidates for surgery; may produce elevated serum cholesterol and low-density lipoprotein levels in addition to other adverse responses listed for bile salts.
chenodiol	Chenix	8–10 mg/kg/day PO initially; gradually increased to 13–17 mg/kg/day if needed to dissolve gallstones	
dehydrocholic acid	Decholin	244–500 mg PO 3×/day after meals	
pancreatic enzymes	Viokase, Pancrease	Dosage highly individualized according to nitrogen and fat content of stools and dietary fat intake	High doses may produce nausea, diarrhea, elevated serum uric acid levels; follow physician's instructions for observation and collection of stools; monitor and record dietary intake
Gallstone Solvent			
Monooctanoin	Moctanin	3–5 ml/h	New drug that dissolves cholesterol gallstones following cholecystectomy; infused continuously through a catheter placed in the common bile duct; treatment continues over 7–21 days; infusion pump must be used to maintain flow rate; adverse responses include pain, nausea, vomiting, and diarrhea.

*These preparations are available with many other proprietary names; check labels for ingredients.

DIGESTANTS

Digestants are drugs that promote the process of digestion (Table 21–6). The primary use of digestants is to replace normal substances that are deficient. For example, pancreatic enzymes may be prescribed for the patient with pancreatitis. Bile acids may occasionally be prescribed for the patient after gallbladder surgery to improve T-tube drainage. Although there are many preparations on the market, their effectiveness as therapy has been questioned by experts. Table 21–6 contains a list of digestants. Adverse responses are few and have been placed in the Notes column next to each preparation.

LAXATIVES AND CATHARTICS

Laxative and cathartics are drugs that increase fecal elimination (Table 21–7). In clinical practice, laxatives are usually considered milder agents whereas cathartics are stronger. Normally, the formation of feces occurs in the large intestine which receives soft semisolid food contents within 2–5 h after eating. The process of digestion and absorption is completed in the large intestine. Gastrocolic and duodenocolic reflexes initiate peristalsis that propels the remnants of digestion through the large intestine where water and electrolytes are absorbed. The content remaining in the colon becomes feces that contains the following components: undigested and digestible food, water, bile and other pigments, microorganisms and their products, cholesterol, salts, mucus, and other secretions. Defecation starts when the colon is stimulated to empty a small amount of feces into the rectum. This results in a desire to defecate. Voluntary contraction of abdominal muscles, descent of the diaphragm, and colon peristalsis combine to empty the colon and rectum. Factors that influence defecation include diet, fluid intake, exercise patterns, abdominal muscle strength, use of prescribed and nonprescribed drugs, established patterns of elimination, and thoughts and feelings about defecation.

There is a wide range of normal with respect to the frequency, size, and consistency of fecal elimination. For example, one person may defecate daily, another weekly, and still another twice daily. A person may use a laxative when he or she is *constipated*: has a reduction in the frequency and bulk of feces and increased hardness of feces. Constipation may develop from disease in the gastrointestinal system or as a side effect of drug therapy. However, in most cases, a person develops constipation as a result of one or more of the following factors: ignoring the initial urge to defecate; inadequate intake of dietary fiber; insufficient fluid intake; lack of exercise; weak abdominal muscles, and lack of established time for defecation.

In some cases a physician may prescribe a laxative to prevent straining by the patient with a hernia, anorectal disease, hemorrhoids, cardiovascular disease. Laxatives may also be prescribed before x-ray examination of the abdomen, kidneys, or gastrointestinal system; before sigmoidoscopy or proctoscopy; and prior to elective surgery on the bowel. Occasionally, laxatives are prescribed as part of the treatment for a patient with drug overdose, other poisoning, or parasites.

I. Actions and uses.
  A. Bulk-forming laxatives bind water and electrolytes to feces to increase its size and water content, increase the speed of passage through the colon. Effects usually occur within 24 h after administration.
  B. Saline and osmotic laxatives increase water content of feces by pulling water into the colon and stimulating peristalsis. Effects are usually noticed within 3–8 h depending on the dose. Larger doses produce liquid or semiliquid stools. For these effects, saline and osmotic laxatives may be ordered preoperatively, before x-ray examination or colon endoscopy, or for the patient with parasites.
  C. Stimulant laxatives stimulate the accumulation of water and electrolytes in the colon and improve peristalsis. The effects usually occur within 1 to 6 h after administration depending on the specific preparation and dose. Laxatives in this group are best used as very short-term agents.
II. Adverse responses.
  A. Bulk-forming laxatives.
   1. Allergic reactions may occur.
   2. Esophageal and intestinal obstruction and fecal impaction may develop in patients with existing gastrointestinal disease or when preparations are accidentally administered dry instead of mixed with water or fruit juice.
   3. Flatulence and stomach rumblings (borborygmi) may occur.
   4. Some bulk-forming laxatives contain large amounts of sodium and cannot be used for patients who retain sodium and water.
   5. Drug interactions include: binding to drugs and reducing intestinal absorption, particularly of cardiac glycosides, Coumadin, nitrofurantoin, and salicylates.
  B. Saline and osmotic laxatives.
   1. System absorption may produce toxicity.
   2. Magnesium intoxication may develop if these preparations are taken by patients with impaired renal function.
   3. Sodium preparations may cause dehydration. Edema may develop in patients with congestive heart failure, renal impairment.
   4. Lactulose may cause abdominal discomfort or cramps, flatulence, nausea and vomiting. Higher doses may produce diarrhea, loss of fluid and potassium, exacerbation of hepatic encephalopathy.
  C. Stimulant laxatives—see also Table 21–7.
   1. Most popular type of laxative associated with laxative abuse.

TABLE 21–7   Laxatives

Nonproprietary Name	Proprietary Name	Adult Dose Range	Notes
Bulk-Forming Agents			
crude bran		6 g PO per day	Add to cereals, salads, and baked goods to increase stool bulk and softness
karaya gum		5–10 g PO per day with water	Allergic reactions have been reported: asthma, dermatitis, rhinitis, urticaria; ask patient about allergies
methylcellulose	Cologel and others	4–6 g PO per day in two to three doses	Administer with at least 1 full glass of water; available as powder or capsule; may also be used for patients with watery diarrhea
polycarbophil and calcium polycarbophil	Mitrolan	1 g PO 4–6×/day with 250 ml of water or	Not recommended for patients taking tetracyclines or those with calcium restriction
psyllium	Effersyllium, Metamucil	3–3.6 g 1–3×/day with 250 ml of water or juice	
Saline and Osmotic Agents			
glycerin		3-g rectal suppository as needed	Promotes defecation within 30 min after insertion; make sure suppository makes contact with rectal walls; used in bowel training programs
lactulose	Cephulac, Chronulac	7–40 g PO syrup mixed with fruit juice	Administer with a full glass of water in addition to fruit juice
		20–30 g PO per day to eliminate intestinal ammonia	Dose for the patient with chronic portal hypertension, hepatic encephalopathy; dose adjusted to cause two to three soft stools per day; do not administer with other laxatives
magnesium citrate	Citro-Nesia and others	240 ml PO	
magnesium hydroxide	Milk of Magnesia	30–60 ml PO	May also be used in smaller dose as antacid; also available in tablets
magnesium sulfate	Epsom salt	5–15 g PO mixed with citrus fruit juice	Intensely bitter taste; may produce nausea
sodium phosphates enema	Fleet enema	118 ml administered as enema	
sodium phosphates oral solution	Phospho-Soda	10–40 ml PO mixed with 1 full glass water	
sorbitol		30 ml of 70% solution PO 120 ml of 25–30% solution administered by enema	
Stimulant Laxatives			
bisacodyl	Dulcolax	10–15 mg PO	Instruct patient to swallow tablets without chewing; do not administer within 1 h of milk or antacids
		10 mg suppository; 10 mg/30 ml enema	Produces stool in 15–30 min after rectal administration; may produce burning, stinging sensation in rectum and irritation of mucous membrane; recommended for short-term use only
cascara sagrada		30 ml PO	Produces soft or semiliquid stool within 8 hours of ingestion
castor oil	Neoloid	15–60 ml PO	Produces one to two copious semiliquid stools within 1–6 h of ingestion; objectionable taste may be masked by mixing with fruit juice
danthron	Dorbane, Modane	37.5–150 mg PO	Same as cascara sagrada above
dehydrocholic acid	Decholin	750 mg–1.5 g PO 3×/day	A bile salt

TABLE 21–7   (cont.)

Nonproprietary Name	Proprietary Name	Adult Dose Range	Notes
docusate calcium	Surfak	50–200 mg PO per day	Docusates are used primarily to keep feces soft; mix oral solutions with milk or friut juice to mask taste; may increase toxicity of other drugs; may produce liver damage, toxicity
docusate potassium	Kasof	Same as above	
docusate sodium	Colace	Same as above	
phenolphthalein	Ex-Lax	30–195 mg PO	Tell patients this drug may turn urine and feces pink
polaxamer 188	Alaxin	240–480 mg PO/day; mix powders according to package insert	Softens stool in 3–5 days
senna pods	Senekot	See package insert	Available as granules, syrup, tablets, or suppository
Other Laxatives			
mineral oil	Nujol and others	15–30 ml PO; 120 ml by rectum as retention enema	May interfere with absorption of fat soluble substances; may produce local irritation and allergic reactions; oral route may cause lipid pneumonia

2. Fluid and electrolyte imbalances, hypoalbuminemia, osteomalacia may develop from depletion of body stores.
3. Allergic reactions may occur.
4. Nausea, vomiting, diarrhea, abdominal cramping, steatorrhea are gastrointestinal side effects.
5. Not recommended during pregnancy since they may stimulate uterine contractions.
  D. *Laxative abuse* is a progressive condition in which a person develops total reliance upon laxatives for defecation. This condition has been associated with spastic colitis, enterocolitis, and misdiagnosis of gastrointestinal disease.
  E. Laxatives may mask symptoms of appendicitis or other serious gastrointestinal disease if administered to a person with undiagnosed abdominal pain, cramps, colic, nausea, or vomiting.
III. Nursing implications.
  A. Gather and record information about the patient's usual patterns of elimination. Minimum information needed includes: usual time, place and frequency, amount and consistency of fecal elimination; changes in bowel habits in any, usual patterns of food and fluid intake, exercise patterns, use of prescribed and nonprescribed drugs including laxatives, possibility of pregnancy.
  B. Seek additional information from the physician or registered nurse before administering a laxative to a patient with abdominal pain, colic, cramps, nausea, vomiting, or for the patient who may be pregnant or nursing.
  C. Administer bulk-forming laxatives with at least one full glass of water or juice. Mix powders according to manufacturer's directions.
  D. Administer saline and osmotic laxatives on an empty stomach with a full glass of water to enhance effectiveness.
  E. Administer rectal suppositories with the flat end first to the length of the index finger against the wall of the rectum. This practice is believed to encourage suppository retention.
  F. Administer castor oil in juice or other liquid to mask objectionable taste.
  G. Use safety measures after administering a laxative. Prevent slips and falls by: anticipating the patient's call for assistance to the bathroom, placing the call bell close at hand and answering the patient's call promptly, placing a bedpan and toilet paper at the bedside if necessary, removing obstacles from the pathway from bed to bathroom.

H. Prevent constipation in hospitalized patients by: maintaining usual pattern and time for defecation when possible; providing privacy and avoiding interruptions while the patient is toileting; encouraging increased fluid intake and high dietary fiber when permitted, demonstrating and assisting the patient to ambulate and exercise; recording daily bowel movements for patients with impaired memory; offering prune juice early when bowel movements first decline in frequency.

I. Teach patients, families, friends, and neighbors to use nondrug measures that prevent constipation: drink 6 to 8 glasses of water daily; eat at least four to eight servings of high-fiber foods daily (bran, whole grains, fresh fruits and vegetables, legumes); take a 15 to 30-minute walk every day; set aside a regular time to defecate without rushing or interruptions; practice abdominal strengthening exercises if necessary.

J. Teach patients, families, friends, and neighbors that a change in bowel habits is a warning signal for cancer that should cause a person to seek medical attention.

K. Advise anyone who asks never to take a nonprescribed laxative when abdominal pain, cramps, colic, nausea, or vomiting is present. Instead, persons with these symptoms should seek medical attention.

L. Advise anyone who reports a regular laxative habit to seek medical assistance.

M. Teach other patients about the wide variety of normal bowel movements.

VITAMIN AND MINERAL SUPPLEMENTS

Vitamin supplements are drugs that resemble natural organic substances acting as essential enzymes for the metabolism of carbohydrates, fats, and proteins. *Mineral supplements* are drugs that resemble natural inorganic substances essential to metabolism. The term *organic* means of animal or plant origin. (See Table 21–8). The amount needed per day to maintain health has been set forth by the National Academy of Science Food and Nutrition Board and called Recommended Daily Allowances (RDA).

Vitamins that have been identified include vitamin A, vitamin B complex (biotin, choline, inositol, niacin, pantothinic acid, pyridoxine, riboflavin, thiamin), vitamin C (ascorbic acid), and vitamins D, E, and K. Recommended daily allowances have also been identified for calcium iodine, iron, magnesium, phosphorus, and zinc.

Normally, vitamins and minerals are present in the foods we eat. However, supplements may be needed for patients where deficiency if present or likely to occur. Inadequate dietary intake, malabsorption, genetic defects, increased body needs, and alcoholism are conditions that may cause a person to develop vitamin or mineral deficiency. Healthy persons who eat a balanced diet that contains the recommended daily allowances for vitamins and minerals do not need supplements. In some cases, self-medication with nonprescribed vitamin and mineral supplements has led to toxicity. When supplements are needed, however, research shows that synthetic preparations have the same effects as those present in food. There is no evidence that natural vitamins, which are usually more expensive, are more beneficial than other kinds.

I. Actions and uses.

A. Vitamin supplements may be ordered to treat or prevent diseases associated with deficiency: night blindness (vitamin A), beriberi (thiamine), pellagra (niacin), rickets (vitamin D), and scurvy (ascorbic acid).

B. Vitamin and mineral supplements may be ordered for the patient who does not eat a balanced diet. For example, the elderly patient on a limited income, the person with anorexia nervosa, alcoholism, psychosis, or on a fad reducing diet; or the comatose patient with a feeding tube may develop deficiency states.

C. Vitamin and mineral supplements may be ordered for the patient with a disease of the gastrointestinal system that interferes with absorption. For example, the patient with diarrhea as a symptom, liver or biliary tract disease, pernicious anemia, or ileostomy may not be able to absorb the RDA.

    D. Vitamin and mineral supplements may be ordered for the patient with increased require-
ments caused by fever, burns, hyperthyroidism, oral contraceptives or neoplastic drugs, tissue wasting, or a genetic abnormality.

    E. In the United States, deficiency states of B complex vitamins usually occur as a multiple de-
ficiency. The patient is more likely to receive a multiple vitamin preparation that contains
most of the B complex vitamins. In some cases, biotin, choline, and inositol have been added
although there is no known deficiency state for these substances.

II. Adverse responses

    A. There are few toxic effects associated with overdose of watersoluble oral preparations (B
complex vitamin supplements). These supplements are generally excreted in the urine. However, anaphylaxis, hypotension, nausea, vomiting, diarrhea, and anorexia have occurred.
Overuse of vitamin C may produce kidney stones.

    B. Vitamin A: hypervitaminosis as outlined below:

        1. Central nervous system: headache, fatigue, drowsiness, irritability, symptoms of in-
creased intracranial pressure.

        2. Gastrointestinal system: anorexia, nausea, vomiting, ascites, liver enlargement and
damage.

        3. Skin: pruritus, dermatitis, erythema, fissures of the lips, generalized peeling of the skin,
disturbed hair growth.

        4. Musculoskeletal system: bone pain, tenderness and enlargement.

        5. Blood: spleen enlargement, hemorrhage, elevated serum calcium.

        6. Birth defects.

    C. Vitamin D: general symptoms of hypercalcemia as outlined below:

        1. Central nervous system: apathy, depression, memory lapses, headache, drowsiness pro-
gressing to syncope, hallucinations, coma, and death.

        2. Gastrointestinal system: anorexia, nausea, vomiting, dysphagia, constipation, abdomi-
nal pain.

        3. Other: weakness and decreased muscle tone, polyphagia, polyuria, kidney stones, cardiac
arrhythmias, hypercalcemia.

    D. Vitamin K: hypervitaminosis as outlined below.

        1. Cardiovascular system: chest pain, dyspnea, flushing, collapse, and death have occurred
from rapid IV administration.

        2. Blood: anemia, polycythemia, spleen enlargement, excessive serum bilirubin has been
noted in infants.

        3. Other: jaundice, liver, and kidney damage.

    E. Calcium: same as vitamin D.

    F. Iron.

        1. Gastrointestinal system: nausea, constipation or diarrhea, dark stools.

        2. Accidental or intentional overdose may produce fever, enlarged lymph nodes, shock, ne-
crosis of stomach and liver, and death.

        3. Not recommended for patients receiving multiple blood transfusions.

        4. IM injections may produce anaphylaxis, pain, discoloration and malignant skin changes
at the injection site, flushing, fever, muscle and joint aches and pains, hypotension.

        5. Drug interactions include: decreased absorption of tetracyclines when taken with iron;
decreased absorption of iron when administered with food, especially milk and eggs.

    G. Magnesium: elevated serum levels may produce nausea, vomiting, diarrhea, hypotension,
central nervous system depression; not recommended for patients with coma or renal impairment.

    H. Potassium supplements: elevated serum levels may produce cardiac arrhythmias, especially
heart block, hypotension, flaccid paralysis, paresthesias, cardiac arrest and death; not recommended for patients with dehydration, potassium-sparing diuretic therapy, heat cramps,
or kidney impairment.

    I. Zinc: nausea, vomiting, gastrointestinal irritation.

TABLE 21–8   Vitamin and Mineral Supplements

Nonproprietary Name	Proprietary Name	Adult Dose Range	Notes
Vitamin Supplements			
ascorbic acid	Vitamin C	100 mg PO, IM, IV	
biotin		5–10 mg PO per day	Water-soluble B complex; recommended supplement for infants with seborrhea, persons with genetic deficiencies, and those on long-term parenteral nutrition
choline	Lecithin	Available as 250 to 650-mg PO tablets	Not recommended for supplement; often added to multivitamin preparations
cyanocobalamin	Redisol, Vitamin B_{12}	10-250 μg PO per day	Dose for deficiency states
		100-200 μg SC, IM, IV per month	Dose for pernicious anemia; PO doses not absorbed unless intrinsic factor is present in stomach
folic acid	Fovite and others	1 mg PO, IM, IV per day initially	
inositol		Available as 250 to 650-mg tablets	Used mainly to supplement infant formulas; not recommended as a supplement for adults
niacin, B_3	Nicobid and others	50–100 mg PO, IM per day	Dose varies with patient's condition
pantothenic acid, B_5	Pantholin	Available as 10 to 545-mg tablets; 10–20 mg PO per day	Not recommended as a supplement; often added to multivitamin preparations
pyridoxine, B_6	Hexa-Betalin	10–600 mg PO, IM, IV per day	Dose depends upon patient's condition; deficiency states most likely to occur as a multiple B deficiency, during pregnancy, when oral contraceptives, isoniazid, or hydralazine are taken
riboflavin, B_2	Riobin-50	5–10 mg PO per day; also available for parental use	Deficiency usually occurs as a multiple B deficiency
thiamine hydrochloride, B_1	Betalin S and others	10–100 mg PO, IM, IV	Dose varies with patient's condition
vitamin A (retinol)	Alphalin and others	10,000–50,000 IU PO per day; 50,000–100,000 IU IM per day	Fat-soluble vitamin; higher doses may be used in severe deficiency states; short-term therapy is recommended to prevent overdose
isotretinoin	Accutane	Available as 10, 20, 40-mg capsules	Vitamin A preparation
tretinoin	Retin-A	Available as solution, cream, gel	Vitamin A topical preparation for the patient with acne vulgaris
vitamin D	Calderol, Hytakerol, Rocaltrol	Dose varies according to preparation ordered; see package insert or check with pharmacist for recommended doses	Fat-soluble vitamin; also available for IM use; may be used for deficiency states, osteomalacia, hypoparathyroidism
vitamin E	Aquasol and others	5–30 IU PO, 60–75 IU IM	Fat-soluble vitamin; currently used for severe multiple deficiency; other uses under investigation
vitamin K			
Menadiol	Synkavite	5–15 mg PO, SC, IM, IV	
Menadione	Menaphthone	2–10 mg PO per day	

TABLE 21–8   (cont.)

Nonproprietary Name	Proprietary Name	Adult Dose Range	Notes
Phytonadione	Aquamephyton	2.5–10 mg PO 0.5–10 mg SC, IM 0.5–10 mg IV at the rate of 1 mg/min	Oral dose may be repeated in 12–24 h. Maximum single dose of 25 mg for SC, IM routes; may be repeated in 6–8 h. IV route used only in emergency hemorrhage; may be repeated in 4h if bleeding continues.
Mineral Supplements calcium carbonate	Os Cal 500	1–1.5 g PO 3×/day with meals up to a maximum of 8 g/day PO	For replacement of deficiences caused by diarrhea, malabsorption, hypoparathyroidism, renal impairment
calcium chloride		500–1000 mg IV every 3 days	Infusion rate should not exceed 1 ml/min; may produce burning and stinging at IV site
calcium gluconate	Kalcinate	1–5 grams PO 3×/day; 0.5–2 g IV every 3 days	Same as above
fluoride	Kari-Rinse, others	10 ml as a rinse to be expectorated	Instruct patient to brush teeth first; use a plastic glass; not recommended for persons on sodium-restricted diets; not recommended where water contains fluoride; used primarily to prevent dental caries
ferrous fumarate	Ferostat and others	100–400 mg PO per day in four divided doses	Used primarily to prevent or treat iron deficiency anemias
ferrous gluconate	Fergon and others	320–640 mg PO per day	
ferrous sulfate	Feosol and others	300–1000 mg PO per day in three to four divided doses	Same as above
iron dextran injection	Imferon and others	100–250 mg IM per day 100 mg IV per day	Anaphylaxis may occur; administer IM injections with Z-tract technique; dilute IV injections; review package insert before administration; see p. 171 for additional information
magnesium	MgPlus	27–133 mg PO per day	Dose highly individualized according to serum levels; also used for eclampsia
manganese	MnPlus	5 mg PO per day	
potassium supplements	Kaon KayCiel K-Lor K-Lyte	15–40 mEq PO, IV per day	Hyperkalemia is a potentially fatal complication; IV doses must be diluted in 1,000 ml of IV fluid and flow rate should not exceed 10–15 mEq/h
zinc supplements	Orazinc Zincate	15–80 mg PO per day	

III. Nursing implications.

  A. Collect and record information about the patient's usually dietary intake as part of the nursing history. Request a nutritional consultation for patients at risk for vitamin or mineral deficiency.

  B. Observe and record the food intake pattern in hospitalized patients. The patient who is NPO or who often misses meals for diagnostic tests, and the patient with impaired consciousness, severe depression, or agitation may easily become deficient in vitamins and minerals. Especially at risk are patients with multiple lengthy surgical procedures on the gastrointestinal tract.

C. Administer fat-soluble vitamins several hours before administering mineral oil in order to maximize absorption.

D. Administer IM vitamin preparations deeply into a large muscle mass.

E. Administer IV vitamin preparations slowly according to the manufacturer's package insert. Rapid IV infusion is associated with an increased incidence of anaphylaxis and hypotension.

F. Administer oral niacin and mineral supplements with or after meals to reduce gastric irritation.

G. Administer oral iron preparations between meals if tolerated because absorption is improved when the patient's stomach is empty.

H. Mix oral potassium supplements with juice, water, or soda to mask objectionable taste.

I. Dilute IV potassium doses in 1,000 ml of IV fluid and administer no faster than 10 mEq/h. This prevents hyperkalemia and pain at the infusion site.

J. Read and follow the manufacturer's package insert when administering magnesium preparations.

K. Administer IM iron preparations using the Z-tract technique.

L. Know where emergency drugs and supplies are located before administering IM iron preparations.

M. Monitor laboratory studies when available to observe patient's response to mineral supplements.

N. Teach patients, families, friends, and neighbors to prevent vitamin and mineral deficiencies by eating a balanced diet. Provide food lists that indicate good sources of essential vitamins and minerals.

O. Advise pregnant women and nursing mothers to consult a physician before taking nonprescribed vitamin or mineral supplements.

P. Advise patients recovering from alcoholism to read labels carefully on nonprescribed liquid vitamin and mineral supplements. Some preparations contain alcohol.

Q. Encourage others not to use nonprescribed vitamin and mineral supplements. Infants and children are more susceptible to overdose.

R. Use food preparation methods that preserve vitamin and mineral content: eat more servings of raw fruits and vegetables, use less water in cooking, cover pots and pans during cooking, use remaining water to make a sauce or gravy.

CASE STUDY 15

Mr. Sam Grayner is a 48-year-old man with peptic ulcer disease. The physician has prescribed cimetidine 300 mg PO quid with meals and at bedtime. Answer the following questions about drug therapy for Mr. Grayner.

1. Compare the actions of cimetidine with other antacids containing aluminum or magnesium hydroxide and similar ingredients.

2. What adverse responses will you be looking for in Mr. Grayner? Compare these to other antacids described in question 1.

3. List five nursing implications associated with the use of cimetidine for Mr. Grayner.

EXERCISE 1

The list below contains examples of typical orders for drug therapy. Answer the following questions about these orders for drug therapy.

- Aluminum hydroxide 5 ml PO p̄ each loose stool.
- Biscodyl 15 mg PO prn in AM.
- Docusate sodium 50 mg PO bid.
- Lomotil 2.4 mg PO now.
- Magnesium hydroxide 30 ml PO hs prn.
- Paregoric 5 ml PO q8h prn × 48 h.

Questions

1. Organize the drugs on the list into two main categories.
2. Describe the patient's symptoms in each category.
3. List two sample patient conditions for each category.
4. Describe major adverse responses for each category.
5. List five major nursing implications for the drugs in each category.

EXERCISE 2

Column A contains examples of nursing implications. Column B contains various potential definitions for each of the examples in Column A. Next to each of the statements in Column A, place the letter of the closest corresponding definition in Column B.

Column A

1. Assess the patient's report of nausea and vomiting. _____
2. Advise pregnant women and nursing mothers to use only supplements prescribed by the physician or obstetrician. _____
3. Encourage the patient to establish and maintain a program of regular exercise. _____
4. Record characteristics of the patient's emesis. _____
5. Assist the patient to choose foods that have high nutritional value and low calorie content. _____
6. Do not leave a vomiting patient unattended. _____
7. Refer the patient to support groups for retraining of eating habits and emotional support. _____
8. Minimize the patient's exposure to nauseating sounds, sights, odors. _____
9. Teach and use food preparation methods that preserve vitamin and mineral content. _____
10. Teach mothers not to use nonprescribed supplements for infants and children. _____
11. Position the patient laterally to prevent aspiration of gastric contents. _____
12. Administer before vomiting begins if possible. _____
13. Offer oral hygiene. _____
14. Teach others about foods contained in a balanced diet. _____
15. Discourage the use of nonprescribed diet aids. _____

Column B

A. An explanation related to the use of appetite suppressants.
B. A nursing implication related to antiemetic drugs.
C. A component of patient teaching when administering vitamin and mineral supplements.

Chapter 22 | DRUG THERAPY AFFECTING THE PATIENT'S ENDOCRINE SYSTEM

EXPECTED BEHAVIORAL OUTCOMES

After completing this chapter you should return to the expected behavioral outcomes and evaluate your ability to:

1. Analyze a specific drug for its effects on a gland and its hormones.
2. Describe at least five nursing implications to be considered when administering insulin to a person with diabetes mellitus, Type 1.
3. Develop an explanation of oral hypoglycemics that would be suitable for the patient or family.
4. List at least six nursing implications to be considered when a patient is receiving drug therapy with corticosteroids.
5. Prepare a list of nursing observations that would indicate adverse responses in a patient receiving a nonsteroidal anti-inflammatory drug.
6. Compare thyroid and antithyroid drugs from the perspective of the patient's condition, actions and uses, adverse responses, and nursing implications.

STRUCTURE AND FUNCTION REVIEW

The endocrine system contains ductless glands. Glands in the system, under the influence of the nervous system, take chemical substances from the bloodstream and manufacture chemical messengers called *hormones*. After manufacturing hormones, endocrine glands secrete them into the bloodstream where they are carried to target organs such as another gland, blood vessels, bones, or the uterus (Fig. 22–1).

Over 50 different hormones are produced by nine different endocrine glands including the hypothalamus, pituitary, and pineal glands located in the skull; the parathyroid and thyroid glands located in the neck; the thymus gland located in the chest; the pancreas located behind the stomach; and the gonads (ovaries and testes) located in the pelvis and genitalia.

Hormone production and secretion are affected by a number of factors including normal rhythmic patterns, body temperature, activity, central nervous system input, and other hormones. According to recent research, a process called *negative feedback loops* is a very important regulator of hor-

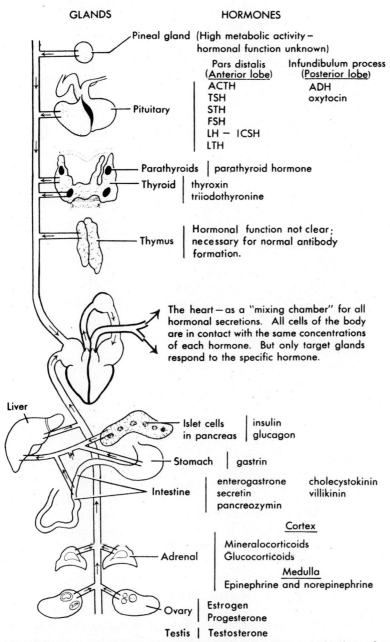

GLANDS   HORMONES

Pineal gland (High metabolic activity –
                 hormonal function unknown)

Pars distalis   Infundibulum process
(Anterior lobe)   (Posterior lobe)
ACTH   ADH
TSH   oxytocin
Pituitary   STH
FSH
LH — ICSH
LTH

Parathyroids │ parathyroid hormone
Thyroid   │ thyroxin
              │ triiodothyronine

Thymus   │ Hormonal function not clear;
              │ necessary for normal antibody
              │ formation.

The heart – as a "mixing chamber" for all
hormonal secretions. All cells of the body
are in contact with the same concentrations
of each hormone. But only target glands
respond to the specific hormone.

Liver

Islet cells   │ insulin
in pancreas   │ glucagon

Stomach   │ gastrin

              │ enterogastrone   cholecystokinin
Intestine   │ secretin   villikinin
              │ pancreozymin

                        Cortex
                Mineralocorticoids
Adrenal   Glucocorticoids
                        Medulla
                Epinephrine and norepinephrine

Ovary   │ Estrogen
        │ Progesterone

Testis │ Testosterone

**FIGURE 22–1   Diagram showing relationship of endocrine glands to the
bloodstream. The bloodstream is always moving, so that small quantities of
hormones enter the blood continuously.** (From Miller, M. A., and Leavell,
L. C.: *Kimber–Gray–Stackpole's Anatomy and Physiology,* 16th ed. Macmillan, New York, 1972.)

mone activity. A rising concentration of hormone in the circulation acts as an inhibitor to further
release of that hormone. Similarly, a falling concentration stimulates additional production and release of that hormone. A disturbance in the negative feedback loop may account for some endocrine
disorders and adverse affects of hormone therapy.

Some hormones and their antagonists have already been described. Table 22–1 contains a list of
hormones described in previous chapters. In this chapter, special consideration is given to glucocorticoid hormones of the adrenal cortex, pancreatic hormones, and thyroid hormones and their antagonists. Generally drug therapy for the patient with a disturbance in the endocrine system is to replace,
augment, or antagonize naturally produced hormones.

TABLE 22–1   Hormones

Hormone	Description	Location
Adrenocorticosteroids	Produced in adrenal cortex; regulate inflammatory processes, metabolism, homeostasis	Chapters 22–24
Aldosterone	Produced in adrenal cortex to regulate extracellular fluid volume	Chapter 19
Androgens	Produced in adrenal cortex, genitalia to regulate male sexual characteristics, reproduction in males	Chapter 19
Antidiuretic hormone (ADH)	Produced in pituitary gland to conserve water	Chapter 19
Epinephrine and norepinephrine	Produced in adrenal medulla to regulate sympathetic nervous system activity	Chapter 17
Estrogens, progestins	Produced in adrenal cortex, genitalia to regulate female reproduction	Chapter 19
Follicle-stimulating hormone (FSH)	Produced in pituitary to regulate fertility	Chapter 19
Insulin	Produced in pancreas to regulate carbohydrate metabolism	Chapter 22
Luteinizing hormone (LH)	Produced in pituitary to regulate fertility	Chapter 19
Oxytocins	Produced in pituitary to stimulate uterine contraction, secretion of breast milk	Chapter 19
Thyroid hormone	Produced in thyroid gland to regulate metabolic and oxygen rates	Chapter 22

CORTICOSTEROIDS

Corticosteroids are drugs that resemble natural glucocorticoid hormone produced by the adrenal medulla (Table 22–2). This hormone produces widespread effects in every body system to regulate human biological responses to changing conditions in the internal and external environment. These widespread effects make possible the use of corticosteroid drugs for diverse clinical conditions. They also account for the variety of adverse responses that may occur in patients receiving corticosteroid therapy.

A particular feature of these drugs is that they can be administered locally or systemically by any route. However, local administration does not prevent the drug from being absorbed systemically to produce side effects. A second feature of corticosteroid therapy is related to its effect on the negative feedback loop described earlier on p. 258. As the blood level of corticosteroid rises during drug therapy, the release of the patient's own hormone is inhibited. Thus, abrupt withdrawal of drug may lead to potentially fatal adrenal failure.

Corticosteroid drug therapy may be used to replace or augment the patient's natural supply of the hormone. In addition, they may be used as an adjunct to other forms of therapy. A particular role of the nurse is related to careful observation for adverse responses in light of the patient's specific clinical condition. In addition, the nurse provides appropriate care related to the patient's specific clinical condition.

   I. Actions and uses.
      A. Corticosteroids stimulate the formation of glucose and its conversion to glycogen. There are associated changes in protein and fat metabolism, redistribution of body fat, and a retention of salt and water.
      B. In the musculoskeletal system, corticosteroids maintain normal muscle mass and strength.
      C. In the cardiovascular system, corticosteroids help to maintain a balance between blood viscosity, blood pressure, cardiac output.

TABLE 22–2   Selected Corticosteroids

Nonproprietary Name	Proprietary Name	Dose Form*	Notes
amcinonide	Cyclocort	0.1% topical application	
beclomethasone	Beclovent Vanceril	Two inhalations 3–4 × /day	Teach patient how to clean inhaler
betamethasone	Celestone	0.6-mg oral tablet or syrup; 6 mg/ml injectable	Some preparations may be injected into joint
	Benisone Uticort Diprosone and others	Available as topical application in various strengths	
clobetasol	Temovate	Topical application—less than 50 g/week	Potent new topical drug for the patient with inflammatory skin conditions; not recommended for applications to face, axilla, genitalia; perineal area; for short-term use only (no longer than 2 weeks)
clocortolone pivalate	Cloderm	0.1% topical application	
cortisol	Cortef Hydrocortisone	5- to 20-mg oral tablets; 25–50 mg/ml injectable; 0.125–2.5% topical application	Also available as enema; some cortisol preparations may be injected into joint
cortisol acetate	Cortef Acetate and others	25–50 mg/ml injectable; 0.5–2.5% topical application	Also available as suppositories and rectal foam
cortisol sodium preparations	Hydrocortone Phosphate Solu-Cortef	50 mg/ml injectable; 100–1,000 mg powder to be diluted for injection	
cortisone acetate	Cortone Acetate	5- to 25-mg oral tablet; 25–50 mg/ml injectable	
desonide	Tridesilon	0.05% topical application	
dexamethasone preparations	Decadron, others	0.25- to 6.0-mg oral tablets; 0.01–0.1% topical application; 0.1% ophthalmic solution	Also, available in elixir for oral administration
	Decadron-LA Decadron Phosphate	2–16 mg/ml injectable; 4–24 mg/ml injectable; 0.1% topical applications; 0.05, 0.1% ophthalmic solution	Also available for inhalation
desoximetasone	Topicort	0.05; 0.25% topical application	
desoxycorticosterone preparations	Doca Acetate and others	5 mg/ml injectable oil	Also available as pellets for SC implant
	Percorten Pivalate	25 mg/ml injectable suspension	
diflorasone	Florone and others	0.05% topical application	
fluocinolone	Synalar and others	0.01–0.2% topical application	
fludrocortisone	Florinef Acetate	0.1-mg oral tablets	
flumethasone	Locorten	0.03% topical application	
fluocinonide	Lidex	0.05 topical application	
fluorometholone	Liquifilm and others	0.1% ophthalmic solution	
flurandrenolide	Cordran	0.025%, 0.05% topical application	
halcinonide	Halog	0.25%, 0.1% topical application	
medrysone	HMS Liquifilm	1% ophthalmic solution	
methylprednisolone preparations	Medrol Depo-Medrol and others	2- to 30-mg oral tablets; 20–80 mg/ml injectable; 0.25%, 1% topical application	Also available as enema
	Solu-Medrol and others	40- to 1,000-mg powder to be diluted for injection	

TABLE 22–2 *(cont.)*

Nonproprietary Name	Proprietary Name	Dose Form*	Notes
paramethasone	Haldrone	1- to 2-mg oral tablets	
prednisolone preparations	Delta-Cortef and others; Econopred and others	1- and 5-mg oral tablets; 25–100 mg/ml injectable	Also available as ophthalmic solution
	Hydeltrasol and others	20 mg/ml injectable	Also available as ophthalmic solution; may be injected into joint
prednisone	Deltasone and others	1- to 50-mg oral tablets; 1 mg/ml oral syrup	
triamcinolone preparations	Aristocort and others	1- to 16-mg oral tablets; 2- and 4- mg/ml oral syrup; 25–40 mg/ml injectable	Some preparations may be injected into joint or bursa
	Kenalog	10 and 40 mg/ml injectable; 0.025–0.5% topical application	Also available for inhalation
Corticosteroid Inhibitors			
aminoglutethimide	Cytadren	250 mg PO every 6 h; gradually increased to a maximum of 2 g/day	Interrupts formation of natural aldosterone; used for hypersecretion in patients with adrenal tumor
metyrapone	Metopirone	750 mg PO every 4 h × six doses	Reduces production of natural cortisol; used for hypersecretion in patients with adrenal tumor, Cushing's syndrome; may produce hypertension
trilostane	Modrastane	30 mg PO 4 ×/day; gradually increased	New drug; controls overproduction of cortisol and other steroid hormones; nausea, flatulence, abdominal cramps, burning of oral and nasal mucous membranes, flushing and headache have been reported; usually discontinued in 2 weeks if patient does not respond

*Dose varies according to specific preparation, patient's condition; smaller doses generally needed for replacement; larger doses generally prescribed for suppression of disease symptoms.

D. In the central nervous system, corticosteroids influence mood, behavior, and excitability of nervous tissue.

E. Corticosteroids increase the formation of red cells and decrease production of certain white cells, particularly those involved in the immune reaction.

F. A striking feature of corticosteroids and the reason they are most often prescribed is their ability to suppress inflammation and its symptoms such as local heat, erythema, tenderness, and swelling.

G. Corticosteroids may be prescribed for their anti-inflammatory effects in patients with rheumatoid arthritis, renal disease, collagen diseases, allergy, bronchial asthma, chronic obstructive lung disease, selected inflammatory eye conditions, skin diseases, ulcerative colitis, chronic hepatitis and cirrhosis, cerebral edema, and cancer. Some of these conditions are thought to be related to *autoimmunity* (see p. 282). In these conditions, corticosteroids suppress the patient's abnormal immune response.

H. Small doses of corticosteroids are generally prescribed for the patient who needs replacement or augmentation. The intended effect is to restore the level of hormone to a normal state.

I. Large doses of corticosteroid are generally prescribed for patients for anti-flammatory, antiallergic, and immunosuppressive effects.

J. Corticosteroid therapy does not cure disease but alleviates symptoms. The appropriate dosage is the lowest possible that alleviates symptoms without producing dangerous adverse responses.

    K. When long-term therapy is used for a patient with chronic illness, alternate-day therapy may be prescribed to reduce adverse responses.

II. Adverse responses.

    A. Abrupt withdrawal of corticosteroids after a period of weeks or months may produce a typical syndrome that includes fever, muscle and joint pains, and malaise.

    B. Abrupt withdrawal of prolonged therapy with higher doses is more likely to produce life-threatening adrenal insufficiency: fainting, weakness, hypotension, shock, and death. Patients on long-term therapy who encounter unexpected stress are also at risk to develop adrenal insufficiency unless the dose of corticosteroid is increased.

    C. Gastrointestinal system: hyperglycemia, glycosuria, peptic ulcers that may perforate and/or hemorrhage.

    D. Musculoskeletal system: characteristic "buffalo hump" at back of the neck, osteoporosis, muscle weakness, central obesity, moon face, compression fractures of the ribs and vertebrae, arrested or inhibited growth in children.

    E. Skin: acne, eccymoses, hirsutism, striae.

    F. Behavior: insomnia, mood changes, nervousness, suicidal tendencies.

    G. Other: cataracts, edema, increased susceptibility to infection, superinfection because early symptoms are masked by the drug.

    H. Drug interactions include:
- Increased effects of corticosteroids when combined with adrenergic drugs (see Table 17–2), anticholinergics (see Table 17–4), tricyclic antidepressants (see Table 16–6), antihistamines (see Table 23–1), meperidine (Demerol), phenylbutazone.
- Increased hypokalemia may occur when corticosteroids are combined with diuretics (see Table 19–3) or amphotericin B.
- Increased likelihood of ulcer formation when corticosteroids are combined with aspirin or other salicylates, indomethacin (see Table 22–3).
- Certain sedative-hypnotics including barbiturates, chloral hydrate, glutethimide (see Table 16–9) decrease the effects of corticosteroids; ephedrine, phenytoin, and rifampin may also decrease corticosteroid effects.
- Corticosteroids decrease the effects of insulin and oral hypoglycemics (see Table 22–4).
- Skin tests and vaccinations are adversely affected because the antibody response is suppressed by corticosteroids.

III. Nursing implications.

    A. Observe, report, and record any information that indicates possible infection before initiating corticosteroid therapy. In most cases, the physician will order appropriate diagnostic tests to determine the location and causative microrganism as well as the antibiotic needed. This step is extremely important because once therapy is initiated, suppression of the patient's inflammatory response may mask usual symptoms. A minimum of information includes: temperature and pulse, presence or absence of cough, fever, diarrhea, unusual drainage, skin lesions, and local signs of inflammation (erythema, edema, warmth, tenderness).

    B. Record initial height, weight, and blood pressure. Monitor changes regularly to estimate fluid retention. Observe for edema in the sacral and tibial areas first.

    C. Monitor laboratory studies if available to observe the effects of corticosteroids on serum sodium, potassium, glucose, red and white blood cells.

    D. Encourage and assist the patient to exercise and ambulate, if permitted, to prevent osteoporosis.

    E. Inspect the skin daily and report petechiae, ecchymoses by their size and location.

    F. Anticipate delayed healing of surgical and other wounds and watch carefully for signs of infection.

    G. Use and teach safety measures that prevent bruising and bleeding. Handle the patient's body gently.

    H. Observe and record patient behavior daily. Report behavioral changes to the registered nurse.

I. Create opportunities for the patient to discuss concerns and questions. Anticipate concerns about altered appearance (moon face, buffalo hump, weight gain, hirsutism). Report the patient's questions and concerns to the registered nurse.

J. Administer oral preparations with or after meals to decrease gastric irritation.

K. Check with the registered nurse or physician so that diagnostic tests and other therapies do not cause delays or missed doses. Work with other health team members to develop a regular dosage schedule.

L. Check the package insert provided by the manufacturer before administering corticosteroids by IV, inhalation, or topical routes. Follow manufacturer's directions. Seek additional information from the registered nurse, pharmacist, or physician if manufacturer's directions are different from the physician's orders.

M. Anticipate that patients on high doses are more likely to develop adverse responses. Teach patients what symptoms should be reported to the physician at once: fever, cough, sore throat, other signs of infection, weight gain, chest or back pain, muscle and joint pain, sleep disturbances, and mood changes.

N. Include the following points in the teaching plan for patients on long-term therapy:

    1. Wear drug identification and physician's name, emergency instructions at all times.

    2. Take the drug exactly as prescribed. Mark calendar if necessary to remember alternate day or weekly dosage regimens so that no doses are missed. Do not stop drug abruptly. If you run out of drug, notify the physician at once.

    3. Avoid alcohol and all other drugs unless they are prescribed by the physician. Tell other physicians, dentists, chiropractors, or other health care providers the name of the drug, dose, and reason for taking it before care is provided.

    4. Use safety measures that avoid accidents and injuries.

    5. Anticipate that additional unexpected stress may require a temporary increase in dose and notify physician.

    6. Maintain a life-style pattern that is relatively free from frequent emotional upheaval and unexpected crises.

    7. Avoid persons with infections.

NONSTEROIDAL AND MUSCULOSKELETAL AGENTS

NONSTEROIDAL ANTI-INFLAMMATORY DRUGS, GOLD COMPOUNDS, ANTIGOUT AGENTS

Nonsteroidal anti-inflammatory drugs (NSAIDs) are agents that reduce inflammation and pain (Table 22–3). The term *nonsteroidal* means that drugs in this group are not related to corticosteroids such as those described on p. 260.

Nonsteroidal anti-inflammatory agents are believed to act by interfering with the manufacture, release, or uptake of *prostaglandins*, hormones manufactured from fatty acids and distributed in a variety of body tissues. All the functions of prostaglandins as chemical mediators are not yet known but they play an important role in fever, inflammation, and pain. Table 16–3 contains a list of additional drugs that have anti-inflammatory effects such as aspirin and phenacetin.

Nonsteroidal anti-inflammatory drugs are frequently prescribed for the patient with osteoarthritis, rheumatoid arthritis, gout, or other musculoskeletal conditions. The patient with osteoarthritis has a local inflammation that involves a gradual wearing out of joints. The patient with rheumatoid arthritis has a systemic progressive disease that involves inflammation and destruction of joints and synovial membranes lining them. The patient experiences fever, pain, swelling, stiffness, and muscle atrophy of the joints affected. Gold compounds may also be prescribed for the patient with rheumatoid arthritis. Antigout agents are the drugs most often prescribed for the patient with gout. The patient with gout has a disorder of purine metabolism that results in elevations of serum uric acid and the deposit of urate crystals in joints of the toe, ankles, knee, or knuckles. Crystals may also settle in the kidney or ear cartilage. The patient experiences pain, tenderness, swelling, and erythema of affected joints.

Other drugs that may be prescribed for the patient with a disorder involving the musculoskeletal system include aspirin (see Table 16–3), corticosteroids (see Table 22–2), or immunosuppressives (see Table 23–2). In addition to drug therapy, the physician may prescribe rest, local heat, exercise, and physical therapy depending upon the patient's specific disease.

I. Actions and uses.
   A. Nonsteroidal anti-inflammatory drugs reduce pain, swelling, and tenderness associated with inflammation for the patient with gout, bursitis, osteoarthritis, rheumatoid arthritis.
   B. Nonsteroidal anti-inflammatory drugs may also be used when the patient has pain associated with dysmenorrhea or soft tissue injuries. These drugs also have antipyretic effects.
   C. Antigout drugs are the drugs of choice for the patient with gout. These agents act in one or more of the following ways: increase the excretion of uric acid by the kidneys; inhibit the formation of uric acid; inhibit the inflammatory response to elevated uric acid levels in the bloodstream.
   D. Gold compounds are believed to suppress the immune responses in the patient with rheumatoid arthritis. Gold therapy (*chrysotherapy*) is used primarily for the patient with rapidly progressing rheumatoid arthritis who is not responding to aspirin or NSAIDs.
II. Adverse responses.
   A. Nonsteroidal anti-inflammatory drugs.
      1. Gastrointestinal system: anorexia, nausea, vomiting, dyspepsia, heartburn, abdominal discomfort or fullness, epigastric pain, constipation or diarrhea, peptic ulcer formation that may lead to perforation and hemorrhage.
      2. Central nervous system: vertigo, blurred vision, insomnia, euphoria, drowsiness, nervousness, tinnitus; frontal headache, depression, hallucinations, psychosis, and suicidal ideas have been reported with indomethacin.
      3. Kidneys: hematuria, nephritis, retention of electrolytes and water, edema.
      4. Blood: serum sickness, leukopenia, aplastic anemia, agranulocytosis, thrombocytopenia.
      5. Skin and mucous membranes: ulcerative stomatitis, skin rashes, pruritus.
      6. Other: pancreatitis and acute asthma have been reported with indomethacin; patients who are allergic to aspirin may also be allergic to NSAIDs.
      7. Drug interactions include:
         • Increased toxicity of anticoagulants, oral hypoglycemics, other anti-inflammatory agents, sulfonamides, and insulin when combined with NSAIDs.
         • Decreased therapeutic effects of furosemide, thiazide diuretics, and antihypertensives may occur when combined with NSAIDs except for tolmetin.
         • Acute renal failure has been reported when indomethacin and triamterene were used together.
   B. Gold compounds.
      1. Skin and mucous membranes—erythema, eczema, exfoliative dermatitis, stomatitis, glossitis, pharyngitis, gastritis, vaginitis, gray-blue pigmentation to skin exposed to sunlight (*chrysiasis*).

TABLE 22–3 Nonsteroidal Anti-inflammatory Drugs, Gold Compounds, and Antigout Agents

Nonproprietary Name	Proprietary Name	Adult Dose Range	Notes
Nonsteroidal Anti-inflammatory drugs			
fenoprofen calcium	Nalfon	300–600 mg PO 3–4×/day to a maximum of 3.2 g/day with meals	Used for the patient with osteoarthritis, rheumatoid arthritis; gastrointestinal side effects are common; may also be used as an analgesic
ibuprofen	Motrin, Rufen, Advil	1,200–2,400 mg PO per day in divided doses	Dose for rheumatoid arthritis, osteoarthritis
		400 mg PO every 4–6 h	Dose for mild to moderate pain, especially dysmenorrhea
indomethacin	Indocin	25 mg PO 2–3×/day; gradually increased to a total daily dose of 100–200 mg PO	Used for patients with ankylosing spondylitis, osteoarthritis, acute gout; special use IV to close patent ductus arteriosus in newborns (special dose required); high potential for toxicity
meclofenamate sodium	Meclomen	200–400 mg PO per day in three to four divided doses with food	Used primarily to relieve pain associated with dysmenorrhea and musculoskeletal conditions; may also be used as anti-inflammatory agent for patients with osteoarthritis, rheumatoid arthritis
mefenamic acid	Ponstel	500 mg PO initially for acute pain; 250 mg PO every 6 h with food	
naproxen	Naprosyn	250–375 mg PO 2×/day	Dose for ankylosing spondylitis, osteoarthritis, rheumatoid arthritis; ototoxicity is an additional adverse response
naproxen sodium	Anaprox	750 mg PO initially; 250 mg PO every 8 h until attack subsides	Dose for acute gout
		500 mg PO initially; 250 mg PO every 6–8 h	Dose for mild to moderate pain associated with dysmenorrhea, bursitis, tendonitis
oxyphenbutazone	Oxalid Tandearil	100 mg PO 3–4×/day	Used for short-term therapy for patients with acute gout, rheumatoid arthritis, osteoarthritis; high potential for toxicity
phenylbutazone	Azolid Butazolidin	300–600 mg PO per day initially; 100–400 mg PO per day as maintenance	Same as oxyphenbutazone
piroxicam	Feldene	20 mg PO per day	Used for the patient with acute gout, ankylosing spondylitis, musculoskeletal pain, osteoarthritis, rheumatoid arthritis; maximum benefits do not occur for 2 weeks
sulindac	Clinoril	150–200 mg PO 2×/day	Used for the patient with ankylosing spondylitis, osteoarthritis, rheumatoid arthritis, acute gout
suprofen	Suprol	200 mg PO every 4–6 h; total dose not to exceed 800 mg/day	

2. Kidneys: proteinuria, hematuria, nephrosis.
3. Blood: thrombocytopenia, leukopenia, agranulocytosis, aplastic anemia.
4. Other: encephalitis, pulmonary infiltrates, peripheral neuritis, hepatitis.
5. Drug interactions include:
    • Increased bone marrow depression if gold compounds are used for patients who have recently had radiation therapy.
    • Increased bone marrow depression if combined with antimalarials, immunosuppressives, oxyphenbutazone, phenylbutazone.
  C. Antigout agents.
    1. Gastrointestinal system: nausea, vomiting, diarrhea, abdominal pain, liver enlargment; hemorrhagic gastroenteritis may occur with acute colchicine poisoning.

TABLE 22-3   *(cont.)*

Nonproprietary Name	Proprietary Name	Adult Dose Range	Notes
tolmetin	Tolectin	400 mg PO 3×/day initially; gradually increased to 600–1,800 mg PO/day in divided doses; maximum daily dose 2 g/day	Two of three doses should be taken on awakening and at bedtime; used for patients with osteoarthritis, rheumatoid arthritis, ankylosing spondylitis
Gold compounds			
aurothioglucose	Solganal	10 mg IM initially; gradually increased to 50 mg IM per week until cumulative dose of 1 g is reached; dose gradually decreased if remission occurs	A gold compound used for patients with rheumatoid arthritis; also suppresses immune system
gold sodium thiomalate	Myochrysine	10 mg IM initially; gradually increased to 25–50 mg IM per week until maximum dose of 1 g is reached; dosage gradually decreased if remission occurs	Same as aurothioglucose
auranofin	Ridaura	6 mg/day PO	New oral drug recommended as adjunct with NSAIDs; may take 3–6 months before benefits occur; less severe adverse responses than IM preparations
Antigout Agents			
allopurinol	Lopurin Zyloprim	100 mg PO per day initially; gradually increased to 200 mg PO per day for maintenance	Reduces uric acid blood levels in patients with gout; force fluids to 4 L/day
colchicine		For acute attacks: 1–1.2 mg PO every 1–2 h during an acute attack until pain disappears or nausea, vomiting, abdominal pain develop. Maximum dose of 10 mg should not exceed; 2 mg IV single dose diluted in 10–20 ml water or 0.9% sodium chloride *For prevention:* 0.5 mg PO 2–3×/week up to 1.8 mg PO per day	Used primarily to relieve acute attacks of gout or prevent their recurrence. Adverse gastrointestinal symptoms common, especially in elderly and those with cardiac, renal, or gastrointestinal disease; high fluid intake is helpful; may reduce sperm formation and cause alopecia as additional adverse responses; store in tightly covered container away from light
sulfinpyrazone	Anturane	100–200 mg PO 2×/day; may be gradually increased to 800 mg PO per day in divided doses	Chronic gout

2. Blood: agranulocytosis, aplastic anemia may occur with long-term colchicine use.
3. Skin: alopecia, urticaria, purpura, pruritus, other skin eruptions may develop.
4. Central nervous system: headache, drowsiness, vertigo; ascending paralysis of central nervous system may develop with acute colchicine poisoning.
5. Other: nephrotoxicity, fever, malaise, muscle aching, peripheral neuritis, cataract.
6. Drug interactions include:
   • Increased anticoagulation when allopurinol is combined with warfarin.
   • Increased frequency of hypersensitivity reactions when allopurinol is combined with thiazide diuretics or ampicillin.
   • Increased potential for theophylline toxicity when combined with allopurinol.
   • Combined therapy with allopurinol and iron is not recommended.

III. Nursing implications.

    A. Gather and record complete information about the patient's age, and previous illnesses. Nonsteroidal anti-inflammatory drugs, gold compounds, and antigout agents are generally not used for patients who are elderly or pregnant, for nursing infants, or for patients with hypertension, or with cardiac, hepatic, renal, blood, or gastrointestinal disease.

    B. Check patient for allergies before administering these drugs. Seek additional information from the registered nurse, pharmacist, or physician before administering drug therapy to a patient with allergy to aspirin. Such a patient may develop a severe cross-sensitivity reaction to NSAIDs, gold compounds, or antigout agents. Bronchoconstriction with asthma is a common hypersensitive response.

    C. Administer oral agents with or after meals if possible to reduce gastrointestinal side effects.

    D. Inspect the patient's skin daily. Report and record rashes, jaundice, bruises, petechia, or purpura. In dark-skinned patients, observe the sclera for jaundice.

    E. Inspect the patient's mouth daily with a flashlight for ulcerations; record findings.

    F. Report gastrointestinal discomfort early and anticipate a change of drug or dose to halt the progression of symptoms.

    G. Observe the patient's urine and stool daily for evidence of bleeding; record findings.

    H. Observe, record, and report behavioral changes that indicate depression, hallucination, and similar adverse responses.

    I. Monitor laboratory studies when available to antipate and understand the patient's clinical responses to drug therapy.

    J. Force fluids if the physician's diet and fluid order permits.

    K. Assist the patient with self-care indicated for conditions involving limited mobility and pain associated with the musculoskeletal system.

    L. Weigh the patient initially and regularly to estimate fluid retention.

INSULIN, ORAL HYPOGLYCEMICS, AND THYROID AGENTS

INSULIN AND ORAL HYPOGLYCEMICS

Insulin and oral hypoglycemics are drugs that lower blood sugar (Table 22–4). They are an essential part of treatment for the patient with diabetes mellitus. Such a person has an insufficient amount of circulating natural insulin to meet body requirements.

Insulin is a hormone produced by beta islet cells in the pancreas and secreted into the bloodstream in response to the ingestion of food, secretion of gastrointestinal and other hormones, and influenced by autonomic nerves and the hypothalamus. Circulating insulin helps to transport glucose and other essential substances from the bloodstream across the cell membrane into the cell. In addition, insulin helps to convert glucose to glycogen for storage.

A person with diabetes is unable to metabolize glucose in the usual way. This results in a rise in blood sugar and a breakdown of proteins and fats for energy. The person with undiagnosed diabetes usually experiences hunger (*polyphagia*), thirst (*polydipsia*), and increased urinary output (*polyuria*). There may also be weight loss, fatigue, and malaise. The blood sugar is elevated and there may be glucose in the urine. As the body meets its energy requirement by breaking down fats and proteins, there is a corresponding rise of ketones, urea, and ammonia in the bloodstream. When the levels of these substances becme high enough, the patient develops a potentially fatal condition known as *diabetic ketoacidosis*. This condition develops over a period of hours or days producing blurred vision, anorexia, nausea, vomiting, thirst, and increasing urination. Drowsiness progresses to stupor and coma and death may occur if the patient remains untreated. Other complications of diabetes mellitus include abnormal changes in blood vessels that lead to an increased potential for blindness, cardiovascular diseases, kidney disease, and peripheral vascular disease.

The causes of diabetes mellitus are not yet known but several distinct types have been identified. The patient with Type 1 (insulin-dependent) diabetes produces little or no insulin because beta islet cells are not functioning. The illness generally develops rapidly, often in young people, produces more severe symptoms and complications, and is more difficult to control. Injections of purified pork, beef, or human insulin are needed daily. The patient with Type 2 (non-insulin-dependent) diabetes produces some insulin from functioning beta islet cells but the secretion from the pancreas is abnormal. This type of diabetes often develops during later years in persons who are overweight and sedentary. Symptoms are less severe, the patient's condition remains more stable, and an oral hypoglycemic agent may be used to stimulate insulin secretion from islet cells. Other types of diabetes that have been identified include: gestational diabetes (develops during pregnancy) and secondary diabetes (develops as a result of other illnesses).

In addition to drug therapy with insulin or oral hypoglycemic agents, diet and exercise play an important and equal role in the control of diabetes. Current research indicates that the patient whose blood sugar remains consistently near normal is less likely to develop complications.

I. Actions and uses.
  A. Insulin preparations are usually composed of purified pork or beef insulin. Currently, human insulin is also available in short- and intermediate-acting preparations.
  B. Insulin is currently thought to act by attaching to special receptors on the cell membrane. This process promotes the transport of glucose across the cell membrane.
  C. Insulin preparations are classified as short-acting, intermediate-acting, or long-acting. All preparations are usually administered SC to persons with Type 1 (insulin-dependent) diabetes.
  D. Intermediate-acting insulins are the ones most commonly used. Short-acting preparations may be ordered several times a day to establish control in newly diagnosed diabetics; they are administered IV for the patient in diabetic ketoacidosis. In addition, short-acting insulins may be added to intermediate preparations when a person has persistent elevations of morning blood sugars but good control at other times. Long-acting preparations are most often used for the patient with persistent elevation of blood sugar at night but good control at other times.
  E. Insulin preparations come in various strengths. Currently, only U100 (100 units of insulin per milliliter) is generally used. U40 and U80 insulins are being eliminated in favor of U100. U500 (500 units of insulin per milliliter) is also available for patients who are resistant to insulin. Special syringes are used to draw up the correct dose. Calibrations on the insulin syringe must correspond exactly to the strength of the preparation to be administered. The dose of insulin is ordered in units also.
  F. In most patients, insulin is administered in the morning before breakfast. Some patients may require additional insulin in the late afternoon.
  G. Oral hypoglycemics are believed to stimulate islet cell tissue to release insulin. For this effect, oral hypoglycemics may be used only for the patient with Type 2 (non-insulin-dependent) diabetes.
  H. Experts recommend that oral hypoglycemics be limited to those patients with Type 2 diabetes who cannot lower the blood sugar with diet, weight loss, and exercise alone.

TABLE 22–4   Insulin, Oral Hypoglycemic Agents

Nonproprietary Name	Proprietary Name	Adult Dose Range	Notes
Short-Acting Insulins—Onset of Action About 1 h			
insulin injection	Regular insulin Actrapid Human* Humulin R*	8–10 U SC 20 min before meals and at bedtime until initial control is established; 2–10 U/1 h by continuous IV infusion for patients in ketoacidosis or hyperosmolar coma; also available as 500 U/ml	Clear in color; may be mixed with other preparations; duration of action about 8 h; only insulin that may be administered IM, IV, and SC
prompt insulin zinc suspension	Semilente insulin	Dose adjusted to patient's blood sugar; administered SC only, available as 100 U/ml	Cloudy in color; may be mixed only with lente insulin; duration of action about 14 h
Intermediate-Acting Insulins—Onset of Action About 2 h			
isophane insulin suspension	NPH insulin Humulin N*	Dose adjusted to patient's blood sugar; basic ingredient of most regimens; administered SC only once daily before breakfast; available as 100 U/ml	Cloudy in color; may be mixed with regular insulin; duration of action about 24 h
insulin zinc suspension	Lente insulin Monotard Human*	Same as NPH	Cloudy in color; may be mixed with semilente; duration of action about 24 h
Long-Acting Insulins—Onset of Action 4 h			
protamine zinc suspension insulin		Dose adjusted to patient's blood sugar; administered SC only; more likely to be used for patients who spill sugar in the urine at night; available in 100 U/ml	Cloudy in color; may be mixed with regular insulin; duration of action about 36 h

II. Adverse responses.
   A. Insulin
      1. Hypoglycemic reactions may develop from too much insulin, unusual exercise, or skipping meals. The patient experiences weakness, inner trembling, nervousness, hunger, tachycardia that may progress to mental confusion, incoherent speech, convulsions, and irreversible brain damage.
      2. Allergic reactions may occur including urticaria and skin rashes. Anaphylaxis and angioedema are rare.
      3. Atrophy or hypertrophy of SC fat may occur at injection sites. This in turn interferes with even absorption.
   B. Oral hypoglycemics.
      1. Hypoglycemic reactions as described above may occur.
      2. Blood: leukopenia, agranulocytosis, thrombocytopenia, anemia.
      3. Gastrointestinal system: jaundice, nausea, vomiting.
      4. Skin: rash, photosensitivity.
      5. Other: headache, paresthesias, tinnitus.
   C. Drug interactions include:
      • Increased risk of hypoglycemic reactions when oral hypoglycemics are used with aspirin and salicylates, alcohol, chloramphenicol, clofibrate, dicumarol, monoamine oxidase inhibitors, probenecid, phenylbutazone, propranolol, or sulfonamides.
      • Alcohol interaction may cause flushing, nausea, and palpitations.
      • Drugs that decrease the effects of insulin include estrogens, progestins, epinephrine and sympathetic agents, corticosteroids, phenytoin, thiazide diuretics.

TABLE 22–4 *(cont.)*

Nonproprietary Name	Proprietary Name	Adult Dose Range	Notes
extended insulin zinc suspension	Utralente insulin		Cloudy in color; may be mixed with regular insulin or semilente; duration of action about 36 h
Oral Hypoglycemics			
acetohexamide	Dymelor	500–1,500 mg PO per day	
chlorpropramide	Diabenese	250–1,000 mg PO per day	
glipizide	Glucotrol	5 mg PO per day initially; 5–40 mg PO per day for maintenance	Administered 30 min before breakfast
glyburide	Diabeta, Micronase	2.5–5 mg PO per day initially; 2.5–20 mg PO per day for maintenance	Usually administered with breakfast
tolazamide	Tolinase	250–1,000 mg PO per day	
tolbutamide	Orinase	1,000–3,000 mg PO per day	
Other Related Drugs			
dextrose 50%		Administered by slow IV injection by a registered nurse or physician to reverse hypoglycemic reaction in the hospitalized patient	
glucagon		1 mg SC to reverse coma associated with hypoglycemia; patient should become conscious in 20 min; may also be administered IM, IV in dose sufficient to reverse hypoglycemia	Glucagon is a natural hormone secreted by islet pancreas cells in response to food and other hormones; actions in general are antagonistic to insulin; used mainly to reverse hypoglycemic reactions when dextrose is not available; and for x-ray examination procedures of intestines; may produce nausea and vomiting

*New insulin preparations that are structurally identical to human insulin.

- Drugs that increase the effects of insulin and enhance the likelihood of hypoglycemic reaction include alcohol and propranolol.
- Changes in serum potassium levels with insulin administration may enhance the likelihood of digitalis toxicity.

III. Nursing implications.

    A. Assist with admission assessment of the hospitalized patient with diabetes. A minimum of information would include: dietary and eating practices, prescribed and nonprescribed drugs taken (include insulin and oral hypoglycemics), exercise pattern, blood or urine testing practices and patterns, condition of skin and mucous membranes, height and weight, vital signs, patterns of urinary and fecal elimination.

    B. Use double-voided urine specimens when urine tests are ordered. Follow the procedure carefully for accurate results; record findings and notify the registered nurse of glucose or ketones in the urine. Check with the pharmacist about drug therapy that may affect the results of urine testing.

    C. Monitor blood glucose to anticipate possible changes in the patient's clinical condition. A normal range of blood glucose is between 80 and 120 mg/ml.

    D. Store and administer insulin at room temperature to prevent atrophy and hypertrophy of SC fat at injection sites.

    E. Use the syringe calibrated to match the strength of insulin prescribed. For example, use only a U100 insulin syringe to draw up a prescribed dose of U100 insulin.

    F. Check the physician's order and the label carefully before drawing up the dose. Insulin and the doses prescribed are more likely to be changed when the patient is hospitalized.

   G. Rotate the vial of insulin gently between the palms of both hands to mix the suspension thoroughly before drawing up the prescribed dose.
   H. Check the dose drawn up in the syringe with another nurse before administering it.
   I. Use the following guidelines to administer insulin on a sliding scale:
      1. Collect a double-voided urine specimen and test it for sugar and acetone if the scale is based upon urine sugar and acetone.
      2. Request the laboratory to collect and report the blood sugar approximately 15–30 min before the dose of insulin is due if the sliding scale is based upon blood sugar.
      3. Compare the findings (urine or blood sugar) to the corresponding dose of regular insulin ordered by the physician.
      4. Administer the dose of regular or short-acting insulin that matches your findings.
   J. Administer the prescribed dose of insulin at the same time daily if possible. The first dose is usually administered about 30 min before breakfast.
   K. Develop a site rotation plan for hospitalized patients that uses injection sites not usually accessible to the patient. For example, injection sites on the upper back, upper outer arms, and buttocks are inaccessible to many patients administering insulin to themselves at home. Using these sites when the patient is hospitalized enables other sites to rest. An acceptable plan is one that does not require the same site to be injected more than once every 6–8 weeks.
   L. Estimate the time of peak action after insulin has been administered and plan to observe the patient more frequently during that time for possible hypoglycemic reaction: 2 to 3 h for short-acting insulins, 8 to 12 h for intermediate-acting insulins, 14 to 20 h or more for long-acting insulins.
   M. Observe and record the patient's dietary intake. Report unfinished meals to the registered nurse or dietitian. Anticipate possible hypoglycemic reactions. In some cases, a snack may be ordered to prevent hypoglycemia.
   N. Know where sugar, candy, and emergency dextrose and supplies for IV administration are located on the nursing unit.
   O. Instruct the patient to report the first signs of nervousness, trembling. These are early indicators of possible hypoglycemic reaction. Report possible hypoglycemia to the registered nurse immediately.
   P. Check hospital or physician's policy when hypoglycemia is suspected. In some cases, there are standing orders for an immediate blood sugar to be drawn as the first step. If the patient is able to swallow, some physicians or hospitals have a specific protocol to be followed. For example, five Lifesavers orally or 8 oz of orange juice containing 2 tsp of sugar may be given to the patient.
   Q. Select other nursing actions that are appropriate for the patient with diabetes.
   R. Participate in patient teaching as requested by the registered nurse. Anticipate that topics for patient teaching will include: a description of diabetes, and of the causes, prevention, and relief of hypoglycemia; urine and blood testing; diet, exercise, insulin administration, oral hypoglycemics, skin care (especially foot care).
   S. Suggest that the patient be assisted at home by a public health nurse if this has not already been done.
   T. Encourage the patient to wear identification with the name and dose of insulin or oral hypoglycemic agent at all times.

THYROID AND ANTITHYROID DRUGS

Thyroid and antithyroid drugs influence the manufacture and release of thyroid hormones such as thyroxine and triiodothyronine (Table 22–5). The thyroid gland is located in the neck at the sides of the trachea. Thyroxine, the principal hormone, is manufactured from amino acids and strongly influenced by iodine intake and thyroid-stimulating and thyroid-releasing hormones from the pituitary gland. The main actions of thyroid hormones are to regulate growth and development and basal metabolism (the rate at which the body uses energy).

Thyroid and antithyroid drugs are prescribed for the patient with either a deficiency of thyroid hormone (*hypothyroidism*) or an oversupply (*hyperthyroidism*). The patient with a deficiency of circulating hormone during fetal life or infancy may develop *cretinism*. This is an abnormal developmental process that includes mental retardation, bradycardia, low body temperature, and characteristic skeletal deformities. The patient who develops hypothyroidism as an adult may have a condition called *myxedema*. Such a person may experience a generalized slowing of bodily functions, tremors and twitching, rough dry skin, coarse hair that falls out easily, swollen, puffy face and hands, and an apathetic mood. Another type of hypothyroidism is related to enlargement of the thyroid gland and undersecretion of thyroxine (*simple goiter*). Patients with an undersupply of thyroid hormone receive thyroid drugs as replacement.

The patient with hyperthyroidism has an overactivity of the thyroid gland that produces a condition called *Graves' disease*. Such a patient may develop exophthalmos (protruding eyeballs), tachycardia and cardiac arrhythmias, nervousness, insomnia, elevated body temperature, weight loss, and digestive disturbances. Another kind of oversupply of thyroid hormone that may cause hyperthyroidism occurs when nodules form in the gland and begin to produce additional thyroid hormone. The patient with hyperthyroidism receives antithyroid drugs.

I. Actions and uses.
  A. Thyroid hormone is usually used to restore normal blood levels of circulating thyroid hormones in patients with hypothyroidism.

TABLE 22–5 Thyroid and Antithyroid Drugs

Nonproprietary Name	Proprietary Name	Adult Dose Range	Notes
levothyroxine sodium	Levothroid, Synthroid	50 μg PO per day for 1–2 weeks; 100 μg PO per day for next 1–2 weeks 50–400 μg PO per day as maintenance dosage 200–500 μg IV for myxedema coma	Dose adjusted to provide full replacement for the patient with hypothyroidism
liothyronine sodium	Cytomel	25 μg PO per day as maintenance dosage for hypothyroidism 10–25 μg IV every 8–12 h or 100 μg IV for myxedema coma	Acts more quickly that other preparations; dose varies according to patient's condition
liotrix	Euthroid, Thyrolar	15–30 mg PO per day gradually increased until replacement dose is reached	A combination preparation that contains both levothyroxine and liothyronine
thyroglobulin	Proloid	60 mg PO per day as maintenance dosage	Dose highly individualized according to patient's condition
thyroid tablets	Thyrar	60 mg PO per day as maintenance dosage	Same as thyroglobulin
thyrotropin	Thytropar	Available in ampules containing 10 IU for SC, IM injection	Used only to test ability of thyroid to respond
thryrotropin-releasing hormone	Thypinone	Available as 500 μg/ml ampules for injection	
Antithyroid Preparations			
methimazole	Tapazole	5–10 mg PO every 8 h	
propylthiouracil		75–100 mg PO every 8 h up to 1,200 mg PO per day may be required	Doses may be prescribed every 4–6 hours if total daily dose exceed 300 mg
radioactive iodine (I131)	Iodotopic Therapeutic	4–10 mg PO total dose	Administered by a physician
sodium iodide—10%		50–150 mg IV per day	
strong iodine solution	Lugol's solution	50–150 mg PO per day	Contains iodine and potassium iodide

B. Antithyroid drugs are used to decrease thyroid function in patients with hyperthyroidism. These drugs may work in one or more of the following ways: inhibit the manufacture of thyroid hormones; damage the thyroid gland; suppress the release of thyrotropin-stimulating and thyrotropin-releasing hormones from the pituitary.

C. Antithyroid drugs may be used alone or in combination with other forms of treatment for hyperthyroidism including: radiation, surgical removal or partial removal of the thyroid gland, radioactive iodide. All forms of treatment are aimed at reducing the output of thyroid hormones.

II. Adverse responses.

  A. Thyroid preparations may produce angina, tachycardia, palpitations and arrhythmias, and general symptoms of hyperthyroidism.

  B. Antithyroid drugs.

   1. Skin: rashes and purpura.

   2. Blood: agranulocytosis and other anemias.

   3. Iodine-specific responses.

       a. Anaphylaxis or allergic responses such as angioedema, cutaneous hemorrhages, fever, joint pains, lymph node enlargement, purpura.

       b. Intoxication may produce brassy taste in the mouth, soreness, burning or mouth, gums, tongue, throat; inflammation of mucous membranes, sneezing and respiratory symptoms; gastritis, diarrhea, vomiting.

   4. Other: joint pain and stiffness, paresthesias, headache, nausea, loss of hair or its pigmentation, drug fever, hepatitis, nephritis.

  C. Drug interactions include:

   • Increased effects of thyroid preparations when combined with epinephrine, antidepressants, clofibrate, phenytoin, phenobarbital.

   • Decreased effects of thyroid preparations when combined with antihypertensives, estrogens and oral contraceptives, propranolol.

   • Increased effects of antithyroid preparations when combined with chlorpromazine, lithium, oral hypoglycemics, phenylbutazone, sulfa drugs, xanthine derivatives.

III. Nursing implications.

  A. Assist in the collection of information for the patient's nursing history.

  B. Administer oral thyroid preparations on an empty stomach if possible to encourage regular and complete absorption.

  C. Monitor laboratory work when possible to anticipate the patient's clinical response to drug therapy.

  D. Check and record the pulse before each dose of thyroid drug. Report a pulse of 100 beats/min or more and/or changes in rhythm and regularity. These are early symptoms of too much thyroid drug.

  E. Instruct the patient taking thyroid hormone to wear drug identification containing the specific preparation and dose.

  F. Instruct the patient not to change preparations without the physician's supervision because hormone content varies with the specific preparation used.

  G. Store thyroid preparations away from light and instruct the patient to do so at home.

  H. Administer antithyroid iodine solutions in a glass of juice, milk, or water and have the patient drink through a straw to prevent straining of the teeth. Iodine preparations have a very unpleasant taste.

  I. Assist the patient with hypothyroidism to use nondrug measures for comfort: additional blankets or clothing for warmth; lotions and minimal soap for dry skin; increased dietary bulk and roughage to prevent constipation.

  J. Assist the patient with hyperthyroidism to use nondrug measures for comfort: frequent rest periods, additional food and fluids, a calm, nonstimulating environment, lightweight clothing, and dark glasses for severe exophthalmos.

  K. Instruct the patient taking thyroid or antithyroid drugs to avoid other drugs and to tell new physicians about the specific preparation and dose being taken.

L. Teach the patient taking antithyroid drugs to report fever and sore throat immediately. These symptoms may indicate the onset of agranulocytosis.

CASE STUDY 16

Mr. Henry Angel is a 25-year-old man who went to his doctor because of weight loss despite persistent hunger, and frequent urination. The physician diagnosed diabetes mellitus, Type 1. After several days of drug therapy with regular insulin U100 according to a sliding scale with the blood sugar, Mr. Angel was placed on lente insulin U100, 20 U SC daily 30 min before breakfast.

QUESTIONS

1. What is the gland and hormone related to diabetes mellitus, regular insulin, and lente insulin?
2. Explain how sliding scale insulin works.
3. What are the nursing implications to be considered when administering lente insulin?
4. When you bring the first does of lente insulin, 20 U, Mr. Angel askes, "Why can't I take those insulin pills every day like my boss does?" How will you respond to Mr. Angel's question?
5. What nursing observations would indicate hypoglycemia; when would you be most likely to observe them; what nursing actions are indicated?
6. List at least one contribution you can make as a student practical nurse to each of the topics associated with patient teaching for Mr. Angel.

EXERCISE 1

Compare thyroid and antithyroid drugs from the perspective of the patient's condition, actions and uses, adverse responses, and nursing implications. A chart is provided to help you organize the information.

	Thyroid drugs	Antithyroid drugs
Patient's condition		
Actions and uses		
Adverse responses		
Nursing implications		

EXERCISE 2

Asking questions about drug therapy is an excellent way to learn. This exercise helps you to formulate questions about drug therapy with corticosteroids or nonsteroidal anti-inflammatory agents. Next to each statement in Column A, formulate a question that is answered by that statement. Some examples have been provided for you.

Column A	Question
Column A	**Question**

Column A

1. The patient with rheumatoid arthritis, osteoarthritis, or gout.
2. Interferes with the activity of prostaglandins.
3. Gastrointestinal disturbances, vertigo, blurred vision, skin rashes.
4. Observe and report signs of infection before administering the first dose.
5. Administer with or after meals.
6. Check the patient for aspirin allergy and report before administering the first dose.
7. Hyperglycemia, buffalo hump, osteoporosis, moon face, adrenal insufficiency.
8. Inspect the skin daily for petechiae, ecchymoses, and pupura and record findings.
9. Anticipate delayed healing of surgical wounds; observe carefully for complications such as infection.
10. Instruct the patient not to stop taking the drug abruptly without notifying the physician.

Question

Who might receive drug therapy with nonsteroidal anti-inflammatory agents?

How can I detect early signs of increased bleeding tendency when administering a corticosteroid?

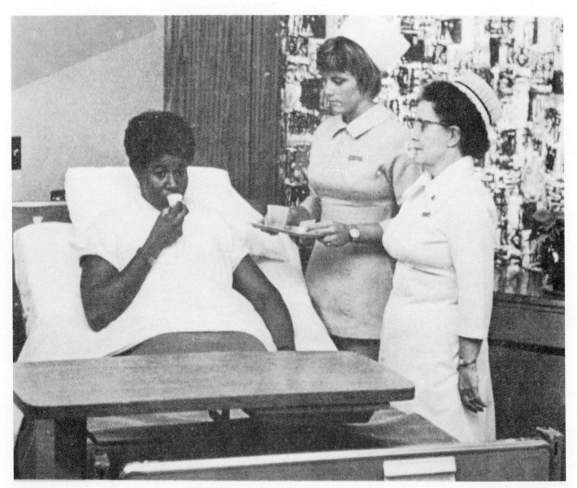

Courtesy of Palm Beach County Practical Nursing Program, The School Board of Palm Beach County, Fla.

Section VI

DRUGS USED FOR SPECIAL CONDITIONS

Chapter 23 | DRUG THERAPY FOR THE PATIENT WITH ALLERGIES

EXPECTED BEHAVIORAL OUTCOMES

After completing the chapter you should return to the expected behavioral outcomes and evaluate your ability to:

1. Relate the specific effects of antihistamines and immunosuppressives to the allergic response and immune response, respectively.
2. Compare antihistamines and immunosuppressives with respect to the patient's condition, actions and uses, adverse responses, and nursing implications.

DESCRIPTION OF ALLERGY

The person with an *allergy* has an overly sensitive response to a substance that normally is not considered harmful. The substances producing this overly sensitive response are called *allergens* or *antigens*. Allergens are usually protein substances such as: food or drugs that are ingested; vaccines, serums, drugs, bee stings that are injected; dust, pollens, powders that are inhaled; and fur, hair, soaps, or other substances that are contacted through the skin. The response that occurs after an allergen is introduced into the body is called allergy or *hypersensitivity*. The allergic response is actually an antigen–antibody reaction that may occur immediately after exposure (*immediate hypersensitivity*) or later on (*delayed hypersensitivity*).

An allergy involves a disturbance in the patient's immune system. The antigen–antibody interaction that takes place during the allergic response does not protect the body from harmful substances as usual but instead causes damage. The special immune cells believed to be active during an allergic response are called immunglobulins E (IgE) and T lymphocytes. The interaction between these cells and the allergen results in the release of histamine, serotonin, acetylcholine, and heparin. These substances act to produce smooth muscle constriction, vasodilatation, pooling of blood in peripheral blood vessels, and leakage of plasma into surrounding tissues. As a result, allergic hypersensitivity may produce many different clincial symptoms such as:

1. Allergic rhinitis or hay faver with the typical reddened, irritated conjunctiva and stuffy nose; may be seasonal or chronic.
2. Asthma, characterized by wheezing and shortness of breath, demonstrates mild or severe bronchial involvement.
3. Gastric disturbances, such as cramping, nausea, and vomiting, can be distressing allergy symptoms.

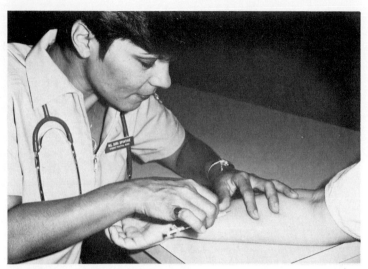

FIGURE 23–1   **Skin testing for allergies.**

4. Headaches can be unilateral, sudden, and severe reactions to foreign proteins.
5. *Anaphylactic shock* is a sudden, devastating manifestation of allergy that may cause death.
6. Angioneurotic edema that is accompanied by laryngeal swelling constitutes a threat to life.
7. Dermatitis, urticaria, or pruritus may occur as an allergic response to insect bites or vegetation poisoning.

In addition, two unusual types of hypersensitivity are currently the subject of much research. The first is *tissue rejection*, a type of delayed hypersensitivity that causes destruction of a transplanted organ in the recipient. A second form of hypersensitivity occurs when the body becomes sensitized to its own tissue. This is called *autoimmunity*. Two diseases that have been linked to an autoimmune process are rheumatoid arthritis and systemic lupus erythematosus.

The physician uses three basic treatment methods for the patient with allergy: avoidance (identifying the allergy and modifying life-style to avoid it), drug therapy for relief of symptoms, and desensitization. See Fig. 23-1.

ANTIHISTAMINES

Antihistamines are drugs that antagonize the actions of histamine (Table 23-1). Histamine is a chemical mediator naturally present in mast cells and basophils; and stored liberally throughout body tissues. During hypersensitivity, histamine is released to produce typical symptoms of allergy as described earlier.

Antihistamines occupy histamine receptor sites on cells. Although histamine is released, it is unable to act on target tissues because receptor sites are already occupied by the antihistamine drug.

   I. Actions and uses.
   A. Antihistamines are helpful in relieving allergic symptoms associated with conjunctivitis, rhinitis and hay fever. Antihistamines are generally not used for patients with bronchial asthma.
   B. Antihistamines are helpful in certain allergic conditions of the skin such as dermatitis, dermatosis, and urticaria. These agents are also helpful in relieving pruritus.
   C. Antihistamines may be used as an adjunct after initial therapy with epinephrine for the patient with angioedema and anaphylaxis.
   D. Antihistamines may be used to prevent allergic responses from blood transfusions and contrast dyes used in diagnostic studies.
   E. Antihistamines may be used for the patient with drug allergy, extrapyramidal side effects (see p. 149), Ménière's disease, and vertigo.

TABLE 23–1   Antihistamines

Nonproprietary Name	Proprietary Name	Adult Dose Range	Notes
Alkylamines			
brompheniramine maleate	Dimetane, others	4 mg PO every 4–6 h; 8–12 mg PO every 12 h sustained release capsule; 5–20 mg IM	Alkylamines are the most powerful group of antihistamines; central nervous system stimulation occurs more often as an adverse response
chlorpheniramine maleate	Chlor-Trimeton and others	4 mg PO every 4–6 h; 8–12 mg PO sustained release capsule twice daily; 5–20 mg IM	
dexchlorpheniramine maleate	Polaramine	1–2 mg PO 3–4 × /day; 4–6 mg sustained release capsule twice per day	
dimethindene maleate	Forhistal	2.5 mg PO 3–4 × /day	
triprolidine	Actidil	2.5 mg PO 3–4 × /day	
Ethanolamines			
bromodiphenhydramine hydrochloride	Ambodryl	25 mg PO 3 × /day	Ethanolamines are more likely to produce sedation as a side effect; gastrointestinal side effects occur less often
carbinoxamine maleate	Clistin	4–8 mg PO every 3–4 h	
dimenhydrinate	Dramamine and others	50 mg PO, IM every 4–6 h	Also used as antiemetic
diphenhydramine hydrochloride	Benadryl and others	25–50 mg PO, IM every 4–6 h	Also used as antiemetic, antipruritic
doxylamine succinate	Decapryn	12.5–25 mg PO every 4–6 h	
Ethylenediamines			
pyrilamine maleate		25–50 mg PO every 4–6 h	Ethylenediamines commonly produce gastrointestinal side effects
tripelennamine citrate	PBZ	37.5–75 mg PO every 4–6 h (liquid)	
tripelennamine hydrochloride	PBZ	25–50 mg PO every 4–6 h; 100 mg PO sustained-release capsule	
Phenothiazines—see also Tables 16–8 and 21–5 for additional information.			
methdilazine	Tacaryl	16–32 mg PO per day in two to four divided doses	A phenothiazine derivative with few side effects; used mainly to relieve pruritus
promethazine hydrochloride	Phenergan and others	25 mg PO, IM, suppository	Produces marked sedation; also used as antiemetic, antimotion sickness agent, preanesthetic
trimeprazine tartrate	Temaril	10 mg PO/day in four divided doses	Produces sedation; used mainly for antipruritic effects
Piperazines			
azatadine maleate	Optimine	1–2 mg PO 2 × /day	Piperazines are especially helpful in relieving pruritus
cyclizine hydrochloride or lactate	Marezine and others	50 mg PO, IM every 4–6 h	Also used for motion sickness
cyproheptadine	Periactin	4–20 mg PO per day in divided doses	
hydroxyzine hydrochloride or pamoate	Atarax Vistaril	25 mg PO, IM every 6–24 h	Also used as antiemetic, preanesthetic
meclizine hydrochloride	Antivert, others	25–50 mg PO every 12–24 h	Also used for vertigo

TABLE 23–1   *(cont.)*

Nonproprietary Name	Proprietary Name	Adult Dose Range	Notes
Other			
cromolyn sodium	Intal	1 capsule: contents inhaled 4×/day	Used to prevent bronchial asthma; see also p. 229.
	Nasalcrom	4% nasal spray: 1 spray in each nostril 3–6×/day	
	Opticrom	4% opthalmic solution: 1–2 gtts 4–6×/day	
terfenadine	Seldane	60 mg PO twice daily	New drug recommended for patients with allergic rhinitis; said to produce less drowsiness

II. Adverse responses.
  A. Central nervous system: sedation, lassitude, fatigue, dizziness, visual disturbances, uncoordination, tremors, insomnia, and headache.
  B. Gastrointestinal system: anorexia, nausea, vomiting, epigastric distress, constipation or diarrhea, and dryness of the mouth and throat.
  C. Respiratory system: dryness of respiratory passages that may lead to cough.
  D. Urinary system: retention, frequency, dysuria.
  E. Allergy: skin rashes, drug fever, photosensitivity.
  F. Blood: leukopenia, agranulocytosis, anemia.
  G. Other: chest tightness, hypotension, tingling of the hands, birth defects.
  H. Poisoning produces central nervous system excitement that includes hallucinations and incoordination leading to convulsions, coma, and death. Fixed dilated pupils, tachycardia, fever, dry mouth, flushed face, and urinary retention may also be present during acute poisoning.
  I. Drug interactions include:
    • Alcohol and other central nervous system depressants (see Chapter 16) increase side effects of drowsiness, lethargy, and respiratory depression when combined with antihistamines.
    • Increased anticholinergic effects when tricyclic antidepressants (see Table 16–6) are combined with antihistamines.
    • Increased antihistamine side effects when combined with monoamine oxidase inhibitors (see Table 16–6).
III. Nursing implications.
  A. Gather and record information about allergies on all newly admitted patients. Notify other appropriate departments of the patient's allergies: dietary, housekeeping, radiology or diagnostic studies, and pharmacy. Display the patient's allergies prominently in several places.
  B. Seek additional information from the registered nurse, pharmacist, or physician before administering an antihistamine to a patient with glaucoma, prostate hypertropy, peptic ulcer, bladder neck obstruction, pregnancy, or to a nursing mother. Antihistamines are generally not recommended for these patients.
  C. Administer oral antihistamines with meals to decrease gastrointestinal side effects.
  D. Administer IM preparations into a large muscle mass such as gluteal muscles.
  E. Know where emergency drugs and supplies are located on your nursing unit, clinic, or doctor's office in case of anaphylaxis.
  F. Before administering a new drug or substance to the skin, ask the patient again about previous allergy. Report possible allergy responses to the registered nurse or physician.
  G. Inspect the patient's skin regularly for rash. Report and record description of skin rashes if applicable.
  H. Ask the patient who receives drug therapy in the outpatient department, clinic, or doctor's office to remain for 20–30 min of observation for possible allergic response.

J. Teach the patient with allergy to avoid others with colds or respiratory infection since these conditions may lead to an acute attack.

K. Teach the patient with allergy general health practices such as eating a balanced diet, getting sufficient rest and sleep, and maintaining emotional balance.

L. Teach the patient with pruritus to scratch the sheets, upholstery, or other textured substance to prevent skin damage.

M. Teach the patient with allergy to read labels carefully on food containers, clothing tags, cosmetic and household products.

N. Teach the patient with allergy to avoid all nonprescribed drugs unless this has been discussed with the physician.

O. Teach the patient taking antihistamines to evaluate drowsiness before driving or participating in activities that require judgment and coordination.

IMMUNOSUPPRESSIVES

Immunosuppressives are drugs that suppress the patient's immune response (Table 23–2). The *immune response* is a natural protection against foreign agents that develop inside the body or enter the body from the outside. When such an agent enters the bloodstream, it comes in contact with a special lymph cell. This contact stimulates the production of antibodies that destroy the foreign agent or render it harmless.

Under certain conditions, this normal protective process becomes harmful to a patient. For example, when a person receives a transplanted organ, the immune response may destroy it as a foreign agent. Thus immunosuppressives may be used to prevent rejection of transplanted organs such as the kidney, heart, bone marrow.

A second use of immunosuppressives is considered investigational at this time. This use is associated with the patient who has a disease linked to autoimmunity. For example, the patient with systemic lupus erythematosus, rheumatoid arthritis, chronic active hepatitis, ulcerative colitis, or nephrotic syndrome may receive an immunosuppressive.

I. Actions and uses.

    A. Immunsuppressives may be administered to prevent rejection in the patient undergoing transplant surgery.

    B. Immunosuppressives may be used investigationally for the patient with a disease linked to autoimmunity.

TABLE 23–2 Selected Immunosuppressives

Nonproprietary Name	Proprietary Name	Adult Dose Range	Notes
azathioprine*	Imuran	3–5 mg/kg initial oral dose; 1–3 mg/kg/day maintenance	Interferes with cell growth and function; used to prevent transplant rejection and is under investigation for the patient with severe rheumatoid arthritis
cyclophosphamide*	Cytoxan	Highly individualized	Believed to suppress immunity by destroying lymphocytes
cyclosporine	Sandimmune	10–15 mg/kg/day initial oral dose; gradually reduced to 5–10 mg/kg/day as maintenance; IV dose about ⅓ of oral dose	Believed to interfere with response of antibodies to antigen; used to prevent transplant rejection and investigationally for the patient with autoimmune idease; toxic to liver and kidneys
prednisone	Deltasone	Highly individualized	Adrenocortical hormone that suppresses immune response by reducing production of immune substances such as immunoglobulins, lymphocytes, macrophages. See Chapter 22, pp. 260–264 for additional information

*These drugs are cytotoxic and have adverse responses that result from the destruction of normal as well as abnormal cells. See Chapter 25 for additional information.

    C. Immunosuppressives also produce fundamental changes in cell growth, reproduction, and function. These changes are usually *cytotoxic* (causing cell death). For these effects, immunosuppressives are frequently used for the patient with neoplasm. See Chapter 25 for additional information.

II. Adverse responses.

    A. Immunosuppressives produce increased susceptibility to infection by interfering with normal body defenses. When infection does occur, it may be very severe and difficult to treat.

    B. Immunosuppressives produce increased susceptibility to tumor formation including malignant tumors.

    C. Immunosuppressives may produce genetic damage.

    D. Certain immunosuppressives are cytotoxic: they destroy cells. Destruction of abnormal cells such as neoplastic cells is helpful. However, destruction of normal cells may produce some or all of the following adverse responses:

- Gastrointestinal disturbances including anorexia, unpleasant taste, nausea, vomiting, diarrhea, biliary stasis, bleeding.
- Skin and mucous membrane alterations including stomatitis, hair loss (alopecia), increased skin pigmentation, other skin alterations.
- Infertility, pulmonary fibrosis, liver and kidney damage.
- Hemorrhagic cystitis causing dysuria, hematuria.

    E. Prednisone is an adrenocortical hormone that produces immunosuppression. For additional information on adverse responses to this drug, see p. 263.

III. Nursing implications.

    A. Collect and record information that may affect nursing care for the patient receiving immunosuppressives. A minimum of information includes temperature, height and weight, condition of skin and mucous membranes, usual eating habits, urinary and fecal elimination patterns, presence or absence of systemic and local signs of infection.

    B. Monitor the patient's laboratory studies as they become available. Anticipate that the physician will order complete blood count (CBC), liver, and renal function studies. The results can be used by the nurse to anticipate clinical side effects.

    C. Use measures that minimize the patient's exposure to infection. Report early signs of infection such as sore throat, cough, rising temperature, malaise, fatigue, unexpected drainage, local signs.

    D. Wash hands thoroughly before and after each patient contact.

    E. Assist the patient with limited mobility to complete oral hygiene and perineal cleansing.

    F. Prevent exposure of the patient to others with infection: family, friends, hospital roommates, hospital staff.

    G. Inspect the patient's mouth daily with a flashlight for erythema or ulceration.

    H. Encourage and assist the patient with specific oral hygiene measures: brushing teeth gently with a soft bristle brush; flossing daily with unwaxed floss; rinsing mouth regularly with water, normal saline, or solutions containing hydrogen peroxide and/or mouthwash. (Lemon and glycerin swabs are avoided since they may irritate and dry mucous membranes.)

    I. Observe gums, skin, urine, and stool daily as possible sources of bleeding. Report and record findings.

    J. Encourage and assist the patient to eat a balanced diet and adequate fluid intake consistent with the physician's order for a specific diet and fluid intake.

    K. Observe the patient for jaundice or crystals in the urine because these findings indicate liver or kidney toxicity, respectively. Report and record findings.

    L. Administer an antiemetic if needed to prevent or relieve nausea and vomiting.

    M. Read package inserts and hospital policies before administering an immunosuppressive agent. In some hospitals, only the registered nurse or physician may administer certain immunosuppressives. Seek additional information from the pharmacist if needed.

    N. Monitor the intravenous flow rate and site in patients receiving immunosuppressives IV; report abnormal findings immediately to the registered nurse.

O. Create opportunities for the patient to discuss concerns and questions about the impact of illness or drug therapy on appearance, relationships, work, and other important areas. Report the patients questions and concerns to the registered nurse.

EXERCISE 1

Compare antihistamines and immunosuppressives as described in this chapter from the perspective of: effects on allergic response and/or immune response; patient's condition actions and uses; adverse responses; nursing implications. A chart is provided to help you organize the information.

Descriptive Categories	Antihistamines	Immunosuppressives
Effects on allergic/ immune response		
Patient's condition		
Actions and uses		
Adverse responses		
Nursing implications		

Chapter 24 | DRUG THERAPY FOR THE PATIENT WITH INFECTION

EXPECTED BEHAVIORAL OUTCOMES

After completing this chapter, you should return to the expected behavioral outcomes and evaluate your ability to:

1. Explain the actions of antimicrobial agents on bacteria, fungi, and viruses.
2. Describe the relationship of a culture and sensitivities test to drug therapy for the patient with infection.
3. Identify two adverse responses common to aminoglycosides and explain how you would observe them in a patient.
4. List at least five nursing actions that enhance the effects of antimicrobial agents.
5. Select an appropriate nursing measure for each of the following adverse responses that may develop in a patient receiving drug therapy for infection: allergy, bone marrow depression, gastrointestinal symptoms, resistance, superinfection.
6. Prepare a written list of instructions for a patient about to be discharged with a prescription for an antimicrobial agent.
7. Describe at least five nursing implications related to the potential for adverse responses in a patient receiving an immunizing agent to prevent infection.

DESCRIPTION OF INFECTION

The person with infection has an inflammation caused by microorganisms. Three different families of organisms may cause disease: bacteria, fungi (plantlike organisms), and viruses (organisms that invade the cell and live there). Bacteria are further described according to their shape, requirement for oxygen, and response to Gram stain.

All microorganisms do not cause disease. Some of them are essential to health. For example, normal flora are bacteria that live on the skin and mucous membranes of the gastrointestinal system, upper respiratory system, and vagina. Normal flora provide a bacterial barrier that prevents the entry of disease causing microorganisms called *pathogens*. Pathogens may enter the body through air, water, food, broken skin or mucous membranes, sexual contact, and hair follicles. Microorganisms may be transmitted by the mother to the fetus through the placenta.

The body contains many defense mechanisms that help to prevent the entry of pathogens, destroy or neutralize them, or prevent their spread. The skin, hair and mucous membranes act as a mechanical barrier. Body secretions such as tears, mucus, gastric secretions, and vaginal secretions trap pathogens. Special cells in body secretions also help to kill or prevent the growth of pathogens. Reflex mechanisms such as sneezing, coughing, swallowing, peristalsis, and movement of cilia help to filter and remove particles or pathogens from the body. Special white blood cells such as phagocytes, antibodies, and microphages ingest, engulf, and destroy pathogens. *Inflammation* is a process that helps to localize infection, destroy pathogens, and remove associated waste products.

Despite numerous and varied body defenses, a person may develop infection if pathogens become too numerous; if pathogens are too virulent (strong); when a person's defenses are too weak; or when pathogens encounter a particular internal environment that favors their reproduction. Anyone may develop an infection but some persons are more likely to become infected than others. For example, persons with the following conditions have increased susceptibility to infection:

1. Burns, trauma, or breaks in the skin or mucous membrane.
2. A reduction of circulation to any body part.
3. Catheters and other tubes that are introduced to body cavities and organs.
4. Diseases that affect blood-forming organs, such as leukemia.
5. Diabetes mellitus and other chronic diseases such as cancer, chronic obstructive lung disease.
6. Drug therapy with immunosuppressives or antibiotics that destroy normal flora.
7. Undernutrition, dehydration, aging, or poor personal hygiene.

ANTIMICROBIALS: GENERAL PRINCIPLES

Antimicrobial agents are drugs that prevent or treat infection caused by bacteria, viruses, or fungi. Several terms may be used to describe various agents. *Antibiotics* are substances produced by microorganisms that suppress and may destroy the growth of other microorganisms. *Antimicrobials* is a general term that refers to all drugs used to kill microorganisms or suppress their growth. *Antifungal agents*, also called *fungicides*, are drugs that destroy or inhibit the growth of fungi such as yeasts and molds. *Antiviral agents* are drugs that inhibit the growth of viruses (parasites that invade the cell and live there).

In general, drug therapy with antibiotics is intended to reduce the number of pathogens to a level that normal body defenses are able to overcome.

   I. Actions and uses.
      A. Antimicrobial drugs act in several ways: destruction of the cell walls of microoganisms to cause death; prevention of reproduction by microoganisms; interference with metabolism of the microorganism.
      B. Antimicrobial agents must be carefully selected according to the specific pathogen and the patient's condition.
      C. Cultures of blood or body fluids are usually obtained first to identify the specific pathogens if possible.
      D. Pathogens identified in the culture are then matched to specific drugs known to be effective. This is called a *sensitivities test*.
      E. Drugs to which the pathogen is sensitive are then matched to the patient's condition. A drug is selected on the basis of its effectiveness in destroying the pathogen and its low potential for toxicity and allergy.
      F. Combination therapy is the use of two or more antimicrobial agents for the treatment of infection. Combination therapy may be used when the patient's infection is caused by several different pathogens, when the specific pathogen cannot be identified, or when a synergistic (additive) action is desired.
      G. All routes of administration may be used. In hospitalized patients with severe infections, the IV route is usually used.
      H. The effects of antibiotics depend upon maintaining a therapeutic level of drug at the site of infection. For this reason, antibiotics are usually ordered at evenly spaced intervals throughout the 24-h period.
      I. Additional factors that influence the specific choice of drug or dose include the patient's age, presence of drug allergy, pregnancy, lactation, kidney disease, nervous system disorders. Such factors tend to enhance the development of adverse responses.

II. Adverse responses.

    A. Allergy: reactions are common and most often seen as skin rashes; anaphylaxis may occur.

    B. Bone marrow depression: certain antimicrobials damage bone marrow and may produce a temporary or permanent deficiency of red or white blood cells; this in turn increases the likelihood of hemorrhage or additional infection.

    C. Gastrointestinal symptoms: nausea, vomiting, and diarrhea are common side effects of most antimicrobial agents.

    D. Nephrotoxicity: some antimicrobials may damage nephrons causing progressive loss of kidney function; there may be a gradual decrease in urine output and/or appearance of abnormal substances like blood or protein; damage may be temporary or permanent.

    E. Ototoxicity: some antimicrobials can damage the auditory nerve causing hearing loss and/or vertigo.

    F. Phlebitis, thrombophlebitis: antimicrobials are generally irritating to veins when administered IV; the site may become red, warm, tender, swollen.

    G. Resistance: pathogens may no longer be killed or inhibited by an antimicrobial that has previously been effective; the patient may develop a recurrence of symptoms.

    H. Superinfection: a new infection that occurs while the patient is being treated for a primary infection; may be caused by the destruction of normal flora by antibiotic therapy; the most common sites are the oropharynx, upper respiratory system, genitourinary system; the patient may develop stomatitis, sore throat, cough, urinary tract infection, vaginitis; diarrhea is also common.

III. Nursing implications.

    A. Assist in the collection of information from the patient with an infection. A minimum of information needed includes local or general symptoms of infection; drug allergies, drug history; presence or absence of pregnancy, lactation, liver or kidney disease, blood disorder.

    B. Use scrupulous technique to collect a culture ordered by the physician. Prevent accidental contamination of the culture specimen with other microorganisms from uninvolved areas such as the nurse's hands or the patient's hands.

    C. Notify the registered nurse or physician if a culture cannot be obtained. Ask specifically if the first dose is to be started without the culture.

    D. Request help from the registered nurse to set a dose schedule that is not interrupted by diagnostic tests or other therapies.

    E. Double-check the patient's allergies before administering the first dose.

    F. Administer most oral doses on an empty stomach to encourage complete absorption if possible.

    G. Administer IM injections deeply into a large muscle mass such as the gluteus; rotate injection sites and massage the injection site well after each dose.

    H. Check the patient's intravenous site about 1 h before the dose of antimicrobial agent is due. Notify the appropriate registered nurse if the site appears red, warm, tender, swollen, or the existing flow rate is irregular or uneven. Early detection and change of the IV site will prevent delays of IV doses.

    I. Do not mix antimicrobials with other drugs or with each other in the same syringe or IV equipment. This practice may cause drugs to precipitate or become inactive.

    J. Inspect the hospitalized patient daily for adverse responses; report positive findings to the registered nurse or physician and anticipate a change in drug or dose; record all findings.

    K. Instruct the outpatient to remain in the clinic or doctor's office for at least 20 to 45 min after receiving a dose of an antimicrobial agent. Check the patient several times for allergy during that waiting period.

    L. Prevent the spread of infection to others by frequent handwashing before and after each patient contact; careful handling and disposal of linens and other clothing; careful handling of the patient's secretions.

    M. Use nondrug measures appropriate for the hospitalized patient with an infection: provide frequent rest periods; encourage good nutritional intake and increase fluids if permitted by the physician; assist the patient with excellent personal hygiene.

N. Teach patients to take antimicrobials exactly as prescribed by the physician.

O. Suggest that the patient call the physician for further instructions if a dose is missed.

P. Teach the patient measures that prevent the spread of infection and measures that encourage the recovery from infection.

Q. Prevent nosocomial (hospital-acquired) infection by providing meticulous physical care to patients; using scrupulous technique during catheterization and catheter care; turning patients who are inactive or immobile, and encouraging coughing and deep breathing in such patients; encouraging and assisting patients to maintain a balanced diet and good fluid intake; encouraging slippers or footwear for all hospitalized ambulatory patients; providing receptacles for bedside disposal of tissues and other bedside waste; encouraging and assisting patients to practice regular and frequent oral hygiene; maintaining the dosage schedule for drug therapy with antibiotics.

AMEBICIDES

Amebicides are drugs that kill certain disease-causing protozoa called *ameba* (Table 24–1). The patient with *amebiasis* has an infection caused by the ingestion of food or water contaminated by human feces containing amebic cysts. Once ameba enter the body, they change form, multiply, and create new cysts. Each of the various forms may cause damage in the body. Erosions and ulcerations in the intestine and dysentery are common forms of amebiasis. However, organisms may also invade other body tissue such as skin, liver, lungs and other respiratory organs.

In the United States, amebiasis is most likely to occur in institutions for the mentally retarded, Indian reservations, migrant labor camps, and among male homosexuals.

I. Actions and uses.

A. Amebicides may exert a direct action on amebic cysts.

B. Some amebicides are effective only against intestinal forms of amebiasis.

C. Other amebicides are affective only against systemic amebiasis.

D. Antibiotics such as paramomycin and the tetracyclines may also be used as a supplement to other amebicides.

E. Laxatives and/or purges of the bowel may be ordered before or after drug therapy in some cases to aid in the elimination of ameba from the intestinal tract.

II. Adverse responses.

A. In the dose necessary for amebiasis, chloroquine has a low potential for toxicity. See p. 297 for additional information.

B. Dehydroemetine and emetine may produce pain, local reaction or abscess formation at the

TABLE 24–1   Amebicides

Nonproprietary Name	Proprietary Name	Adult Dose Range	Notes
chloroquine	Aralen Sulfate Plaquenil Sulfate	1 gram PO per day for 2 days; then 500 mg per day for 2–10 weeks	A second-choice agent for the patient with systemic amebiasis; antimalarial effects; see p. 297 for adverse response
dehydroemetine or emetine preparations		1–1.5 mg/kg/day SC or IM up to a maximum of 90 mg/day × 5 days	An older drug for systemic amebiasis; gradually replaced by metronidazole. High potential for toxicity; available from Centers for Disease Control
diloxanide furoate	Furamide	500 mg PO 3 ×/day × 10 days; a second course may be needed	Used for intestinal amebiasis
metronidazole	Flagyl	750 mg PO 3 ×/day × 5–10 days; also available for IV administration	Drug of choice for amebiasis; also has powerful bacteriocidal effects; may turn urine reddish-brown; gastrointestinal side effects are common; drug–alcohol interaction may occur

injection site; systemic potentially fatal toxicity including adverse effects on the heart and blood vessels, neuromuscular system, gastrointestinal system, or central nervous system.

    C. Diloxanide furoate may produce flatulence, pruritus, urticaria, and vomiting.

    D. Metronidazole may produce anorexia, nausea, vomiting, diarrhea, epigastric distress, and abdominal cramping. Headache, metallic unpleasant taste, glossitis and stomatitis, neuromuscular effects may also occur. Combined with alcohol, metronidazole may produce an interaction that includes flushing, abdominal cramping, vomiting, headache, tachycardia.

III. Nursing implications.

    A. Review the nursing implications presented above on pp. 290–291.

    B. Collect stools for examination for ova and parasites as ordered by the physician, and send to the laboratory for examination while warm.

    C. Follow package insert directions completely and carefully when preparing metronidazole for IV administration.

    D. Report adverse responses.

    E. Explain the alcohol–drug interaction of metronidazole to the patient and instruct him or her not to drink alcohol during therapy.

AMINOGLYCOSIDES

I. Actions and uses.

    A. *Aminoglycosides* are a group of chemically related drugs used primarily for the patient with infection caused by aerobic gram-negative bacteria such as Pseudomonas strains, Proteus, Staphyloccoccus aureus (Table 24–2).

    B. Aminoglycosides act to interfere with the manufacture of proteins by bacteria.

    C. Aminoglycosides are usually administered IM or IV to ensure complete absorption. Oral administration of some drugs is also used.

    D. Aminoglycosides are eliminated slowly in the urine.

    E. In general, a course of antimicrobial therapy with aminoglycosides lasts about 10 days.

    F. Kanamycin and neomycin may be ordered preoperatively to remove normal flora from the bowel before intestinal surgery.

II. Adverse responses.

    A. Ototoxicity: damage to the auditory nerve and vestibular apparatus in the ear may produce tinnitus, high-frequency hearing loss, headache, nausea, vomiting, disequilibrium, ataxia. Toxicity increases as dose increases.

    B. Nephrotoxicity: damage to kidney structures may produce a rise in plasma creatinine, falling plasma levels of potassium, calcium, phosphates. This in turn may cause retention of the drug and increase its toxic effects in the ear. Toxicity increases as dose increases.

    C. Acute muscular paralysis and apnea have occurred following administration of amimoglycosides by all routes. Patients with myesthenia gravis or chronic obstructive lung disease are more susceptible than others.

    D. Resistance to aminoglycosides is a common adverse response in hospitalized patients.

    E. Optic nerve damage, peripheral neuritis, paresthesias, hypersensitive reactions, blood disorders, and anaphylaxis are rare adverse responses.

    F. Drug interactions include:

       • Inactivation of aminoglycoside if accidentally combined in the same syringe or IV preparation with carbenicillin, ticarcillin.

       • Increased nephrotoxcity when combined with diuretics such as ethacrynic acid and furosemide, other nephrotoxic agents.

       • Increased likelihood of acute muscular paralysis and apnea when combined with other neuromuscular blocking agents like those listed in Table 16–5.

III. Nursing implications.

TABLE 24–2   Aminoglycosides

Nonproprietary Name	Proprietary Name	Adult Dose Range	Notes
amikacin	Amikin	15 mg/kg/day divided into two to three equal doses; for IM, IV administration	Same as gentamycin; also useful for resistant nosocomial infections in hospitalized patients; nephrotoxic, ototoxic
gentamicin	Garamycin	3–5 mg/kg/day IM, IV in three evenly spaced dose intervals; also available as ointment, cream, ophthalmic ointment or solution, intrathecal injection (without preservative)	Useful for patients with urinary tract infections, pneumonia, meningitis, infected burns, peritonitis and osteomyelitis caused by gram-negative aerobic bacteria; irreversible ototoxicity; nephrotoxic
kanamycin	Kantrex	8–12 g PO per day divided into 6-h intervals; 15 mg/kg/day IM in two to three evenly spaced and divided doses Total dose should not exceed 15 g	Used for patients with tuberculosis as adjunct therapy; also administered orally to prevent hepatic coma, also used as a second-choice agent for other gram-negative infections; ototoxic and nephrotoxic; skin reactions, intestinal malabsorption, superinfection has occurred.
neomycin	Mycifradin, Myciguent, Neobiotic	4–12 g PO per day in divided doses Ointments and creams are applied 2–3×/day	Dose for surgical bowel preparation; see kanamycin for additional uses and adverse responses; neomycin is not for parenteral use
neomycin and polymixin B sulfate solution for irrigation	Neosporin G.U. irrigant	1 ml of solution is added 1,000 ml of 0.9% sodium chloride and instilled into the bladder over a 24-h period	Dose for continuous bladder irrigation
netilmicin	Netromycin	Same as gentamicin	Useful for patients with infections that have become resistant to gentamicin
streptomycin		1–2 g IM per day in two divided evenly spaced doses	May also be used for patients with bacterial endocarditis, tularemia, plague, tuberculosis
tobramycin	Nebcin	IM, IV doses are same as gentamicin	Same as gentamicin
	Tobrex	Ophthalmic ointments and solutions	

A. Review nursing implications on pp. 290–291.

B. Check the patient for ototoxicity before administering each dose of aminoglycoside. Report tinnitus and any other disturbances of hearing or equilibrium to the registered nurse before administering a dose. Anticipate ototoxic effects with high doses.

C. Monitor laboratory reports as available to anticipate possible adverse kidney responses. Serum creatinine and blood urea nitrogen (BUN) are the tests most often ordered. Anticipate nephrotoxicity with higher doses.

D. Prevent nephrotoxicity by forcing fluids to 3 to 4 L/day if permitted by the physician.

E. Administer IV doses over a period of 30 to 60 min to prevent acute muscular paralysis and apnea.

F. Use measures that prevent the development of nosocomial (hospital-acquired) infections in hospitalized patients.

ANTHELMINTICS

Anthelmintics are drugs that rid the body of parasitic worms (helminths) (Table 24–3). Three different families of worms may cause infection in humans: roundworms (nematodes), flatworms (cestodes), and flukes (trematodes). Infections caused by parasitic worms (helminthiasis) affect over 2 billion people worldwide. Overcrowding, poor sanitation, increased world travel, and inadequate personal hygiene are a few factors known to contribute to the high incidence of this infection.

Once parasitic worms enter the body, they may remain in the patient's gastrointestinal system to cause malnutrition, diarrhea, and other gastrointestinal symptoms. Parasitic worms may also invade body tissue such as the lungs, liver, muscle, brain and spinal cord, skin, eyes and other tissue. The patient's symptoms may range from mild discomfort to life-threatening, depending upon the part of the body affected.

I. Actions and uses.

　A. Some anthelmintics act locally to expel worms from the gastrointestinal tract.

TABLE 24–3　Anthelmintics

Nonproprietary Name	Proprietary Name	Adult Dose Range	Notes
diethylcarbamazine	Hetrazan	2 mg/kg/PO 3×/day after meals 10–30 days	Dose and frequency may vary according to specific roundworm infection; corticosteroids may be administered to minimize severe adverse responses
mebendazole	Vermox	100 mg PO initial dose, repeated in 2 weeks; or 100 mg PO AM and PM for 3 consecutive days	Dose frequency varies with specific roundworm; cannot be used during pregnancy or for patients with previous allergic reaction; low potential for adverse responses
metrifonate	Bilarcil	5–15 mg/kg PO every 2 weeks × three doses	Used only for patients with a specific fluke infection; available only from Centers for Disease Control; patients should not receive neuromuscular blocking agent for 48 h after treatment
niclosamide	Niclocide	2 g chewed and swallowed with small amount of water	Patient must be fasting before drug is administered; a purge of the bowel is usually ordered from 1 to 2 h after dose; low potential for adverse responses; used for flatworm infections
niridazole	Ambilhar	25 mg/kg PO per day × 7 days	Adverse responses not usual; urine turns dark and has unpleasant odor; may lead to cancer; usually not ordered for patients with epilepsy, psychosis, neurosis, severe debilitation; used as alternative agent for flatworm and fluke infections
oxamniquine	Vansil	12–60 mg/kg PO per day from 1 to 3 days; after meals	May turn urine an orange-red color; used for fluke infections
piperazine citrate	Antepar Vermizine	75 mg/kg PO per day for 2 consecutive days	Not used for the patient with epilepsy; low potential for toxicity
praziquantel	Biltricide	25–40 mg/kg PO; single or multiple doses depending upon specific parasite	Used for flatworm and fluke infections
pyrantel pamoate	Antiminth	11 mg/kg—1 g PO suspension administered as a single dose; repeated in 2 weeks for selected parasitic infections	Used for intestingal pinworm, hookworms; low potential for adverse responses; not recommended during pregnancy and for children under 2 years
thiabendazole	Mintezol	25 mg/kg—3 g maximum PO per day for 1 to 5 days depending on specific parasite; administered after meals	Used for roundworms, hookworms; adverse responses are common and may be severe

   B. Other drugs act systemically on tissues invaded by parasitic worms.
   C. Anthelmintics have several potential actions: dislocation of parasites from the site of the infection, or alteration in cell membranes of parasites so that normal body defenses can kill them.
  II. Adverse responses.
   A. Gastrointestinal system—anorexia, abdominal or epigastric distress, diarrhea, nausea, vomiting.
   B. Central nervous system: headache, malaise, fatigue, drowsiness, dizziness, confusion, fever, eye changes, insomnia.
   C. Skin: pruritus, alopecia, rash.
   D. Cardiovascular system: tachycardia; bradycardia and hypotension with thiabendazole only.
   E. Blood: leukocytosis, agranulocytosis.
   F. Other: angioedema, facial flush, chills, lymph node enlargement, joint pains, unpleasant odor to urine.
 III. Nursing implications.
   A. Assist in the collection of information from the patient with possible helminthiasis. A minimum of information includes residential environment; recent outbreaks of infection in schoolchildren; residents of institutions, neighborhoods; individual patient symptoms; recent travel, personal hygiene practices; cooking and food handling practices.
   B. Collect stool for ova and parasites as ordered by the physician and send to the laboratory while warm.
   C. Administer most anthelmintics after meals. One exception is niclosamide; the patient must be fasting when this drug is administered.
   D. Report adverse responses; anticipate an order for drug therapy to relieve severe but temporary adverse responses.
   E. Prevent the spread of infection by excellent personal hygiene; avoiding raw fish and undercooked pork; using disposable bags when outdoor bathrooms are not available for defecation; covering foods to prevent contamination with flies.
   F. Teach the patient measures that prevent the spread of infection at home.
   G. Teach the patient with intestinal parasites to wash clothing, bed linens, and towels with hot water until the follow-up stool samples are clear. Toilet seats at home should also be disinfected daily.
   H. Encourage the patient with intestinal parasites to bring the entire family in for treatment and to return for follow up studies to prevent recurrence.

ANTIFUNGAL AGENTS

  I. Actions and uses.
   A. *Antifungal agents* kill or inhibit the growth of plantlike yeasts and molds that cause disease (Table 24–4).
   B. Systemic agents are used for patients with systemic infections: histoplasmosis, coccidioidomycosis, blastomycosis, candidiasis.
   C. Systemic agents are often used with other unrelated drugs because patients who receive antineoplastic agents and immunosuppressives are more likely to develop serious systemic fungal infection.
   D. Antifungal agents may be applied locally for infections involving the skin, hair, nails, mucous membranes (see Chapter 27).
  II. Adverse responses.
   A. Gastrointestinal system: nausea, vomiting, diarrhea, anorexia, enterocolitis, hepatomegaly.
   B. Central nervous system: headache, chills, fever, convulsions, generalized pain, flushing, parkinsonism.

TABLE 24–4   Antifungal Agents

Nonproprietary Name	Proprietary Name	Adult Dose Range	Notes
Systemic Agents			
amphotericin B	Fungizone	1 mg in 20 ml 5% dextrose in water is administered IV over 20–30 min as a test dose	Monitor vital signs during test dose and every 30 min for 4 h
		0.3 mg/kg in 500 ml of 5% dextrose and water IV over 4–6 h	Dose varies according to patient's condition
		May also be injected into a joint or spinal canal	All routes have a high potential for toxicity
flucytosine	Ancobon	50–150 mg/kg PO every 6 h	Lower potential for toxicity but not as effective in most cases as amphotericin B; used mainly in combination with amphotericin B
griseofulvin	Fulvicin U/F Grifulvin V	500 mg–2 g PO per day at 6-h intervals	Used primarily for fungal infections of the skin, hair, nails if topical therapy is not successful; side effects common
hydroxystilbamidine isethionate		225 mg in 200 ml of 5% dextrose in water or isotonic saline is administered IV over 2–3 h every day	Also effective against protozoa; too rapid infusion may cause hypotension, gastrointestinal side effects common; protect IV solution from light
ketoconazole	Nizoral	200–400 mg PO per day	Used for patients with histoplasmosis
miconazole	Monistat IV	200–3,600 mg IV per day	High potential for toxicity; useful primarily for severely ill patients who do not respond to other agents; preparations are also available for vaginal and topical application
nystatin	Mycostatin Nilstat and others	500,000–1 million U PO 3–4×/day	Dose for oral candidiasis
		1–2 vaginal tablets per day × 14 days	Dose for vaginitis; many other preparations available for topical application

    C. Allergy: anaphylaxis, urticaria, angioedema.

    D. Nephrotoxicity.

    E. Blood: thrombocytopenia, anemia, leukopenia.

    F. Drug interactions include:

       • Increased nephrotoxicity when combined with other nephrotoxic agents.

       • Increased bone marrow depression when combined with antineoplastic drugs.

       • Barbiturates and sedative-hypnotics decrease the effects of griseofulvin.

       • Antacids, anticholinergics, cimetidine decrease the effects of ketoconazole.

III. Nursing implications.

    A. Review the nursing implications on pp. 290–291.

    B. Read package insert carefully and completely before administering or monitoring a patient receiving a systemic antifungal agent.

    C. Report the first evidence of an adverse response. Some responses become more severe as the dose of drug increases.

    D. Prevent fungal infections in susceptible hospitalized patients by: inspecting the mouth, perineum, and skin daily and recording findings, assisting the patient with frequent scrupulous oral hygiene, careful drying of skin folds and perineal area during the bath.

ANTILEPROSY AGENTS

Antileprosy agents are drugs that inhibit the growth of *Mycobacterium leprae*, the causative agent of leprosy (Hansen's disease) (Table 24–5). The patient with leprosy has a chronic infection that attacks and destroys superficial tissues, especially the skin, peripheral nerves, and nasal mucous membranes. In early stages, the patient with leprosy may have skin lesions such as macules or plaques. In later stages, the patient frequently develops blindness and crippling of the hands and feet from destruction of peripheral nerves. Other skeletal deformities develop according to the area affected. The causative agent is believed to enter the body through the skin or nasal mucous membrane.

About 10 to 20 million people worldwide are affected with leprosy. In the United States, the infection is more common in California, Hawaii, Florida, New York, and Texas.

I. Actions and uses.
   A. Antileprosy agents inhibit the growth of *Mycobacterium leprae*.
   B. A combination regimen that includes all of the drugs in Table 24–5 is generally recommended. The regimen usually includes daily doses of dapsone and clofazimine. In addition, monthly doses of clofazimine and rifampin are ordered.
   C. Drug therapy usually continues for a minimum of 2 years.
II. Adverse responses.
   A. Clofazimine: red discoloration to skin, enteritis.
   B. Dapsone.
      1. Blood: hemolytic anemia is common.
      2. Gastrointestinal system: anorexia, nausea, vomiting.
      3. Sulfone reaction: fever, malaise, exfoliative dermatitis, enlarged lymph nodes, anemias, jaundice with liver destruction may occur 5 to 6 weeks after treatment.
      4. Nervous system: headache, nervousness, insomnia, blurred vision, peripheral neuropathy, paresthesia, psychosis.
      5. Other: drug fever, hematuria, pruritus and skin rashes; infectious-mononucleosis-type syndrome that may be fatal; resistance of organisms.
   C. Rifampin.
      1. Gastrointestinal system: nausea and vomiting, jaundice and liver damage, epigastric distress, abdominal cramps, diarrhea.
      2. Nervous system: fatigue, drowsiness, headache, dizziness, confusion, ataxia, generalized numbness, pain in extremities, muscle weakness.
      3. Hypersensitivity: fever, pruritus, skin eruptions, sourness of mouth and tongue.
      4. Other: anemias and kidney damage.
      5. Drug interactions include:
         • Decreased effectiveness of digitalis derivatives, oral anticoagulants, clofibrate, ketoconazole, metaprolol, prednisone, propranolol, quinidine, oral hypoglycemic agents.
III. Nursing implications.
   A. Review the nursing implications on pp. 290–291.
   B. Report and record adverse responses.
   C. Assist the patient with self-care measures as needed.

ANTIMALARIALS

Antimalarials are drugs that either kill or inhibit the growth of four species of plasmodium, the causative agent of malaria (Table 24–6). The patient with malaria has an infection that enters the bloodstream from a bite from an infected female Anopheles mosquito. The patient develops chills, fever, headache, muscle pains, anemia, jaundice, and liver enlargement. A characteristic feature of malaria is paroxysms of shaking chills lasting from 20 to 60 min alternating with high fever (104 to 107°F), and diaphoresis lasting from 3 to 8 h. Malaria affects over 125 million people in over one hundred countries of Africa, Central and South America and Asia. In the United States, recent increases in malaria are associated with an increase in world travel, the return of large numbers of military personnel from Southeast Asia, and the arrival of refugees from other countries.

I. Actions and uses.
   A. Antimalaria agents kill or inhibit the growth of plasmodium organisms.

TABLE 24–5   Antileprosy Agents

Nonproprietary Name	Proprietary Name	Adult Dose Range*	Notes
Clofazimine	Lamprene	50 mg PO per day; plus 300 mg PO per month under supervision	Patient may develop red discoloration of skin; available only from National Hansen's Disease Center in Louisiana
Dapsone	DDS	50–100 mg PO per day	Dose may be individualized according to patient's response
Rifampin	Rifadin Rimactane	600 mg PO per month under supervision	Also used a antitubercular agent (see Table 24–7)

*Recommended doses for combination therapy of leprosy; doses may vary when a single agent is used.

    B. Antimalaria agents may be used for prevention in travelers and others who live in endemic areas.

    C. Antimalaria agents may also be used for treatment of acute attacks and prevention of recurrence in persons who already have malaria.

    D. Combination therapy is common both to discourage the development of resistant organisms and reduce toxicity.

II. Adverse responses.

    A. Resistance is an important obstacle to the successful treatment of malaria with all drugs in Table 24–6.

    B. Gastrointestinal system: mild upset, epigastric distress, abdominal cramps.

    C. Nervous system: transient headache, visual disturbances.

    D. Skin: discoloration of nailbeds and mucous membranes, skin eruptions.

    E. Psychiatric disturbances such as hallucinations and depression have been reported.

    F. Anemias have been reported with primaquine, especially in black and dark-skinned white persons.

    G. Quinine poisoning produces disturbances in vision and hearing, gastrointestinal symptoms, hot flushed skin, diaphoresis, fever, headache, confusion and coma, and potentially fatal respiratory depression.

III. Nursing implications.

    A. Review nursing implications on pp. 290–291.

    B. Report and record adverse responses.

    C. Assist the patient with self-care as indicated.

ANTITUBERCULAR AGENTS

Antibubercular agents are drugs that kill or inhibit the growth of *Mycobacterium tuberculosis*, a bacillus that causes tuberculosis (Table 24–7). The patient with tuberculosis has an infection that most often affects the lungs. Other organs that may become infected are the kidneys, bones, lymph nodes, and meninges. The disease is transmitted from one person to another by the inhalation of fresh droplet nuclei containing tubercle bacilli. The patient develops the usual symptoms of infection but also has night sweats that are characteristic of tuberculosis. If untreated, the patient develops progressive lung damage and related diseases such as pneumonia and bronchiectasis. After about 2 weeks of treatment with the appropriate drugs, the disease is no longer considered contagious. However, drug therapy must be continued for a minimum of 18 to 24 months to prevent recurrence of infection from dormant tubercle bacilli that may become reactivated.

    Tuberculosis was once a leading cause of death worldwide. Effective drug therapy has been a key factor in reducing the incidence of infection. Early detection of tuberculosis and improved standards of living are two other important influences on the decline of tuberculosis.

I. Actions and uses.

    A. First-line agents for the treatment of tuberculosis include ethambutol, isoniazid, pyrazinamide, rifampin, and streptomycin.

TABLE 24–6 Antimalarials

Nonproprietary Name	Proprietary Name	Adult Dose Range*	Notes
chloroquine phosphate	Aralen Phosphate	500 mg PO per week before or after meals	Dose for travelers starts 1 week before exposure and continues for 6 weeks after exposure; also used to prevent recurrence of acute attacks
		1 g PO initially; 500 mg PO in 6–8 h; 500 mg PO per day for 2 days; 2.5 g total in 3 days	Dose for acute attacks
chloroquine hydrochloride injection		250 mg IM every 6 h × 24 h; half the dose is injected into each buttock	Used only for the patient in coma from acute attack; oral administration is started as soon as possible
hydroxychloroquine sulfate	Plaquenil Sulfate	400 mg PO per week before or after meals	Same as chloroquine phosphate
		800 mg PO initially; 400 mg PO in 6–8 h; then 400 mg PO per day for 2 days; 400 mg is equivalent to 500 mg chloroquine	
mefloquine		1,500 mg PO single dose; 500 mg PO per week for 1 year	Used mainly for patients who become resistant to chloroquine; still investigational in the United States
primaquine phosphate		15 mg PO per day for 14 days; 45 mg PO may be added to regimen for chloroquine	Used mainly as a radical cure for specific forms of relapsing malaria; used in combination with chloroquine
pyrimethamine	Daraprim	25 mg PO 2 ×/day for 3 days	Dose for an acute attack is combined with sulfadiazine 500 mg 4 ×/day × 5 days
pyrimethamine 25 mg and sulfadoxine 500 mg	Fansidar	1 tablet PO per week	Dose for travelers starts 1 week before exposure and continues for 6 weeks after exposure; may also be used to prevent recurrence
quinine sulfate		650 mg PO 3 ×/day after meals for 10–14 days; also available for IV administration in emergencies; some experts recommend 6 weeks of treatment	Used mainly for patients with severe malaria resistant to chloroquine; used in combination with either primaquine and a sulfa drug or tetracyclines; high potential for toxicity; lower doses may be prescribed to relieve nocturnal leg cramps
totaquine		600 mg PO 3 ×/day after meals	Quinine-type drug; same as quinine

B. Second-line agents may be needed if the patient develops resistance to first-line drugs or is unable to take first-line drugs. Second-line drugs include amikacin, aminosalicylic acid, capreomycin, cycloserine, ethionamide, and kanamycin.

C. Combination therapy is common with either two or three drugs. Regimens for drug therapy may vary with the patient's condition and specific strain of tubercle bacillus.

D. Drug therapy is usually prolonged. Patients usually must take drugs for a minimum of 18 to 24 months.

E. Drug therapy may be ordered to prevent tuberculosis in patients who have been exposed, those with a positive tuberculin test, and those with inactive tuberculosis.

II. Adverse responses.

A. Resistance to drugs is common. This response is more likely when the strain of mycobacterium has not been identified or when a patient does not take prescribed drugs as ordered.

B. Hypersensitivity responses include: fever, rash, urticaria, pruritus.

C. Musculoskeletal system: arthralgia of knees, wrists, elbows, back; muscle twitching, paresthesias.

TABLE 24–7   Antitubercular Agents

Nonproprietary Name	Proprietary Name	Adult Dose Range	Notes
First-Line Agents			
ethambutol	Myambutol	15 mg/kg/day PO	Often used in combination with isoniazid; low potential for adverse responses
isoniazid	Nydrazid and others	5 mg/kg/day PO, IM; maximum dose is usually 300 mg/day	Often used in combination with either ethambutol, rifampin, or streptomycin; most effective drug for tuberculosis; used alone for prevention
pyrazinamide		20–35 mg/kg/day PO in three to four evenly spaced dose intervals; maximum dose per day is 3 g	Liver damage a common and serious side effect; used mainly for short-term therapy in underdeveloped countries
rifampin	Rifadin Rimactane	600 mg/day PO either 1 h before or 2 h after a meal	Higher doses may be used for the patient with meningitis; most effective drug for tuberculosis; low potential for adverse responses; may cause orange and red discoloration of skin, urine, feces, saliva, sweat, and tears
rifampin 300 mg and isoniazid 150 mg	Rifamate	See isoniazid and rifampin doses above.	
streptomycin		1 g/day for 2 months; reduced to 1 g 2×/week. IM route is most often used.	Usually used only in combination with other drugs; see also p. 289
Second-Line Agents			
amikacin	Amikin	15 mg/kg/day divided into two to three equal doses; IM, IV	An aminoglycoside that is nephrotoxic and ototoxic; see p. 293 for additional information
aminosalicylate sodium	Teebacin	8–12 g/day PO divided into three to four equal doses taken after meals	
capreomycin sulfate	Capastat Sulfate	20 mg/kg—1 g/day IM for 60–120 days; then 1 g IM 2–3 ×/week	Nephrotoxic, ototoxic; used only in combination with other drugs
cycloserine	Seromycin	250–500 mg 2×/day PO	Drug–alcohol interaction may cause seizures; not used in patients with epilepsy, anxiety, depression
ethionamide	Trecator—SC	250 mg PO 2×/day; gradually increased to a maximum of 1 g daily with meals	Postural hypotension, stomatitis, impotence, gynecomastia, alopecia, acne, menstrual disturbances, and additional adverse responses
kanamycin	Kantrex	1 g PO per day	An aminoglycoside that is nephrotoxic and ototoxic; see p. 293 for additional information

  D. Blood: anemia, agranulocytosis, pyridoxine deficiency anemia with isoniazid.
  E. Central nervous system: dizziness, ataxia, optic neuritis, stupor, euphoria, memory impairment, florid psychosis, excessive sedation, tinnitus.
  F. Gastrointestinal system: dry mouth, jaundice, liver damage, epigastric distress, nausea and vomiting.
  G. Kidneys: urinary retention, kidney damage.
  H. Other: lupuslike syndrome (isoniazid), flulike syndrome (rifampin).
  I. Drug interactions include:
    • A reduction in therapeutic effects of clofibrate, flurazepam and its relatives, digitoxin, ketoconazole, metoprolol, propranolol, quinidine, oral hypoglycemics, when combined with rifampin.
    • An increase in plasma concentration of phenytoin when combined with isoniazid.

- Increased central nervous system depression when barbiturates are combined with isoniazid.

III. Nursing implications.
  A. Review the nursing implications on pp. 290–291.
  B. Assist in the collection of information about the patient with possible tuberculosis.
  C. Seek additional information from the registered nurse, physician, or pharmacist before administering antitubercular agents to patients with liver or kidney disease.
  D. Teach the patient to use measures that prevent the spread of infection.
  E. Encourage and assist the patient to find ways to continue drug therapy exactly as prescribed in order to prevent resistance or recurrence of active tuberculosis.

ANTIVIRAL AGENTS

I. Actions and uses.
  A. *Antiviral agents* inhibit the growth of viruses or cause their death (Table 24–8). *Viruses* are parasites that invade the cell and live there.

TABLE 24–8   Antiviral Agents

Nonproprietary Name	Proprietary Name	Adult Dose Range	Notes
acyclovir	Zovirax	200 mg PO 5×/day for 10 days then 200 mg PO 3–5× per day for up to 6 months	Dose for acute genital herpes infection and prevention of recurrent infection
		1.25 cm² (½-in.) ribbon of 5% ointment/25 cm² (4 square in.) of skin	Dose for application to skin only; not for use in eyes or vagina; glove or fingercot should be used for application; for herpes viral infections involving skin lesions; burning may occur
		5 mg/kg IV every 8 h; dose is administered over a 60-min period	IV route is generally used for seriously ill patients who are immunosuppressed; watch for local phlebitis, diaphoresis, renal dysfunction, mental changes and report
amantadine hydrochloride	Symmetrel	200 mg PO per day	Used to treat or prevent influenza A
idoxuridine	Herplex Stoxil	ophthalmic ointment 0.5%: every 4 h during the day and once at bedtime. ophthalmic solution 0.1%: 1 drop every hour during the day and every 4 h at night when improvement is obvious	Primarily used for the patient with herpes simplex keratitis; may produce eye irritation, pain, pruritus, inflammation or edema of eyelids, photophobia
ribavarin	Virazole	12–18 h/day for 3–7 days; administered by aerosol; requires small particle aerosol generator (SPAG)	New broad-spectrum drug currently limited to patients with respiratory syncytial virus; not recommended during pregnancy; adverse responses include aggravation of chronic cardiac and pulmonary conditions
trifluridine	Viroptic	1% ophthalmic solution	Used for the patient with herpes simplex eye infection that does not respond to vidarabine or idoxuridine
vidarabine	Vira A	15 mg/kg/day IV in 2.5 L of IV solution infused over 12–24 h for 10 days	Used for the patient with encephalitis caused by herpes simplex virus; may also be used for the patient with herpes zoster
	Vira A Ophthalmic	3% ophthalmic ointment every 3 h to a maximum of 5×/day	Used for the patient with herpes simplex keratitis; less irritating to eye than idoxuridine ointment

   B. Acyclovir is an antiviral agent used specifically for the patient with herpes, Types 1 and 2. This includes genital herpes and nongenital herpes infections.

   C. Amantadine is an antiviral agent used specifically for the patient with influenza A; it may also be used as prevention.

   D. Idoxuridine is used specifically for eye infections caused by the herpes simplex virus.

   E. Vidarabine is used for herpes simplex infections.

   F. Acyclovir and vidarabine may be used for patients with shingles caused by the varicella-zoster virus or chicken pox caused by varicella virus. Treatment is usually reserved for patients with severe infection and existing immune deficiencies.

II. Adverse responses.

   A. Topical acyclovir ointment may produce local irritation and burning when applied to genital lesions.

   B. Oral acyclovir may produce occasional nausea, headache, amnesia.

   C. Intravenous acyclovir may produce local phlebitis, rash, diaphoresis, nausea, vomiting, hypotension, and kidney dysfunction.

   D. Idoxuridine ophthalmic may produce photophobia, pain, irritation, pruritus, inflammation or edema of eyelid.

   E. Amantadine may produce insomnia, difficulties in concentrating that may increase to confusion, hallucinations, seizures, and coma if toxicity develops.

   F. Vidarabine may produce nausea, vomiting, diarrhea, rash, weakness, thrombophlebitis at the IV site. Central nervous system responses are similar to those with amantadine and more likely with high doses.

III. Nursing implications.

   A. Review nursing implications on pp. 290–291.

   B. Use gloves or special applicators when administering drug therapy for the skin or eyes.

   C. Monitor intravenous flow rates carefully to prevent toxicity associated with overly rapid infusion rates.

   D. Prevent herpes Whitlow, an infection common to nurses, by wearing two gloves while suctioning the nasopharynx, oropharynx, or trachea.

CEPHALOSPORINS

I. Actions and uses.

   A. *Cephalosporins* are chemically related drugs that kill or inhibit the growth of gram-positive and gram-negative cocci, round-shaped bacteria (Table 24–9).

   B. Cephalosporins may be seen as falling into three categories that reflect both the time of development and the actions on specific bacteria. First-generation drugs are more effective for gram-positive bacteria. Second-generation drugs are also effective for gram-negative bacteria. Third-generation drugs are more effective for gram-negative bacteria and not as effective for gram-positive organisms.

   C. Cephalosporins are able to penetrate a variety of body tissues and fluids including joints, bile, synovial fluid, cerebrospinal fluid, and aqueous humor of the eye. This characteristic enables cephalosporins to be used for many infections such as meningitis and pneumonia, osteomyelitis.

   D. Cephalosporins may also be used for the patient whose infection has become resistant to other drugs.

   E. Cephalosporins may be used before and after surgery to prevent infection.

   F. Cephalosporins are well absorbed from oral and parenteral routes and are excreted by the kidneys.

II. Adverse responses.

   A. Hypersensitive reactions are more common than others. Anaphylaxis, bronchospasm, or urticaria may develop immediately. Rash, fever, and lymph node enlargement may occur as a delayed reaction. Persons who are allergic to penicillins are more likely to have an allergy to cephalosporins. This type of allergy may be termed *cross-sensitivity*.

B. Other: nephrotoxicity, diarrhea, alcohol–drug interactions; platelet dysfunction that may produce bleeding; anemia, nausea and vomiting; resistance to the drug.

C. Intramuscular injections are painful and may cause severe local reactions such as induration, tenderness, and sterile abscess.

D. Drug interactions include:
- Increased nephrotoxicity when aminoglycosides (see Table 24–2) are combined with cephalosporins.
- Increased effectiveness of most cephalosporins when combined with probenicid.
- Tetracyclines decrease the effectiveness of cephalosporins.

III. Nursing implications.

A. Review general nursing implications on pp. 290–291.

B. Report penicillin allergy to the registered nurse or physician before administering the first dose. Anticipate a possible change of drug.

C. Administer oral preparations with a full glass of water on an empty stomach if possible to encourage complete absorption.

D. Consult package insert and prepare solutions for intramuscular, intravenous administration as directed.

E. Administer IM injections deeply into a large muscle mass and rotate injection sites.

F. Observe the patient for adverse responses before administering each dose of cephalosporin. Minimum observations would include the skin for evidence of rash; the IM injection site for induration, erythema, tenderness; urinary output, and signs of superinfection, especially in the mouth.

G. Use Testape instead of Clinitest tablets if the patient's urine must be checked for glucose.

H. Caution the patient not to drink alcohol when taking a cephalosporin. Alcohol–drug interactions have occurred with several agents.

I. Follow the manufacturer's directions for storage of cephalosporins. Most drugs must be stored away from concentrated light. Some preparations must be refrigerated after reconstitution.

PENICILLINS

I. Actions and uses.

A. Penicillins are a group of chemically related drugs that kill or inhibit the growth of gram-positive and gram-negative bacteria depending upon the specific drug used (Table 24–10).

B. Some penicillins can be absorbed orally but others are absorbed only by parental routes.

C. Penicillins may be used for pneumococcal, streptococcal, staphylococcal, or gonococcal infections of the lungs, joints, bones, ears, meninges, pericardium, and urethra.

D. The patient with other infections including syphilis, diphtheria, and anthrax may be placed on penicillin.

E. Penicillins may be used as prevention for the patient with a chronic or potentially recurring infection such as rheumatic fever, gonorrhea, or syphilis.

F. Patients with congenital or acquired heart disease may take penicillin before dental or heart surgery.

G. The dose of a penicillin drug depends upon the specific infection for which the patient is under treatment.

H. The many penicillins available reflect the ability of susceptible organisms to become resistant to drugs that were once effective.

II. Adverse responses.

A. Resistance: bacteria produce two enzymes that are capable of inactivating various antibiot-

TABLE 24-9 Cephalosporins

Nonproprietary Name	Proprietary Name	Adult Dose Range	Notes
First-Generation Drugs			First-generation drugs are effective for infections caused by gram-positive bacteria
cefadroxil	Duricef, Ultracef	0.5–1 g PO every 12 h	Used primarily for urinary tract infections
cefazolin	Ancef, Kefzol	1 g IM, IV every 6–8 h	Especially effective for infections caused by *Escherichia coli*, Klebsiella, and staphylococci
cephalexin monohydrate	Keflex	250 mg–1 g PO every 6 h	
cephalothin sodium	Keflin	1–2 g IM, IV every 4–6 h	First-generation cephalosporin; especially effective for infections caused by staphylococci
cephapirin sodium	Cefadyl	500 mg—1 g IM, IV every 4–6 h	
cephradine	Anspor, Velosef	250 mg–1 g PO every 6 h; 2–4 g/day IM, IV in four equal doses at 6-h intervals	Only cephalosporin available for both oral and parenteral routes
Second-Generation Drugs			Second-generation drugs are effective for infections caused by gram-positive and/or gram-negative bacteria
cefaclor	Ceclor	250 mg–1 g PO every 8 h	
cefamandole	Mandol	1–2 g IM, IV every 4 h	May inhibit production of vitamin K by normal intestinal flora; watch for signs of bleeding
cefonicid	Monocid	1–2 g IM, IV every 24 h	New drug; only second-generation agent available for once-a-day administration; may produce nausea, vomiting, and a flulike syndrome as additional adverse responses
ceforanide	Precef	1 g IM, IV every 12 h	New drug active against a broad spectrum of gram-positive and gram-negative bacteria; nausea and vomiting are additional adverse responses
cefoxitin sodium	Mefoxin	2–3 g IM, IV every 4–6 h	
cefuroxime	Zinacef	3 g IM, IV every 8 h	
Third-Generation Drugs			Third-generation drugs are effective for infections caused by gram-negative bacteria
cefoperazone	Cefobid	2–4 g IM, IV per day in divided doses every 12 h	
cefotaxime sodium	Claforan	2 g every 4 h	
cefotetan	Cefotan	1–2 g IM, IV twice daily	New drug especially for patients with either gynecologic or mixed abdominal infection
ceftazidime	Fortaz	500 mg–2 g IM, IV every 8–12 h	New drug
ceftizoxime	Cefizox	3–4 g IM, IV every 8–12 h	
ceftriaxone sodium	Rocephin	1–2 g IM, IV every 24 h	New drug; only third-generation agent available for once-a-day administration
moxalactam disodium	Moxam	2–6 g/day IM, IV in divided doses every 8 h for up to 14 days	

TABLE 24–10   Penicillins

Nonproprietary Name	Proprietary Name	Adult Dose Range	Notes
amdinocillin	Coactin	Up to 10 mg/kg IM, IV every 4 h	Used primarily for urinary tract infections cause by *E. coli*, Klebsiella, and Enterobacter
amoxicillin	Augmentin Amoxil	0.75–1.5 g PO per day in three divided doses	Used for common infections such as sinusitis, otitis media, and lower respiratory infections
ampicillin	Amcill Omnipen, Polycillin and others	2–4 g PO per day in divided doses every 6 h; 6–12 g/day IV in four divided doses	Effective for infections caused by *K. influenzae*, *E. coli*, Neisseria. Parenteral solutions must be administered within 30–60 min after reconstitution
azlocillin	Azlin	8–18 g IV per day in four to six divided doses.	Effective for infections caused by Pseudomonas, Streptococci
bacampicillin hydrochloride	Spectrobid	800–1,600 mg PO per day in two divided doses	Ampicillin relative; see ampicillin for susceptible bacteria
carbenicillin	Geopen, Pyopen	30–40 g IM, IV in divided doses every 4–6 h	Carbenicillins are effective for infections caused by Pseudomonas and Proteus bacteria, all preparations may produce additional adverse responses of congestive heart failure, hypokalemia, and bleeding
carbenicillin indanyl sodium	Geocillin	2–4 g PO per day in four divided doses	Used primarily for the patient with urinary tract infection caused by certain strains of Proteus and Pseudomonas bacteria
carbenicillin phenyl sodium	Carfecillin	Same as above	Same as above
cloxacillin	Cloxapen Tegopen	250–500 mg PO every 6 h	Semisynthetic penicillin; effective against infections caused by Staphylococci that produce penicillinase
cyclacillin	Cyclapen W	0.75–1.5 g PO per day in three divided doses	Ampicillin relative; see ampicillin, above, for susceptible bacteria
dicloxacillin	Dynapen, Veracillin, others	250 mg or more PO every 6 h	See Cloxacillin above.
hetacillin	Versapen	See ampicillin PO	See ampicillin above.
methicillin	Staphcillin	4–12 g IV in four to six divided doses	Semisynthetic penicillin that resists destruction from penicillinase-producing staphylococci; each dose must be prepared fresh; not for continuous IV infusions
mezlocillin	Mezlin	6–18 g IV per day in four to six divided doses	Azlocillin relative, effective against gram-negative bacteria
nafcillin	Nafcil Unipen	6–12 g PO, IV per day in six divided doses every 4 h	Especially effective for infections caused by resistant strains of *Staphylococcus aureus*
oxacillin	Bactocill Prostaphlin	2–4 g PO per day in four divided doses; 2–12 g IM, IV per day every 4–6 h	see nafcillin
penicillin G-benzathine suspension	Bicillin LA and others	1.2–4.8 million U IM	Long-acting preparation; never administer IV
penicillin G-potassium or sodium	Aqueous Penicillin G	6–20 million U/day IV every 2–4 h or by continuous IV infusion	Penicillins are used for pneumococcal and streptococcal infections, diphtheria, and others
penicillin G-procaine suspension	Duracillin Mycillin	300,000–600,000 U IM every 12 h; larger doses may be used for some patients	Large doses may produce additional adverse responses associated with procaine; dizziness, headache, tinnitus, hallucinations, seizures; never administer IV
penicillin V potassium	Pen-Veek V-cillin K and others	250–500 mg PO every 6 h for 7–30 days	
piperacillin	Piperacil	12–24 g IM, IV per day in three to six divided doses	see azlocillin
ticarcillin disodium	Ticar	200–300 mg/kg IM, IV in four to six divided doses	Semisynthetic penicillin similar to carbenicillin; see carbenicillin

ics—penicillinase and beta-lactamase. Penicillins vary in their ability to be destroyed by these enzymes.

B. Hypersensitive reactions are the most common adverse response to penicillin drugs. Anaphylaxis and angioedema may develop immediately. Later forms of allergic response include rash, fever, bronchospasm, exfoliative dermatitis, serum sickness, vasculitis, and nephritis.

C. Bone marrow depression leading to various anemias and hepatitis has been reported with nafcillin and oxacillin.

D. Bleeding has been reported as a result of platelet dysfunction that may occur with penicillin G, carbenicillin, or ticarcillin.

E. Oral preparations may cause nausea, vomiting diarrhea.

F. IM injections may cause pain and sterile inflammatory reactions at the injection site; IV administration may produce phlebitis or thrombophlebitis at the IV site.

G. Drug interactions include:
- Increased effectiveness of penicillins when combined with gentamicin or probenicid.
- Decreased effectiveness of penicillins when combined with erythromycin or tetracyclines.
- Destruction of selected oral penicillins when administered with acid foods or drugs: cranberry or orange juice, ascorbic acid, methenamine hydrochloride, ammonium chloride.

III. Nursing implications.

A. Report penicillin allergy to the registered nurse or physician before administering the first dose.

B. Observe the patient for adverse responses before administering each dose of a penicillin. Minimum observations include the skin for evidence of rash or pruritus, pain, or local irritation at the IM, IV injection sites; superinfection particularly in the mouth; signs of congestive heart failure or bleeding when carbenicillin or ticarcillin is used.

C. Administer oral preparation on an empty stomach to encourage complete absorption.

D. Administer IM, IV solutions of ampicillin within 1 h of reconstitution.

E. Monitor laboratory studies if available when preparations are ordered that contain sodium or potassium.

F. Follow the general nursing implications listed on pp. 290–291.

SULFONAMIDES

I. Actions and uses.

A. *Sulfonamides* inhibit the growth of a wide range of gram-positive and gram-negative bacteria (Table 24–11).

B. Sulfonamides are absorbed rapidly through the gastrointestinal system and distributed in all body tissues. The drugs are metabolized in the liver and excreted mainly in the urine.

C. Sulfonamides are most often used for patients with urinary tract infection, bacillary dysentery, meningococcal infections. Topical preparations are applied to burns to prevent infection.

D. Selected oral preparations are not absorbed well from the gastrointestinal tract. Such preparations may be used to reduce normal intestinal flora before intestinal surgery. They may also be used for the patient with ulcerative colitis or regional enteritis.

E. Sulfonamides may be used for prevention of streptococcal infection or rheumatic fever in susceptible persons who are allergic to penicillin.

II. Adverse responses.

A. Urinary system: kidney damage, crystals in the urine, stones in the kidneys, ureters, or bladder.

B. Blood: acute hemolytic anemia, agranulocytosis, aplastic anemia, thrombocytopenia.

TABLE 24–11 Sulfonamides

Nonproprietary Name	Proprietary Name	Adult Dose Range	Notes
sulfacytine	Renoquid	500 mg PO initial dose; then 250 mg PO 4×/day	
sulfadiazine		2–4 g PO initial dose; then 2–4 g PO per day in three to six divided doses	
sulfamethizole	Thiosulfil and others	500–1,000 mg PO 3–4×/day	Used for urinary tract infections
sulfamethoxazole	Gantanol	1–2 g PO initial dose; then 1 g PO every 8–12 h	
with phenazopyridine	Azo-Gantanol	Same as above	Added ingredient turns urine an orange-red color
sulfasalazine	Azulfadine and others	1–3 g PO per day	Not well absorbed in gastrointestinal tract; used mainly for patients with ulcerative colitis, regional enteritis
sulfisoxazole	Gantrisin and others	2–4 g PO initially; then 1 g every 4–6 h	
with diolamine		100 mg/kg/day IV in three to four divided doses	Must be infused slowly; read manufacturer's directions. Also available as 4% ophthalmic solution or ointment
with phenazopyridine	Azo Gantrisin	Same as oral dose above	Added ingredient turns urine an orange-red color
trimethoprim-sulfamethoxazole	Bactrim Septra	160 mg trimethoprim and 800 mg sulfamethoxazole PO every 12 h for 10–14 days	Several preparations are available with different doses of each ingredient; especially effective against bacteria that become resistant to other sulfonamides. Used mainly for recurrent urinary tract infections, acute bacterial respiratory tract infections, gastrointestinal shigellosis, and susceptible genital infections
Topical Sulfonamides			
mafenide acetate	Sulfamylon cream	Apply once or twice daily a 1 to 2-mm-thick layer over burned skin	Used for prevention of infection in a patient with burns; cleaning and debridement may produce intense pain, allergy, and fluid loss at the site of application, superinfection with candida may occur
silver sulfadiazine	Silvadene	Apply cream 1–2×/day in a 1- to 2-mm-thick layer over burned skin	Used for prevention of infection in patients with burns; cleaning and debridement
sulfacetamide sodium	Isopto Cetamide, Sulamyd Sodium	1–2 drops of ophthalmic solution 10–30% every 2 h for acute eye infections and 3–4×/day for chronic infection	An ophthalmic ointment (10%) is also available for use at bedtime

    C. Hypersensitivity reactions: skin rash, urticaria, exfoliative dermatitis, drug fever, serum sickness, pruritus, skin photosensitivity, bronchospasm, anaphylaxis.

    D. Gastrointestinal system: anorexia, nausea, vomiting, hepatitis.

    E. Other: arthritis, thyroid disturbances, neuropsychiatric disturbances, peripheral neuritis.

    F. Drug interactions include:
   - High potential for toxicity of oral anticoagulants, oral hypoglycemics, phenytoin anticonvulsants if combined with sulfonamides.

  III. Nursing implications.

    A. Report allergies to the registered nurse or physician before administering the first dose.

    B. Administer oral sulfonamides on a full stomach to minimize gastric irritation.

  C. Consult package insert and follow manufacturer's directions before administering parenteral sulfonamide.

  D. Cleanse and debride the skin as ordered by the physician before administering a sulfonamide cream to burned skin.

  E. Observe the patient for adverse responses before administering each dose of a sulfonamide.

  F. Encourage and assist the patient to drink 3 L of fluid per day to prevent the formation of kidney stones.

  G. Review and use the general nursing implications listed on pp. 290–291.

TETRACYCLINES

 I. Actions and uses.

  A. *Tetracyclines* are a group of chemically related drugs that inhibit the growth of a wider range of gram-positive and gram-negative bacteria (Table 24–12). For this reason, tetracyclines are also described as *broad-spectrum antibiotics*.

  B. Tetracyclines are used for infections caused by rickettsiae such as Rocky Mountain spotted fever and certain typhus organisms.

  C. The patient with pneumonia caused by mycoplasma, chlamydia, and other sexually transmitted diseases such as gonorrhea and syphilis may be treated with tetracyclines.

  D. The patient with proteus or pseudomonas infection of the urinary tract, chronic obstructive lung disease, or intestinal disease may be placed on a tetracycline drug.

  E. The patient with acne may benefit from low doses of tetracycline.

 II. Adverse responses.

  A. Gastrointestinal system: epigastric burning and distress; nausea and vomiting, abdominal cramps and diarrhea; pseudomembranous colitis; jaundice and liver damage.

  B. Skin: photosensitivity, rash, urticaria, exfoliative dermatitis, vaginitis, pruritus ani.

TABLE 24–12 Tetracyclines

Nonproprietary Name	Proprietary Name	Adult Dose Range	Notes
chlortetracycline hydro-chloride	Aureomycin	1% ophthalmic solution 1–2 drops 2–6 ×/day in conjunctival sac	Review directions on p. 104 for instillation of eye drops
demeclocycline hydro-chloride	Declomycin	150–300 mg PO every 6 h	
doxycycline hyclate	Vibramycin, others	100 mg PO per day in divided doses, 100 mg PO 1–2 ×/day for severe infection	
		100–200 mg IV infusion	Mix drug with at least 1 ml of IV solution for every 5 mg of dose ordered
methacycline hydrochloride	Rondomycin	150–300 mg PO every 6–12 h	
minocycline hydrochloride	Minocin	200 mg PO initial dose; then 100 mg PO every 12 h	
	Minocin IV	IV dose same as PO	Mix drug with at least 1 ml of IV solution for every 5 mg of dose ordered
oxytetracycline hydro-chloride	Terramycin and others	1–2 g PO per day	
		500 mg–1 g IV every 12 h	See instructions for IV minocycline
tetracycline hydrochloride	Achromycin and others	1–2 g PO per day	
		500 mg–1 g IV every 12 h	See instructions for IV minocycline
		Ophthalmic solution 1% 1–2 drops 2–6 ×/day in conjunctival sac	Also available as ophthalmic ointment; review p. 104 for instillation of eye drops

    C. Nephrotoxicity.

    D. Bones and teeth: brown discoloration of teeth; depression of bone growth (especially in children and infants who received the drug in utero).

    E. Hypersensitivity reactions: angioedema, anaphylaxis, cross-sensitivity to other tetracyclines.

    F. Superinfections, especially in the oropharynx and vagina, are common.

    G. Blood: leukocytosis, purpura.

    H. Drug interactions include:

      • Inactivation of tetracyclines when they are taken with milk, iron preparations, sodium bicarbonate, or antacids containing calcium, aluminum, or magnesium.

      • Additive anticoagulant effects when combined with anticoagulants.

      • Increased nephrotoxicity when combined with other nephrotoxic agents.

      • Decreased effectiveness of penicillins when combined with tetracyclines.

      • Increased hypoglycemia when insulin or oral hypoglycemics are combined with tetracyclines.

    I. Adverse responses may occur in the newborn if the mother takes tetracyclines during pregnancy.

    J. Intramuscular injections are absorbed poorly and produce local irritation. For this reason, the IM route is not recommended.

III. Nursing implications.

    A. Review general nursing implications on pp. 290–291.

    B. Report allergy to tetracyclines or possible pregnancy before administering the first dose. Anticipate possible change of drug.

    C. Administer oral preparations on an empty stomach if possible. Do not administer with foods, liquids, or other drugs that contain calcium, aluminum, iron or magnesium. Milk, cheese, iron supplements, and antacids are examples of substances that must be avoided.

    D. Observe the patient for adverse responses before each dose and report and record findings.

    E. Observe the diabetic patient taking insulin or oral hypoglycemics for hypoglycemic reactions. Instruct the patient to anticipate a possible reaction and report symptoms immediately.

    F. Administer IV preparations slowly to avoid thrombophlebitis.

MISCELLANEOUS ANTIMICROBIALS

I. Actions and uses.

    A. *Bacitracin* is a topical antimicrobial agent that inhibits growth of a variety of gram-positive bacteria (see Table 24–13 for bacitracin and other miscellaneous antimicrobials). Ophthalmic solutions and ointments and skin powders and ointments are available.

    B. *Chloramphenicol* is a broad-spectrum antibiotic that inhibits the growth of a variety of gram-positive and gram-negative bacteria. Because it is highly toxic, this drug is now used only for the patient with typhoid fever or serious anaerobic infections (bacterial meningitis, rickettsial infections) when other agents fail.

    C. *Clindamycin* is an antibiotic that inhibits the growth of anaerobic gram-positive cocci bacteria. This drug is especially useful in combination with an aminoglycoside (see Table 24–2) for the patient with lung abscess, intra-abdominal or pelvic abscess, or peritonitis.

    D. *Colistin* and *polymixin B* are antibiotics effective for gram-negative bacteria including Enterobacter, *E. coli*, and Salmonella.

    E. *Erythromycin* is an antibiotic that inhibits the growth of a small number of gram-positive bacteria such as certain strains of Streptococcus. This drug may be used for patients with mycoplasmic pneumonia, Legionnaire's disease, Chlamydia infections, diphtheria.

TABLE 24–13   Miscellaneous Antibiotics

Nonproprietary Name	Proprietary Name	Adult Dose Range	Notes
bacitracin	Baciguent	Skin powders and oint-ments; ophthalmic oint-ment	Used for skin and eye infections caused by susceptible bacteria
chloramphenicol	Chloromycetin, Mychel	1 g PO IV every 6–8 h for 1–4 weeks	Dose depends on the patient's specific in-fection
clindomycin	Cleocin	150–450 mg PO every 6 h; 600–1,200 mg IM, IV per day in two to four evenly divided doses	Larger IV doses may be ordered for severe infections
colistin	Coly-Mycin S	5–15 mg/kg PO per day	
erythromycin	E.-Mycin, Ilotycin, Ilosone, others	1–2 g PO per day in four di-vided doses every 6 h	
	Ilotycin, Glucep-tate, Erythrocin lactobionate-IV	0.5–1 g IV every 6 h	IM injections not recommended
imipenim-cilastatin	Primaxin	250–500 mg IV dose every 6–8 h; total daily dose should not exceed 50 mg/kg	New broad-spectrum antibacterial for pa-tients with infections of unkown causes or those with hospital acquired infection; not effective in cerebrospinal fluid; may produce myoclonus, confusion, and sei-zures in addition to nausea and vomiting, fever, hypotension, urticaria; do not ad-minister concurrently with other anti-biotics
spectinomycin hydrochloride	Trobicin	2–4 g IM single dose; 2 g IM 2 ×/day for 3 days	Usual dose for acute gonorrhea Dose for disseminated gonorrhea
Vancomycin hydrochloride	Vancocin HCl	500 mg–1 g IV every 6–12 h	Dose is diluted and injected over 30- to 60-min period
		500 mg PO every 6 h oral solution	Dose for antibiotic-associated colitis only

   F. *Spectinomycin* is an antibiotic that selectively inhibits the growth of organisms that cause gonorrhea. The drug is injected IM for patients with genital or rectal gonorrhea who are al-lergic to penicillins.

   G. *Vancomycin* is an antibiotic that inhibits the growth of gram-positive organisms. The drug is used primarily for the patient with a serious infection that has become resistant to other drugs.

   H. Drugs in this miscellaneous category can be considered second- or third-choice agents for most infections. They are used when organisms become resistant to other drugs or when the patient is allergic to the first-choice drug.

II. Adverse responses.

   A. Bacitracin: occasional hypersensitivity reaction at the site of topical application.

   B. Chloramphenicol: hypersensitivity including anaphylaxis and angioedema; bone marrow failure that is frequently fatal; nausea, vomiting, and diarrhea; perineal irritation; visual dis-turbances; drug interactions cause severe toxicity of chlorpropamide, dicumarol, phenytoin, tolbutamide if combined with chloramphenicol; phenobarbital decreases effectiveness of chloramphenicol.

   C. Clindamycin: diarrhea, potentially fatal pseudomembranous colitis, skin rash, anaphylaxis, thrombocytopenia, elevated liver function studies; this drug may increase effects of neuro-muscular blocking agents.

   D. Colistin and polymixin B: nausea and vomiting; hypersensitivity is rare.

   E. Erythromycin: allergic reactions including fever and rash; jaundice and hepatitis; epigastric distress with oral route; local irritation with IM, IV routes; rare auditory nerve damage; drug interactions include enhanced potential for toxicity of carbamazepine, corticosteroids, di-goxin, theophylline when combined with erythromycin.

    F. Spectinomycin: urticaria, fever, chills, dizziness, nausea, insomnia.

    G. Vancomycin: hypersensitivity reactions including anaphylaxis, skin rashes; ototoxicity and nephrotoxicity; phlebitis and pain at injection site; nephrotoxicity increases when vancomycin is combined with aminoglycosides, ethacrynic acid, or furosemide.

III. Nursing implications.

    A. Anticipate that patients receiving drugs listed in Table 24–13 have either developed resistance to other drugs or have allergy to other drugs.

    B. Monitor laboratory studies when available to anticipate the patient's clinical response to drug therapy.

    C. Observe the patient before each dose for adverse drug responses specifically related to the drug ordered.

    D. Administer oral erythromycin 1 h before or 2 h after meals if possible.

    E. Follow manufacturer's directions for preparing and administering parenteral doses.

    F. Review and use the general nursing implications listed on pp. 290–291.

IMMUNIZING AGENTS

  I. Actions and uses.

    A. *Immunizing agents* provide a recipient with resistance to a specific infection (Table 24–14).

    B. *Antitoxins* are antibodies that neutralize toxins produced by certain disease-causing microorganisms. Antitoxins provide temporary short-term passive immunity.

    C. *Immune serums* containing human antibodies may be collected from human donors and administered to provide temporary passive immunity to persons who have been exposed to certain infections. *Immunoglobulins* is another term used to describe five different types of natural human antibodies.

    D. *Toxoids* are immunizing agents composed of toxins from specific microorganisms that have been changed to make them harmless. Although harmless, toxins are still able to stimulate the production of natural antibodies in the recipient. Thus toxoids produce active acquired immunity that is usually permanent.

    E. *Vaccines* are immunizing agents composed of suspensions of attenuated (weakened) or dead bacteria, rickettsiae, or viruses. The vaccine stimulates the production of natural antibodies in a recipient. This results in *active acquired immunity* which is permanent.

    F. Immune serums and antitoxins are generally administered either to prevent a specific disease following exposure or to reduce the severity of disease.

    G. Several immunizing agents may be given together in a single administration such as diphtheria; tetanus pertussia; diphtheris, pertussis, tetanus (DPT) vaccine; measles, mumps, rubella (MMR) vaccine.

  II. Adverse responses.

    A. Hypersensitivity reactions may develop immediately or several days or weeks later. Anaphylaxis and angioneurotic edema are examples of immediate hypersensitive reactions. *Serum sickness* is a delayed hypersensitive reaction that may produce fever, rash, aching joints, and enlargement of lymph nodes.

    B. Fever, malaise, aching occur often after an immunizing agent has been administered.

    C. Pain, erythema, and tenderness and/or a lump that persists for weeks or months at the injection site.

    D. Guillain-Barré syndrome (progressive ascending paralysis) is a rare complication of some vaccines; other rare adverse responses include shock, lethargy, convulsions, encephalopathy.

  III. Nursing implications.

    A. Assist in the collection of information from the patient. Report allergies to horse serum, eggs, and other proteins to the registered nurse or physician before administering an immunizing agent. Also report possible pregnancy, use of corticosteroids and immunosuppres-

TABLE 24–14   Immunizing Agents

Immunizing Agent	Proprietary Name	Dose Range	Notes
Antitoxins—Passive Immunity			
antirabies serum		55 U/kg	A horse serum used as second-choice agent; used with rabies vaccine to prevent rabies after animal bites.
botulism antitoxin		100,000 Units IV as directed	Used for the patient with botulism caused by *Clostridium botulinum*
diptheria antitoxin		1,000 U IM, IV for prevention 20,000 U IM, IV for treatment	A horse serum used with antibiotics; used for the unvaccinated person who has been exposed to diptheria
tetanus antitoxin		1,500 NIH U SC for prevention 40,000 NIH U SC for treatment	A horse serum used as a second-choice agent for the unvaccinated person with a wound that is susceptible to *Clostridium tetani*
Human Immune Serum Globulins—Passive Immunity			
hepatitis B Immune globulin	H-B1G Hyper HEP and others	0.06 ml/kg IM immediately after exposure and repeated in 1 month	Administered to prevent hepatitis B after exposure
diptheria and tetanus toxoids; diptheria, pertussis, tetanus (DPT) vaccine		0.5 ml IM every 4–8 weeks × three doses; booster dose 7–12 months later and again at age 5–6 years	Dose for infants and children up to age 6
tetanus toxoid, adsorbed		0.5 ml IM every 5–6 weeks × two doses; booster dose 1 year later, then every 10 years	Dose for adults
tetanus and diptheria toxoids, adsorbed		0.5 ml IM every 4–6 weeks × two doses; booster dose 1 year later; then every 10 years	Dose for adults and children 7 years and older
Vaccines—Active Immunity			
BCG vaccine		0.1 ml intradermally	Skin test for tuberculosis sensitivity
cholera vaccine		0.5 ml SC, IM every 1–4 weeks × two doses, then every 6 months if necessary	Used for travelers to Africa, Asia, Middle East. Immunization period is short
hepatitis B	Heptavax-B	one ml IM every month × two doses; repeated in 6 months	Used for patients at risk for developing hepatitis B: physicians and surgeons, nurses in dialysis units, dentists, IV drug users, male homosexuals, patients on dialysis
immune serum globulin (gamma globulin)	Gammar Immu-G and others		Various doses may be administered to prevent hepatitis A and B, measles, varicella after exposure; may also be used with antibiotics for several bacterial infections and to replenish deficiencies
rabies immune globulin	Hyperab	20 U/kg IM	Administered to prevent rabies after animal bites
rh D immune globulin	Rho-GAM	Dose varies; administered IM	Administered after delivery, abortion or miscarriage to prevent future Rh incompatibility when the mother is Rh negative and the father is Rh positive; also used to prevent transfusion reaction with errors in blood transfusions

TABLE 24–14   *(cont.)*

Immunizing Agent	Proprietary Name	Dose Range	Notes
tetanus immune globulin	Hyper-Tet and others	250 U IM for prevention; 3,000–6,000 units IM for treatment	Used with tetanus toxoid to prevent tetanus in unvaccinated clients who have wounds susceptible to *Clostridium tetani*
Toxoids—Active Immunity diphtheria and tetanus toxoids, adsorbed		0.5 ml im every 4 weeks × two doses; additional dose 1 year later; repeated before child enters school	Dose for infants and children up to age 7 who are unable to receive pertussis vaccine at the same time
influenza vaccine	Fluax Fluogen	Dose varies according to manufacturer's directions	Administered only to high-risk patients who are not allergic to eggs: the elderly, those with chronic diseases; does not provide immunity to all influenza viruses
measles vaccine	Attenuvax	0.5 ml SC × one dose	May be administered after the age of 1 year; do not administer to women who are pregnant
measles and rubella vaccines	M-R-Vax II	Entire single-dose vial is administered SC	Dose to prevent measles and rubella (German measles) in children 15 months to puberty
measles, mumps, and rubella vaccines		Entire single-dose vial is administered SC	Dose to prevent measles, mumps, and rubella in children 15 months to puberty
meningitis vaccines	Meningovax AC, or C Menomune A/C or A/C/Y or C, W-135	0.5 ml SC adult dose	Administered to high-risk persons who live in areas with a high incidence of meningitis
mixed respiratory vaccine	MRV	0.05 ml SC gradually increased every 4–7 days to a maximum of 1 ml, then a maintenance dose 0.5 ml SC every 1–2 weeks	Administered to prevent the development of allergy to bacteria. May be helpful to persons with bronchial asthma, rhinitis, urticaria
mumps vaccine	Mumpsvax	Entire contents of single-dose vial SC	Administered to adults and children at least 1 year old to prevent mumps
pertussis vaccine		0.5 ml SC every 4 weeks × three doses; booster doses same as DPT	Dose to prevent pertussis (whooping cough) in children
plague vaccine		1 ml IM initially; 0.2 ml 1 month later; 0.2 ml 6 months after initial dose	Used for travelers and high-risk persons in areas with high incidence of plague; also used in disasters; for laboratory workers
pneumococcal vaccine polyvalent	Pneumovax Pnu Imune	0.5 ml SC, IM	Contains strains of most pneumococci that cause infections in the United States; administered to high-risk persons: elderly individuals, those with chronic disabling conditions
poliomyelitis vaccine (Salk)	IPV	1 ml SC every 4–6 weeks × three doses; fourth dose in 6–12 months and booster doses every 5 years	Inactivated polioviruses are administered to persons whose immune systems are depressed by disease or drugs
poliovirus vaccine (Sabin)	Orimune	0.5 ml or 2 drops PO every 6–8 weeks × three doses; booster dose at 4–6 years	Contains weakened polio viruses that can be placed on a sugar cube or mixed with chlorine-free water, milk, or simple syrup

TABLE 24–14   *(cont.)*

Immunizing Agent	Proprietary Name	Dose Range	Notes
rabies vaccine	Imovax WYVAC	IM doses are administered in a series	Used for persons who have been bitten by a potentially rabid animal; may also be used as prevention for laboratory workers, animal keepers, veterinarians
Rocky Mountain spotted fever vaccine		1 ml SC, IM every week-× three doses	Administered to prevent Rocky Mountain spotted fever in persons who work in areas where prevalent
rubella and mumps vaccines	Biavax 11	Entire volume of single-dose vial SC	Administered to prevent rubella and mumps in children over 1 year old
rubella virus vaccine	Meruvax	0.5 ml SC	Usually administered with other vaccines in combination preparation; do not administer to patients who are allergic to neomycin
smallpox vaccine	Dryvax	Interadermal multiple puncture	Recommended only for health care personnel and travelers
typhoid vaccine		0.5 ml SC every 4–6 weeks × two doses; booster doses every 3 years if exposure continues	Dose regimens may vary; recommended only for travelers and other high-risk persons
typhus vaccine		0.5–1 ml SC every 4 weeks × two doses	Used only for persons who live or travel in high-risk areas: Africa, Asia, South America; do not administer to persons allergic to eggs
yellow fever vaccine		0.5 ml SC single dose	Used only at WHO (World Health Organization) yellow fever vaccination centers; cannot be administered to persons allergic to eggs

Abbreviations: BCG, bacillus Calmette–Guérin; NIH, National Institutes of Health.

sives, drug therapy for cancer, phenytoin. Patients in these situations usually do not receive immunizing agents.

B. Check the expiration date and read manufacturer's directions carefully and completely before administering an immunizing agent.

C. Take vital signs before administering an immunizing agent. Report fever to the registered nurse or physician.

D. Know where emergency drugs, equipment, and supplies are located in the clinic, doctor's office, emergency room, or nursing unit before administering an immunizing agent.

E. Use recommended methods of administering trivalent oral polio vaccine to infants and children.

F. Administer DPT vaccine in the lateral thigh of infants.

G. Administer MMR vaccine SC within 8 hours after reconstitution with the manufacturer's diluent.

H. Assist the physician with sensitivity tests as directed before administering antitoxins.

I. Inject immune serum globulin deep IM into a large muscle mass such as the gluteus. Use two or more sites if the volume to be injected exceeds 4 to 5 ml.

J. Use the following guidelines to teach others about immunizing agents: consult Table 24–14 for recommended immunizations and intervals; assist patients to maintain accurate and complete immunization records for themselves and their children; report adverse responses other than mild fever, malaise, pain at the injection site.

K. Instruct the patient to remain in the clinic, doctor's office, emergency room, or hospital room for 30 min after receiving an immunizing agent. Observe frequently for hypersensitivity.

CASE STUDY 17

Mr. David Mason is a 68-year-old man with benign prostatic hypertrophy (BPH). Three days ago Mr. Mason had a transurethral resection of the prostate (TURP) under general anesthesia. On the third postoperative day, you begin your initial observation and assessment in the morning and collect the following information:

- Temperature, pulse, respiration (TPR) 100.2°F, 106, 24.
- Foley catheter drains cloudy pink urine without clots.
- Patient reports malaise and myalgia.

Questions

1. Underline the information in the case study that directly relates to infection and explain the reason for each selection.
2. What additional information and assessment is indicated for Mr. Mason?

The physician notes your observations recorded in the nursing notes and suspects infection. Several diagnostic tests are ordered.

3. What diagnostic tests do you anticipate?
4. Describe how you would explain each of the diagnostic tests to Mr. Mason.

The physician orders gentamicin 80 mg IM every 8 h × 7 days. Serum blood urea nitrogen (BUN) and creatinine are also ordered every 3 days.

5. Explain the actions and uses of gentamicin.
6. Describe how you would explain the need for blood tests every 3 days to Mr. Mason.
7. Relate each of the major adverse responses to gentamicin to a nursing action that detects or prevents it.
8. List other drugs in the same chemical family as gentamicin.

CASE STUDY 18

Mrs. May Anoki is a 35-year-old woman who is leaving the hospital after an appendectomy. The physician's discharge orders include:

- Ampicillin 1 PO every 6 h for 10 days.

The registered nurse asks you to give the patient the drug after it arrives from the hospital pharmacy and instruct Mrs. Anoki about taking the drug at home.

Questions

1. Imagine that you are Mrs. Anoki. List the questions you might have about taking ampicillin in the space below.
2. Now consider what you know about ampicillin as a practical nursing student studying about drug therapy. Add any additional questions that are important to the list you started in question 1. Consider questions Mrs. Anoki might not ask but might need to ask after discharge.
3. Use your final complete list of questions to develop a set of written instructions for Mrs. Anoki. The written instructions should provide answers to each of the questions on your list. Use a separate piece of paper for your written instructions.

EXERCISE 1.

Complete each of the following sentences related to drug therapy for the patient with infection.

1. Antimicrobial agents are drugs that _____.
2. The physician usually orders a culture and sensitivity test before the initial dose of an antimicrobial drug because _____.
3. Three nursing actions related to the collection of specimens for culture and sensitivities are:
   a. _____.
   b. _____.
   c. _____.
4. Three specific nursing implications related to the administration of cephalosporins for infection include:
   a. _____.
   b. _____.
   c. _____.
5. Three nursing implications that enhance the effects of tetracyclines in a patient with infection include:
   a. _____.
   b. _____.
   c. _____.

EXERCISE 2.

The list below contains examples of common immunizing agents. First, organize the list according to the common types of agents presented in the chapter. Next, describe the major features of each type of immunizing agent. Then, describe one major adverse response associated with each type of immunizing agent. Last, provide one example of a nursing implication for each type of immunizing agent. A chart is provided to help you organize the information.

- Tetanus antitoxin
- Gamma globulin
- Rabies immune globulin
- Tetanus and diphtheria toxoids
- Measles, mumps, rubella vaccine
- Poliomyelitis vaccine (Sabin)

Type of Immunizing Agent	Examples	Major Characteristics	Adverse Responses	Nursing Implications

Chapter 25 | DRUG THERAPY FOR THE PATIENT WITH CANCER

EXPECTED BEHAVIORAL OUTCOMES

After completing this chapter, you should return to the expected behavioral outcomes and evaluate your ability to:

1. Describe the effects of antineoplastic drugs for the patient with cancer on malignant and nonmalignant cells.
2. List at least five nursing measures that increase the patient's comfort and sense of well-being during cancer chemotherapy.
3. Select an appropriate nursing action for each of the adverse responses that a patient may develop during IV therapy.

DESCRIPTION OF CANCER

The patient with *cancer* has a malignant tumor that contains rapidly growing and multiplying abnormal cells that contribute nothing to the body but use its resources. Neoplasms are classified primarily by the type of tissue that gives rise to the tumor. *Carcinomas* are solid tumors that arise from epithelial tissue such as skin, mucous membrane and serous membrane. *Sarcomas* are solid tumors that arise from connective tissues such as bone, cartilage, fat, and tendons. *Leukemias* are cancers of the bone marrow. *Myeloma* is a cancer of the bone marrow that produces an abundance of abnormal plasma cells. *Lymphomas* are cancers of lymph tissues and lymph nodes. In most types of cancer, abnormal cells spread to other parts of the body either by extension of the solid tumor or by transportation in the bloodstream or lymph.

The cause of cancer is not known. It is currently thought to be a group of diseases that have different causes. Some factors are known to favor the development of cancer. Irritation of a body part over time may result in the formation of malignant cells. Pipe smoking and cigarette smoking are examples of personal habits that cause irritation to the lip and lungs, respectively. Persons with a low resistance to infection are more likely to develop malignancy. For example, persons receiving immunosuppressives to prevent organ rejection are at risk to develop cancer. Some cancers have been associated with viruses. High-dose radiation, overexposure to sunlight, certain chemicals and drugs, alcohol use, high fat diets and low dietary fiber intake have all been linked to higher rates of cancer.

Cancer is the second leading causes of death in the United States and the incidence is rising. Treatment is much more likely to be effective when malignancy is detected early. A key role of the nurse is assisting in early detection. Early symptoms can be recalled be remembering the acronym TROUBLE:

- *T*hickening or lump, particularly in the breast.
- *R*egular appearance of wart or mole changes in color, size, shape.

- *O*ral sore or any other sore that does not heal.
- *U*nusual changes in bowel and bladder habits.
- *B*leeding or discharge, irregular vaginal bleeding.
- *L*aryngitis, hoarseness, or persistent cough.
- *E*ating problems such as indigestion or persistent difficulty in swallowing.

The patient with cancer may be treated with surgery, radiation, drug therapy, or a combination of therapies that are directed toward one or more of the following objectives: removing the tumor, killing tumor cells, improving body defenses, shrinking tumor size, relieving pain.

Drug therapy for cancer is usually called *chemotherapy*. The purpose of most chemotherapy is to slow the growth and multiplication of malignant cells. Drugs used in chemotherapy are called *antineoplastic agents*. Combination therapy is common and special protocols have been established for various types of cancers. Five main groups of antineoplastic drugs are used in chemotherapy of cancer: alkylating agents, antibiotics, antimetabolites, hormones, and miscellaneous drugs. A key to understanding the effects of chemotherapy on a person with cancer is remembering that all body cells are affected, not only malignant cells.

Nursing implications are similar for all drug therapy for the patient with cancer. For this reason, nursing implications have been placed in a separate section that follows information about various groups of drugs.

ALKALOIDS

I. Actions and uses.
  A. *Alkaloids* are natural drugs that come from a species of myrtle, the periwinkle plant (Table 25-1).
  B. Alkaloids interfere with the natural life cycle of the cell, preventing cell division and reproduction.
  C. Alkaloids may be used for the patient with metastatic tumors, Hodgkin's disease, lymphomas.
II. Adverse responses.
  A. Neurotoxicity—peripheral neuropathy, numbness and tingling of extremities, foot drop, loss of neuromuscular reflexes, ataxia, muscle cramps, nerve pain, mental depression, fever.
  B. Gastrointestinal system: anorexia, nausea, vomiting, diarrhea, lesions of the mouth, severe constipation.
  C. Blood: leukeopenia, anemias.
  D. Other: alopecia, cardiac ischemia, dermatitis, polyuria, dysuria, cellulitis, and thrombophlebitis if IV drug leaks into surrounding tissues.

TABLE 25–1   Alkaloids

Nonproprietary Name	Proprietary Name	Adult Dose Range	Notes
vinblastine sulfate	Velban	5.5–7.4 mg/m²/week IV; maximum of 18.5 mg/m²/week	Dose may be adjusted according to patient's response; most often used with bleomycin (see Table 25–3) and cisplatin (see Table 25–5) for the patient with metastases to testicle
vincristine sulfate	Oncovin	2 mg/m²/week IV	Used as part of several drug protocols for childhood leukemia, non-Hodgkin's lymphoma, brain tumors, carcinoma of male and female reproductive systems
vindesine sulfate	Eldisine	3–4 mg/m²/week IV	Optimum dose schedules still under investigation; used for the patient with lymphoma, certain leukemias

ALKYLATING AGENTS

I. Actions and uses.
  A. *Alkylating agents* slow down activity, growth, and multiplication of cells (Table 25–2).
  B. *Nitrogen mustards* are a group of chemically related alkylating agents that may be used alone or with other drugs for the patient with Hodgkin's disease, lymphoma, leukemias.
  C. *Nitrosoureas* are a group of chemically related alkylating agents used for the patient with meningeal leukemia, metastatic brain tumors, Hodgkin's disease, lymphomas, melanomas, carcinomas of breast, bronchi, gastrointestinal system, and kidneys.
  D. *Triazene drugs* are used primarily for the patient with malignant melanoma.
II. Adverse responses.
  A. Blood: bone marrow depression that affects most types of cells, resulting in increased susceptibility to infection and increased likelihood of abnormal bleeding.
  B. Reproductive system: temporary or permanent infertility in men and women, amenorrhea in women, depression of sperm manufacture in men.
  C. Skin and mucous membranes: damage to hair follicles resulting in temporary hair loss (alopecia), skin eruptions and damage; damage to mucous membranes of eyes, skin, respiratory tract; herpes zoster, pulmonary fibrosis.

TABLE 25–2 Alkylating Agents

Nonproprietary Name	Proprietary Name	Adult Dose Range	Notes
Alkyl sulfonates			
busulfan	Myleran	2–8 mg PO initially; then 1–3 mg PO per day as maintenance if needed	Used for patients with chronic leukemia; hyperuricemia is an additional adverse response; patient may receive allopurinol; cataracts, gynecomastia may also occur
Nitrogen Mustards			
chlorambucil	Leukeran	4–10 mg PO per day for 3–6 weeks	
cyclophosphamide	Cytoxan	2–50 mg/kg/day PO, IM IV	Dose varies according to kind of cancer; may also be administered into pleura or peritoneum
mechlorethamine hydrochloride	Mustargen	0.4 mg/kg IV total dose	May also be injected into a body cavity
melphalan	Alkeran	6 mg PO per day for 2–3 weeks; then 2–4 mg PO per day as maintenance if necessary	Especially useful for patients with multiple myeloma, carcinoma of breast or ovaries; nausea and vomiting rare; alopecia, liver and kidney damage do not occur but bone marrow depression is common
uracil mustard		1–2 mg PO per day for 3 weeks; repeated after a week of rest	Alternate regimen is 3–5 mg PO per day for 7 days, then 1 mg /day for 3 weeks; nausea, vomiting, diarrhea, dermatitis, bone marrow depression
nitrosoureas			
carmustine	BICNU	100–200 mg/m^2 IV infusion over 1–2 h; repeated 6 weeks later	Used for patient with Hodgkin's disease, lymphomas, myelomas
lomustine	CEENU	130 mg/m^2 PO; repeated 6 weeks later	
streptozocin	Zanosar	500 mg/m^2 IV daily for 5 days; course repeated every 6 weeks	Used primarily for patient with metastases to islet cells in pancreas; potentially fatal kidney toxicity, liver toxicity is common
triazenes			
dacarbazine	DTIC-DOME	3.5 mg/kg IV daily for 10 days; repeat every 28 days	

    D. Gastrointestinal system: nausea and vomiting, liver toxicity, oropharyngeal ulcerations.

    E. Nervous system: convulsions, progressive muscular paralysis.

    F. Urinary system: hemorrhagic cystitis.

ANTIBIOTICS

I. Actions and uses (Table 25–3).

    A. Selected antibiotics are too toxic too be used for the patient with infection. However, these drugs do inhibit the growth of rapidly multiplying cells.

    B. Antibiotics have been used alone or in combination with other drugs for the patient with rhabdomyosarcoma, Kaposi's and soft tissue sarcoma, choriocarcinoma, metastatic tumors in the lungs and testicles, and Wilm's tumor in children.

II. Adverse responses.

    A. Gastrointestinal system: anorexia, nausea and vomiting, diarrhea, proctitis, oral ulcerations.

    B. Blood: bone marrow depression.

    C. Skin: alopecia, skin rashes, swelling, ulcerating skin lesions, hyperpigmentation, erythema, pruritus.

    D. Lungs: potentially fatal pulmonary fibrosis, dyspnea, rales, lung infiltrates, cardiorespiratory collapses.

    E. Nervous system: fever, headache.

TABLE 25–3 Antibiotics

Nonproprietary Name	Proprietary Name	Adult Dose Range	Notes
bleomycin sulfate	Blenoxane	10–20 U/m^2 IM, IV 1–2×/week; total course does not exceed 400 U	May also be administered SC, via intra-arterial injection; used with other drugs for the patient with cancer of testicles; also used for palliation of head and neck cancers; high potential for adverse responses of skin and lungs
dactinomycin	Actinomycin D, Cosmegen	10–15 μg/kg IV × 5 days; repeated every 3–4 weeks; total dose is usually 2.5–5 mg	Used for children with rhabdomyosarcoma or Wilm's tumor; adults with various sarcomas, choriocarcinomas; ulcerations of mucous membranes and bone marrow depression are more common than other adverse responses
daunorubicin	Cerubidine	3–60 mg/m^2 IV 1–3×/week	Used primarily for patients with acute lymphocytic or granulocytic leukemia; cardiotoxicity a serious adverse response; tell patient that drug turns the urine red
doxorubicin hydrochloride	Adriamycin	60–75 mg/m^2 by IV infusion; repeated after 21 days	Used for patients with acute leukemia and solid tumors; used with several other agents in various protocols for lymphomas, ovarian cancer, breast cancer, various sarcomas, cancers of the bronchi, bladder, metastatic thyroid cancer; cardiotoxic
mithramycin	Mithracin	25–30 mg/kg/day IV or alternate days × eight to ten doses	Limited use for patients with advanced cancers of testicles, hypercalcemia; highly toxic to bone marrow, liver, kidneys; hemorrhage is common; report epistaxis immediately
mitomycin	Mutamycin	2 mg/m^2 IV daily for 5 days, repeat every 2 days until total dose of 20 mg/m^2 has been reached	Total dose may also be given as a single dose; for temporary benefits in patients with advanced cancers of head and neck, breast, lung, pancreas, bladder, colon, cervix; lung and kidney damage more common

    F. Other: hypotension, cardiotoxicity may produce tachycardia, arrythmias, dyspnea, congestive heart failure, cardiomyopathy.

ANTIMETABOLITES

  I. Actions and uses.

    A. *Antimetabolites* kill cells by entering the cell and either depriving it of nutrients necessary to cell life or stimulating the formation of abnormal DNA (Table 25–4).

    B. Antimetabolites may be used for patient with selected acute or chronic leukemias, Hodgkins's disease, lymphomas, choriocarcimona, other advanced cancers.

    C. In some protocols, "rescue" agents are added to drug therapy to prevent fatal damage to normal cells. Leucovorin (folinic acid) and thymidine are examples of rescue agents.

  II. Adverse responses.

    A. Blood: bone marrow depression producing leukopenia, various anemias, thrombocytopenia with bleeding.

    B. Skin and mucous membranes: alopecia, dermatitis, nail changes, hyperpigmentation, skin atrophy.

    C. Gastrointestinal system: stomatitis, diarrhea, hemorrhagic enteritis, liver damage, anorexia, nausea, vomiting, dysphagia.

    D. Respiratory system: interstitial pneumonitis.

    E. Reproductive system: damage to manufacturing of ova and sperm.

    F. Kidneys: nephrotoxicity.

    G. Nervous system: Neurotoxicity, cerebellar syndrome, seizures.

TABLE 25–4   Antimetabolites

Nonproprietary Name	Proprietary Name	Adult Dose Range	Notes
azathioprine	Imuran	3–5 mg/kg/day PO, IV initially; 1–3 mg/kg/day as maintenace	Immunosuppressive used primarily to prevent transplant rejection; also used for the patient with severe rheumatoid arthritis; antineoplastic effects still under investigation
cytarabine	Cytosar-U	100–200 mg/m² IV daily for 5–7 days	Used primarily for patients with acute leukemia; used in combination with other agents
floxuridine	FUDR	24 mg/kg IV daily for 4 days; then 12 mg/kg IV every other day for two to four doses	May also be administered via arterial infusion to local tumors of liver, head, and neck
fluorouracil	5-FU Adrucil	12 mg/kg IV daily for 4 days; then 6 mg/kg every other day for two to four doses; maximum daily dose is 800 mg	Also available as topical agent (Efudex) for patients with premalignant skin lesions and psoriasis; used for the patient with certain breast and gastrointestinal cancers
mercaptopurine	Purinethol	100–200 mg PO per day initially; maintenance dose of 1.2–2.5 mg/kg daily	Used for patients with acute leukemia, choriocarcinoma, and a host of other chronic diseases including psoriasis, rheumatoid arthritis; also used in combination with other drugs
methotrexate	Folex Mexate	2.5–10 mg/day PO, IM	Used for patient with acute leukemia, choriocarcinoma, and a host of other chronic diseases including psoriasis, rheumatoid arthritis; also used in combination with other drugs
thioguanine	TG	2–3 mg/kg PO daily	Used mainly with other agents to produce remissions for patients with acute granulocytic leukemias

MISCELLANEOUS AGENTS

I. Actions and uses.
  A. Drugs in this group are not related chemically but have limited activity and high potential for toxicity (Table 25-5).
  B. Drugs in this group are often used either in conjunction with other agents as part of a specific protocol, or as alternative drugs for patients who do not respond favorably to other drugs.
  C. Hormones such as those described in Chapters 19 and 22 may also be used for the patient with cancer. Adrenocorticosteroids (see Table 22-2) androgens (see Table 19-1), and estrogens (see Table 19-5) are most often used.
II. Adverse responses.
  A. Blood: bone marrow depression, leukopenia, thrombocytopenia, immunosuppression, hemorrhage.
  B. Skin and mucous membranes: dematitis, oral ulcerations.
  C. Gastrointestinal system: anorexia, nausea, vomiting, jaundice and liver toxicity, pancreatitis, diarrhea.
  D. Nervous system: somnolence, lethargy, psychic disturbances, peripheral neuropathy, seizures, fever.
  E. Kidneys: nephrotoxicity, electrolyte imbalances.
  F. Lungs: interstitial pneumonia.
  G. Hypersensitivity: anaphylaxis.
  H. Cardiovascular system: arrhythmias, hypotension.
  I. Drug interactions include:
   • Patients taking procarbazine are instructed to avoid alcohol, tricyclic antidepressants, adrenergic agents, and foods containing high levels of tyramine such as those listed on p. 135.

NURSING IMPLICATIONS

  1. Determine the responsibilities of the licensed practical nurse/licensed vocational nurse (LPN/LVN) in your hospital/agency/clinic for the patient receiving chemotherapy. Chemotherapy by oral routes may often be administered by registered nurses and/or LPN/LVN's. Chemotherapy by other routes usually requires special training for registered nurses. Consent for chemotherapy is usually obtained in writing by the physician.
  2. Weigh the patient and measure his or her height. This and other measurements help the physician to calculate the correct dose.
  3. Report all of the patient's or family questions and concern to the registered nurse or physician. Administer an antiemetic if ordered before and after chemotherapy.
  4. Encourage and assist the patient to eat a balanced diet and drink sufficient fluids. Consult the dietician for modification of diet that may improve intake.
  5. Assist in the application of a head tourniquet or scalp ice bags if these are used to prevent or reduce alopecia.
  6. Inspect the patient's mouth daily with a flashlight; report inflammation, lesions, bleeding from gums. See Fig. 25-1.
  7. Encourage and assist the patient with scrupulous oral hygiene that includes: twice-daily brushing with a soft-bristled brush; daily flossing with unwaxed floss; oral rinsing with equal parts hydrogen peroxide and water every 4 h and after meals; remove dentures often and clean; remove dentures entirely if they irritate the patient's mouth.
  8. Omit brushing and flossing if there is actual or potential bleeding from gums; instead cleanse teeth with toothettes or cotton-tipped applicators moistened with dilute solutions of hydrogen peroxide and water, normal saline, or Cepacol mouthwash; avoid lemon and glycerin swabs; increase oral rinses.

TABLE 25–5 Miscellaneous Agents

Nonproprietary Name	Proprietary Name	Adult Dose Range	Notes
cisplatin	Platinol	10 mg/m² IV every 4 weeks	Dose may be reduced when used with other drugs; ototoxicity and kidney damage are additional adverse responses; used mainly for cancers of testicles, ovaries, bladder, head, and neck
etoposide	VePesid	50–100 mg/m² daily for 5 days; repeated every 3–4 weeks	Used for patients with lung cancer, Hodgkin's disease, and other lymphomas and sarcomas
hydroxyurea	Hydrea	80 mg/kg PO every third day or 20–30 mg/kg PO daily for 6 weeks	Used mainly for patients with chronic granulocytic leukemia
L-asparaginase	Elspar	200–1,000 IU/kg/day IM, IV for 10–28 days	Used mainly for the patient with acute lymphoblastic leukemia who does not respond to other drugs; produces hypersensitivity, severe toxicity of the liver, pancreas, kidneys, central nervous system, and clotting mechanism
leuprolide	Lupron	1 mg SC daily	New synthetic hormone specifically for patients with prostatic cancer; may produce hot flashes, gynecomastia, nausea and vomiting, peripheral edema
mitotane	Lysodren	8–10 grams PO per day in three to four doses for 3 months	Use limited to patients with inoperable carcinoma of adrenal cortex; damages adrenal cortex; corticosteroid must be taken; do not administer spironolactone at the same time
procarbazine hydrochloride	Matulane	2–4 mg/kg PO daily for 1 week; then 4–6 mg/kg PO daily until good response or toxicity appears; 1–2 mg/kg PO daily as maintenance	Used mainly with other drugs as part of a protocol for Hodgkin's disease

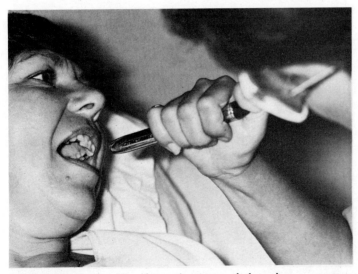

FIGURE 25–1 Checking the patient's mouth for adverse responses to drug therapy for cancer.

9. Inspect the patient's body openings daily for signs of infection or bleeding.

10. Wash the hands often before and after caring for the patient to prevent infection.

11. Encourage and assist the patient with meticulous personal hygiene to prevent infection. Assist with perineal cleansing if necessary and dry skin folds well; use electric razor if bleeding is likely.

12. Monitor visitors and others with colds or other infection who might come in contact with the patient.

13. Monitor appropriate laboratory studies to anticipate the patient's clinical responses to drug therapy. Laboratory studies most frequently ordered include complete blood count (CBC), liver and kidney function tests, serum electrolytes.

14. Inspect intravenous administration sites daily for erythema, warmth, tenderness, swelling. Report adverse findings to the appropriate registered nurse. When monitoring IV chemotherapy, report immediately any signs of infiltration (decrease or stop of flow), swelling, or report of pain. Many chemotherapy drugs cause severe damage if they leak into SC tissue.

15. Suggest scarves, wigs, hats to the patient who develops alopecia as a result of cancer chemotherapy.

16. Encourage and support the patient having chemotherapy by listening, by providing meticulous physical care, identifying and praising patient's strengths, talking to patient about a range of topics that include life both inside and outside the world of cancer, asking specifically about the patient's concerns.

CASE STUDY 19

Miss Helen Toma is a 33-year-old woman with Hodgkin's disease who is receiving chemotherapy with a special regimen abbreviated as MOPP. Drugs in the MOPP regimen include: Mechlorethamine, vincristine (Oncovin), Prednisone, and Procarbazine.

Answer the following questions about drug therapy for Miss Toma.

1. Underline drugs in the case study that are antineoplastic agents.
2. Circle drugs in the case study that are hormones.
3. Next to each drug in the MOPP regimen listed below, describe its effects on nonmalignant cells. Use the space provided to write your answer.

Drug	Effect on Malignant Cells	Effect on Normal Cells
mechlorethamine		
vincristine (Oncovin)		
prednisone		
procarbazine		

4. For each of the major adverse responses associated with Miss Toma's chemotherapy, select a nursing action to detect or prevent it. Use the space below to organize your information.

Adverse Response	Nursing Action for Detection or Prevention

5. Describe five nursing actions you could take to increase Miss Toma's comfort and well-being during chemotherapy. Do not repeat nursing actions you have already identified in question 4. Use the space below to describe the nursing action you select.

a. _____.

b. _____.

c. _____.

d. _____.

e. _____.

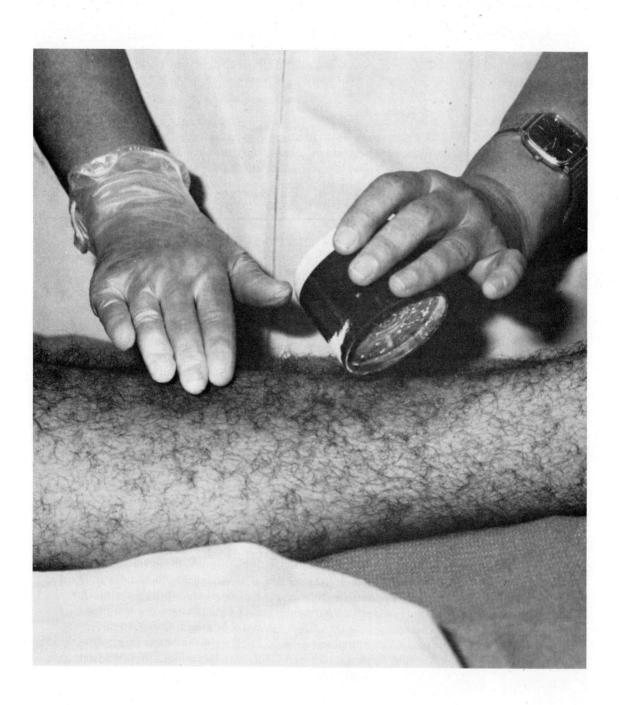

Section VII

MISCELLANEOUS DIAGNOSTIC AND THERAPEUTIC AGENTS

Chapter 26 | DRUG THERAPY WITH INTRAVENOUS FLUIDS

EXPECTED BEHAVIORAL OUTCOMES

After completing this chapter, you should return to the expected behavioral outcomes and evaluate your ability to:

1. Identify common factors that may lead to fluid and electrolyte imbalance in hospitalized patients.
2. Describe essential characteristics of a complete order for IV therapy.
3. List at least five nursing actions appropriate for the patient receiving drug therapy with IV fluids.
4. Select an appropriate nursing action for each of the adverse responses that a patient may develop during IV therapy.

FLUID AND ELECTROLYTE BALANCE

In order for the body cells to function normally, the volume and composition of body fluids must remain fairly constant. Total body fluids comprise from 50 to 70% of body weight. Approximately 35% of all body fluids are located in the extracellular compartment (bloodstream and between cells). Approximately half is located in the intracellular compartment (inside cells). The remaining amount of body water is located in bones, body secretions, cerebrospinal fluid, and aqueous humor of the eye.

The composition of body fluids varies considerably but contains similar substances called *electrolytes*. Electrolytes are electrically charges particles that play a vital role in cell life, help to maintain fluid balance, and help to maintain normal acidity–alkalinity inside the body fluids (acid-base balance). The major electrolytes in all body fluids are sodium, potassium, calcium, magnesium, bicarbonate, chloride, phosphate, and sulfate.

Whenever illness causes excessive losses or gains of total body fluid or its constituents, a patient may develop fluid and/or electrolyte imbalance. A person may develop a fluid or electrolyte imbalance from insufficient intake and/or excessive losses. Examples of common situation that may lead to fluid and electrolyte imbalance in hospitalized patients include fever and diaphoresis, vomiting, diarrhea, nasogastric suction, NPO restriction for diagnostic tests or surgery, anorexia. The patient with kidney disease may develop severe fluid and electrolyte imbalance when the kidneys are unable to form urine or concentrate it in the usual way.

The patient with excessive losses of chlorides or bicarbonates from diarrhea may develop *metabolic acidosis*. The patient with excessive of hydrogen ions from vomiting may develop *metabolic alkalosis*. The patient with excessive losses of salt and water may develop *dehydration*. The person with hyponatremia has too little sodium circulating in the bloodstream. The person with *hypokalemia* has too little potassium circulating in the bloodstream.

TABLE 26–1   Intravenous Fluids and Electrolytes

Nonproprietary Name	Proprietary Name	Adult Dose Range	Notes
dextrose (glucose)	2.5%–50%	Available in volumes of 50, 100, 250, 500, or 1,000 ml	50% solution used only for the patient with hypoglycemic reaction
dextrose and saline	5% dextrose in 0.22% sodium chloride 5% dextrose in 0.45% sodium chloride	Available in volumes of 250, 500, or 1,000 ml	
potassium chloride	2 mEq/ml		40–100 mEq added to at least 1,000 ml of IV fluid; administer over 24 h no faster than 10–15 mEq/h
Ringer's lactate		500, 1,000 ml	Contains all major electrolytes
sodium chloride	0.9%—isotonic 0.45%—hypotonic 3–5%—hypertonic	Available in volumes from 50 to 1,000 ml	

Intravenous fluids (Table 26-1) may be used to replace fluids and electrolytes or restore fluid and electrolyte balance in these and other conditions.

I. Actions and uses.
  A. Various concentrations of hypotonic or isotonic physiologic saline may be ordered IV for the patient with dehydration or hyponatremia.
  B. Hypertonic saline may be ordered for the patient in crisis with Addison's disease (adrenal insufficiency).
  C. Various concentrations of dextrose (glucose) may be ordered to replace fluids lost and provide energy.
  D. Combination solutions containing various amounts of both dextrose and saline may be ordered.
  E. Ringer's lactate injection may be ordered when the patient has mild acidosis.
  F. A complete IV administration order is provided by the physician and contains the following components.
    1. Volume of fluids to be administered.
    2. Composition of fluids to be infused.
    3. Drug and dose to be added to the IV fluids if desired.
    4. Flow rate stated as a volume per hour or per minute.
II. Adverse responses.
  A. Allergy: the patient may have an allergy to the IV fluid, the IV administration set, or the needle or cannula used for venipuncture.
  B. Circulatory overload: sudden onset of dyspnea, cough, tachycardia, pallor or cyanosis; edema caused by too-rapid administration of IV fluids or inability of kidneys to eliminate fluids.
  C. Diuresis: increased formation and excretion of urine caused by additional fluids in circulation.
  D. Electrolyte imbalance: an adverse response to the volume or type of fluids prescribed; the patient's symptoms depend upon the type of imbalance.
  E. Infection: fever, chills, tachycardia, malaise, and other symptoms caused by the entry of pathogens into the bloodstream via the IV cannula or needle.
  F. Infiltration: a cold, hard, painful lump at the IV administration site, swelling at the IV site; a change in the flow rate (irregular or slow) caused by the leakage of IV fluids into surrounding tissue outside the vein.
  G. Inflammation: erythema, warmth, tenderness, swelling at the IV administration site means a phlebitis caused by the irritation of IV fluids, needle, or cannula along the vein wall.
III. Nursing implications.
  A. Compare the label on every container of IV fluids to the physician's written order before administering.

B. Prepare a label with the patient's name and date of infusion according to local custom and place the label on the IV container after the physician's order has been verified with the container; do not cover up the label already on the container.

C. Seek additional information from the physician when the written order is incomplete or unclear.

D. Compare the label on the IV container to the patient's identification bracelet for correct identification.

E. Hang IV fluids without introducing microorganisms into the closed system.

F. If licensed practical nurses/licensed vocational nurses (LPN/LVNs) do not hang or prepare IV infusions in your hospital, notify the appropriate registered nurse at least 1 h before the next IV container is to be hung.

G. Calculate the IV flow rate using the following formula:

$$\frac{\text{volume to be infused} \times \text{drop factor*}}{\text{time in minutes}} = \text{drops per minute}$$

*Drop factor is stated on the IV Administration set as drops/ml.

H. Adjust the height of the IV administration pole so that the container of fluid is 12 to 18 in. above the patient's head. Intravenous fluid flows in by gravity.

I. Monitor the patient every hour during IV therapy. A minimum observation includes the patient's color, respiratory rate, and pulse; condition of the IV administration site; IV flow rate, amount remaining in the container compared to that expected. (See Figure 26-1.)

J. Report excessively fast flow rates to the registered nurse at once. If an adjustment of flow rate is permitted, use the following formula to calculate the adjusted flow rate:

   1. Take the amount to be infused over the next hour.

   2. Subtract the volume of fluid excess from the amount given in item 1 above. (This is the difference between what you expected and what remains.)

   3. The result becomes the new volume to be infused over the next hour.

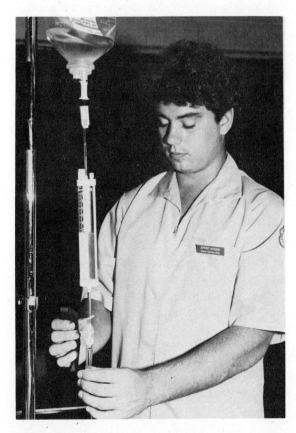

FIGURE 26-1 Checking the flow rate as part of monitoring the patient receiving IV therapy.

   4. Use IV flow rate formula to calculate the adjusted flow rate for the next hour. (The time in minutes will be 60 min.)

   5. Consult the registered nurse to ensure that the adjusted flow rate is a safe one for the particular patient.

   6. Return after the adjusted flow rate hour and determine if further adjustment is needed.

   7. Do not adjust flow rates without consulting the registered nurse.

K. Report excessively slow flow rates to the registered nurse. If an adjustment of flow rate is permitted, use the following formula to calculate the adjusted flow rate:

   1. Take the amount of IV fluids to be infused over the next hour.

   2. Add the *volume of fluid deficit* to the amount in item 1 above. (This is the difference between the amount remaining in the bottle and the amount you expect to be there.)

   3. The result becomes the new volume to be infused over the next hour.

   4. Use the IV flow rate formula to calculate the adjusted flow rate for the next hour. (The time in minutes will be 60 min.)

   5. Consult the registered nurse to ensure that the adjusted flow rate is a safe one for the particular patient.

   6. Return after the adjusted flow rate hour to determine if further adjustments are indicated.

   7. Do not adjust flow rates without consulting the registered nurse.

L. Report other adverse responses to the registered nurse.

M. Anticipate the patient's need for easy access the bathroom or bedpan.

N. Record intake and output according to hospital policy.

O. Change the IV dressing according to hospital policy and procedure.

P. Plan ahead if your hospital has a special intravenous therapy team. Notify the team early if there are problems with the IV administration site.

CASE STUDY 20

Mr. Frank Ivy is a 55-year-old man who returned from the operating room after a resection of the colon. During the initial postoperative observations and assessment, the following information was gathered:

---

   1. Drowsy but responds appropriately to verbal stimuli.

   2. Nasogastric tube drains dark-brown liquid.

   3. Abdominal dressing dry and intact.

   4. Lactated Ringer's IV solution running at 125 ml/h; 400 ml remains.

The physician's postoperative orders include:

- NPO.
- Nasogastric tube to low suction; irrigate q4h prn with normal saline.
- Complete present IV administration of Lactated Ringer's solution by 4 PM.
- Then, 5% dextrose in 0.45% saline with 20 mEq KCL.

The registered nurse assigns you to care for Mr. Ivy and tells you to "watch the IV."
Answer the following questions about IV therapy for Mr. Ivy.

   1. Underline factors in the case study that may lead to fluid and electrolyte imbalance in Mr. Ivy.

   2. What additional information do you need to complete the postoperative assessment of IV therapy for Mr. Ivy? Use the space below to record your answer.

   3. What additional information do you need to carry out the postoperative orders for IV therapy for Mr. Ivy? Use the space below to record your answer.

4. List five nursing actions that you will take to "watch the IV" as directed by the registered nurse. Use the space below to record your actions.

   a. _____ .
   b. _____ .
   c. _____ .
   d. _____ .
   e. _____ .

5. For each of the adverse responses listed below, describe the corresponding related observations and select a nursing action for detection or prevention.

Adverse Response	Related Observations	Nursing Action for Detection and Prevention
Circulatory overload		
Diuresis		
Infection		
Infiltration		
Inflammation		

6. The record below indicates a part of the IV monitoring related to the IV flow rate. For each of the hours that the IV flow rate is not on time, calculate the adjusted flow rate using a drop factor of 10 gtt/ml. Show all work in the space provided

Patient: Frank Ivy	Room: 402	Date:	
IV fluid ordered: 5% dextrose in 0.45% saline		Flow rate ordered: 125 ml/h	
Hour	Amt. Expected in IV Container	Amt. Actual in Container	Adjusted Flow Rate
5 PM	875 ml	800 ml	
6 PM	750 ml	750 ml	
7 PM	625 ml	700 ml	
8 PM	500 ml	500 ml	
9 PM			

5 PM calculations:

6 PM calculations:

7 PM calculations:

8 PM calculations:

Chapter 27 | DRUGS APPLIED TO THE SKIN, EYE, AND EAR

EXPECTED BEHAVIORAL OUTCOMES

After completing this chapter, you should return to the expected behavioral outcomes and evaluate your ability to:

1. Select a nursing action appropriate for each of the adverse responses that a patient may develop when drugs are applied locally to the skin or mucous membrane.
2. List nursing actions appropriate for the patient receiving topical drug therapy.

REVIEW OF STRUCTURE AND FUNCTION

The *skin* is an organ that covers the body and protects underlying tissues, regulates body temperature, excretes waste products, and maintains water and electrolyte balance. The skin protects the body from pathogens and also serves as the organ for touch.

Mucous membrane is continuous with skin and lines various canals and body cavities. Mucous membranes secrete *mucus*, a lubricating substance that protects membranes from foreign bodies and waste.

I. Actions and uses.
   A. *Topical agents* are drugs applied to the skin or mucous membranes. Many topical agents have already been described in previous chapters. (See Chapters 16–18, 20, 22, 24.) This chapter focuses on drug therapy with other substances.
   B. Topical agents may also be applied to mucous membranes linings of the ears (Table 27-3) and eyes (Table 27-2).

II. Adverse responses.
   A. Drugs applied topically may be absorbed and produce systemic side effects.
   B. Incorrect administration may introduce infection in the ear, eyes, or nose.
   C. Topical drugs may produce local hypersensitivity reactions.
   D. Topical drugs for the skin may stain the patient's clothing.

III. Nursing implications.
   A. Report the patient's allergies before administering the first dose of a topical agent.
   B. Wash the hands before and after each topical application.

    C. Use careful technique for instilling ear, eye, and nose drops. Review this chapter if needed.

    D. Use an applicator or a glove when applying topical drugs to the skin.

    E. Determine whether or not previous applications must be removed from the skin or skin lesion, before the new application.

    F. Determine whether or not the skin or lesion is to covered after the application.

    G. Observe, report, and record adverse responses.

IV. Common skin disorders.

    Included in the common skin disorders are the following:

    A. *Acne* is a condition that takes on several forms the most common of which is *acne vulgaris*, characterized by comedones (pimples), pustules, and nodules, usually appearing on the face, neck, and upper trunk of teenagers.

    B. *Burns* are an injury to the skin (or deeper tissues) caused by heat, chemicals, electricity, the sun's rays, and radiologic equipment.

    C. *Dermatitis* is an inflammation of the skin that may be brought about by a number of irritants.

    D. *Eczema* is a condition characterized by blistering, itching, swelling, scaling, and oozing of the skin, usually due to allergy.

    E. *Erysipelas* is an infection of the skin caused by Streptococcus. It usually is found on the face and neck. The symptoms include edema, redness, and heat.

    F. *Erythema* is a symptom rather than a disease. It is a redness of the skin caused by the engorgement of the peripheral capillaries.

    G. *Impetigo* is a skin condition characterized by a pustule rash usually caused by Streptococcus, sometimes in conjunction with Staphylococcus.

    H. *Pruritus* is a symptom rather than a disease. It is common in many skin diseases, and in some systemic diseases such as diabetes mellitus. It is characterized by itching in various degrees.

    I. *Psoriasis* is characterized by bright red patches with silvery scales, usually occurring on the scalp, and areas around the elbows and knees.

    J. *Tinea* is infection of the skin. There are many types such as *T. barbae*, of the beard; *T. capitis,* of the scalp; *T. corporis*, or ringworm; *T. pedis*, of the foot.

    K. *Urticaria* is a vascular, usually reddened, elevated rash attended by severe itching frequently resulting from an allergy. Hives.

    L. *Vitiligo* is a condition in which there is a progressive loss of skin pigment that causes patchy areas of pink or white skin.

    M. *Warts* are small hard rough growths appearing on the skin and caused by a virus. *Plantar warts* occur on the soles of the feet and can be very painful because of the pressure constantly exerted on the feet.

TABLE 27–1   Drugs Applied to the Skin

Drug (Proprietary Name)	Therapeutic Use	Precautions and Comments
	Antibiotics are drugs that kill or inhibit bacterial growth	
Antibiotics		
bacitracin (Baciguent)	Powder or ointment is applied to skin infected with gram-positive organisms	Hypersensitivity reactions may occur
gentamicin	Used for impetigo, infected skin lesions	May cause irritation and pruritis
mafenide (Sulfamylon Cream)	Sulfa drug; cream is applied 1–2 ×/ day to burn to prevent infection	Burn must be cleaned and debrided before each application; may cause allergy, pain, fluid loss through burned areas
neomycin sulfate (Mycifradin)	Ointment may be applied to skin infected with impetigo, wound infections	

TABLE 27–1 *(cont.)*

Drug (Proprietary Name)	Therapeutic Use	Precautions and Comments
Antibiotics		
polymixin B (Aerosporin)	Ointment may be applied to abscesses, infected burns, ulcers and wounds	
silver sulfadiazene (Silvadene)	See mafenide above.	See mafenide

Antiseptics are substances that kill or prevent the growth of microorganisms when applied to living tissue such as skin or mucous membranes.

Antiseptics		
acetic acid	Solution may be used for surgical dressings, bladder irrigations, vaginal douches to suppress Pseudomonas	
benzalkonium chloride (Zephiran)	An older solution for cleansing skin and instruments; no longer recommended	
chlorhexidine	Solution is applied to skin or mucous membrane before minor surgery, dental surgery	
ethanol or isopropyl alcohol	Solution most often used to cleanse skin before needle insertion	May cause dry, scaly skin; do not apply to wounds and broken skin
iodine	Solution is applied to skin or mucous membranes to destroy microorganisms; also used to clean wounds and skin abrasions	Hypersensitivity reactions including fever and skin eruptions
nitrofurazone (Furacin)	Creams, soluble dressings and other preparations especially helpful in preventing burn infection; may also be used for selected surgical dressings	
povidone-iodine	Applied to skin or mucous membrane to destroy microorganisms; used as preoperative scrub	Hypersensitivity reactions may occur

Ectoparasiticides are drugs that kill head and body lice.

Ectoparasiticides		
benzyl benzoate	Lotion for the patient with scabies	Apply lotion to body except for face; apply second coat after first has dried; wash residue off after 24 h
crotamiton (Eurax)	Cream or lotion for the patient with scabies	May cause irritation to inflamed skin.
lindane (Kwell)	Cream, lotion, or shampoo for the patient with scabies, head, body or pubic lice	Apply thin layer over entire body and remove in 8–12 h; keep away from face and eyes; may stimulate central nervous system
malathion (Prioderm)	Lotion for the patient with head lice and nits	Rub into scalp and leave for for 8–12 h; then shampoo and comb hair; repeat in 7–9 days if necessary
sulfurated lime solution	Ointment or solution for the patient with scabies or pediculosis	

Emollients are substances, usually fatty or oily, used to keep the skin soft and pliable. Some of these substances may also be used to protect. Listed below are some of these drugs.

Emollients		
ammonium lactate (Lac-Hydrin)	Reduces excessive epidermal hardening	New lotion that promotes retention of water in the skin; for external use only; not recommended for eyes, lips, or mucous membranes; may produce burning, erythema, peeling, stinging as adverse responses
glycerin	Frequently used to lubricate instruments that are to be passed into body openings	May be in the form of rectal suppositories

TABLE 27–1 (*cont.*)

Drug (Proprietary Name)	Therapeutic Use	Precautions and Comments
	Emollients	
lanolin, wool fat	Keeps the skin soft and pliable	
petrolatum	Both protective and emollient qualities; may be used to dissolve and remove skin debris	In certain forms used as a laxative
	Topical Enzymes debride wounds, burns, ulcers by digesting protein.	
Topical Enzymes		
collagenase (Biozyme-C)	Ointment used to debride severely burned areas and dermal lesions	Apply to lesion every day and cover with sterile dressing
elase	Ointment used to debride surgical wounds, burns	Local sensitivity may occur; report allergy to fibrinolysin or deoxyribonuclease (ingredients in the ointment)
papain (Panafil White)	Same as above	Keep away from eyes; cover lesions with gauze, apply twice daily
sutilains (Travase)	Ointment used to debride surgical wounds, burns, decubitus ulcers, varicose ulcers	Keep away from eyes; may produce pain; paresthesia, bleeding, dermatitis
trypsin (Granulex)	Aerosol used to debride ulcers, varicose ulcers, burns	Apply at least twice daily
	Nonsystemic fungicides are drugs that kill or inhibit the growth of fungi when applied locally.	
Nonsystemic Fungicides		
acrisorcin (Akrinol)	Cream for the patient with tinia versicolor	Apply twice daily to affected lesions for up to 6 weeks after they clear; keep away from eyes; may produce local erythema, burning, and stinging
benzoic and salicylic acids ointment (Whitfield's ointment)	Ointment for the patient with tinea pedis or capitis	Apply for several weeks or months until infected skin is shed; mild irritation may occur
ciclopirox Olamine (Loprox)	1% cream for the patient with candidiasis and various tinea infections	May produce hypersensitivity
clotrimazole (Lotrimin)	Lotion for the patient with various tinea infections	Also available for oral use, vaginal application
econazole (Spectazole)	1% cream for the patient with various tinea infections, skin candidiasis	Apply twice daily for 4–5 weeks
haloprogin (Halotex)	1% cream, spray, powder, or lotion for the patient with various tinea infections, ringworm	Apply twice daily for 2–4 weeks
miconazole nitrate (Micatin, MonistatDerm)	2% cream, spray, powder, or lotion for the patient with various tinea infections, ringworm	Apply twice daily for 14 days; use only lotion between skin folds; may produce burning, itching, irritation
tolnaftate (Aftate; Tinactin)	1% cream, powder, aerosol, solution for the patient with various fungal infections	Apply twice daily
undecylenic acid	Soap, powder, ointment foam, and solution for the patient with tinea pedis	
	Keratolytics are drugs that loosen and soften thickened skin and promote desquamation (the shedding of scales and sheets of skin).	
Keratolytics		
benzoic acid	Keratolytics are applied to the skin	
propylene glycol and salicylic acid (Karalyt)	and covered with plastic for patients with psoriasis, chronic dermatitis or dermatitis, other	
resorcinol	hyperkeratotic conditions	

TABLE 27–1   (cont.)

Drug (Proprietary Name)	Therapeutic Use	Precautions and Comments
Melanizing agents are drugs that add or remove pigment from the skin.		
Melanizing Agents		
hydroquinone	Creams, lotions, and solutions that bleach and lighten small areas of darkened skin (freckles, melasma of pregnancy)	Burning and stinging may occur; do not use near eyes or open cuts; not for children under 12
methoxsalen (Oxsoralen)	Oral capsules and topical lotions that increase the amount of melanin in patients with vitiligo when they are exposed to ultra-violet light	Burns, nausea, pruritis, and blisters may occur; lotion is applied by physician followed by 5 min exposure to ultraviolet light. Special protection for eyes is needed. Higher rates of skin cancer have been reported
monobenzone (Benoquin)	Ointment that removes remaining pigment for patients with vitiligo who wish to be one color	Mild erythema and dermatitis may occur
trioxsalen (Trisoralen)	Oral tablets that increase the amount of melanin in patients with vitiligo when they are exposed to ultraviolet light	Occasional nausea or gastric irritation
Protectants are substances that cover the skin or mucous membranes to protect them from irritation.		
Protectants		
dextranomer (Debrisan)	Beads that are placed in infected wounds, decubitus and varicose ulcers, infected burns for de-bridement.	Application and removal of beads may cause bleeding, burning, erythema, and pain
dimethicone	Creams, lotions, ointments, and sprays may be applied to the skin to provide waterproof protection	
Stomahesive	Placed around the stoma of an os-tomy to protect the skin from urine or intestinal contents	

TABLE 27–2   Ophthalmic Agents*

Drug	Adult Dose Range	Therapeutic Use	Precautions and Comments
Miotic Drugs Used on the Eyes (Contract the Pupils)			
betaloxol (Betoptic)		Used in treatment of glaucoma; reduces ocular pressure	New drug; not recommended for patients with sinus bradycardia, heartblock, or congestive heart failure
carbachol (Carbacel)	1.5% solution 1.5% ointment as ordered	As above	May cause aching of eyes and head
demecarium bromide (Humorsol)	0.125%–0.25% solution as ordered	As above	Avoid overflow into nasal and pharygeal spaces
ecothiophate	As ordered	As above	
bevobunolol (Betagan)		As above	New drug not recommended for patients with COPD, asthma, bradycardia, heart block, CHF
physostigmine	0.5% solution gtt 1–2 as ordered	As above	
pilocarpine	1–2% solution gtt 1–2 as ordered	As above	
timolol (Timoptic)	0.25–0.5% solution gtt 1–2 twice daily	As above	Does not constrict pupils

TABLE 27–2   (cont.)

Drug	Adult Dose Range	Therapeutic Use	Precautions and Comments
Mydriatic Drugs Used on the Eyes (Dilate the Pupils)			
atropine sulfate	1% solution gtt 1 as ordered	Used to dilate the pupils	
cyclopentolate	0.5% solution gtt 2 1% solution gtt 1 as ordered	Used in refractions	
epinephrine	1–2% solution 1% ointment as ordered	Dilates pupils	May cause intraocular pressure
homatropine hydrobromide	1% solution gtt 5 as ordered	Used to dilate the pupils	
hydroxyamphetamine	1% solution 1–2 gtt or as ordered	Dilates pupils	Also effective in shrinking of nasal mucosa
tropicamide	0.5–1% solution 1–2 gtt as ordered	Dilator of relatively short duration	

Abbreviations: CHF, congestive heart failure; COPD, chronic obstructive pulmonary disease.

*See also tables listing antibiotics in Chapter 24; see Table 22–2 on corticosteroids.

TABLE 27–3   Otic Agents

Drug	Therapeutic Use	Precautions and Comments
chloramphenicol otic solution 0.5%	Otitis media	Instill 2–3 drops into affected ear
polymixin B	Superficial infections of external ear	Instill 3–4 drops into affected ear 3–4 ×/day

EXERCISE

Complete the following sentences that describe drugs administered locally.

1. Drugs may be applied to the _____ or _____
   of the _____.
2. Four potential adverse responses to drugs administered locally include:
   a. _____.
   b. _____.
   c. _____.
   d. _____.
3. Elase is a topical enzyme that may be used for _____.
4. Kerolytics like Karalyt may be used for the patient with psoriasis because they _____.
5. One adverse response to methoxsalen for the patient with vitiligo is _____.
6. Stomahesive is considered a protectant because it _____.
7. Before inserting an enema tip into a patient's rectum you would lubricate it with _____.
8. Bacitracin is an _____ that may be applied to the _____.
9. Lindane is a drug used for _____.
10. Before you apply mafenide (sulfamylon cream), you should
    a. _____.
    b. _____.
    c. _____.
11. Pilocarpine is a miotic drug that may be used _____.
12. An otic solution is a topical agent applied _____.

13. _____ is an antiseptic commonly used as a preoperative scrub.
14. *Pruritus* means _____.
15. Haloprogin may be applied as a spray by the person with _____.
16. _____ is an antiseptic that may be ordered as a bladder irrigation.
17. Homatropine is a mydriatic drug that may be used to _____.
18. Hydrogen peroxide may be used in clinical practice to _____.
19. Vitiligo is _____.
20. One nursing action that should be taken before applying substances to the skin or mucous membrane is _____.

Chapter 28 | MISCELLANEOUS DIAGNOSTIC AGENTS

EXPECTED BEHAVIORAL OUTCOMES

After completing this chapter, you should return to the expected behavioral outcomes and evaluate your ability to:

1. Discuss at least five nursing implications for the patient receiving a diagnostic drug and/or contrast agent.

DIAGNOSTIC AIDS

Diagnostic aids are drugs administered to the patient for a diagnostic test. The nurse who works in a clinic, doctor's office, laboratory, or radiology department may administer selected diagnostic aids. Nurses who work with hospitalized patients may also administer drugs for diagnostic tests. All nurses may participate in the collection of information and specimens for diagnostic studies. In addition, the licensed practical nurse/licensed vocational nurse (LPN/LVN) may observe and report symptoms of drug allergy and/or drug interactions in some patients receiving drugs for diagnosis.

A summary of the nursing implications related the use of drugs for diagnosis can be located in Table 28–1. Table 28–2 contains a summary of selected drugs used in diagnostic tests and related additional nursing implications. Table 28–3 contains a summary of selected contrast agents used to highlight various body parts so that they can be visualized by x-ray examination or a scanner.

TABLE 28–1   Nursing Implications for Patients Receiving Drugs for Diagnosis

1. Record allergies prominently on the front of the chart. Be sure the patient is wearing an allergy identification band before a diagnostic test. Record allergies on the requisition for a laboratory test or x-ray and/or notify the department if necessary.
2. Describe in advance to the patient, any sensations that can be expected after a diagnostic drug is administered. Seek additional information from the registered nurse, physician, laboratory technologist, or radiology technologist.
3. Read manufacturer's instructions completely and carefully before administering a drug for diagnosis. Seek additional information from the registered nurse, pharmacist, or physician if necessary.
4. Know where emergency drugs, supplies, and equipment are located before administering a diagnostic drug in the clinic, doctor's office, diagnostic department, or nursing unit.
5. Report adverse responses at once to the appropriate nurse or physician.
6. Provide appropriate aftercare following administration of a diagnostic agent to prevent complications such as fecal impaction with some agents.
7. Record the diagnostic aid used on the patient's chart.

TABLE 28–2 Diagnostic Drugs

Drug	Diagnostic Use	Comments/Precautions
acetylcholine	Injected IV to improve visualization of tumors in the kidney	
adrenocorticotropin hormone (ACTH; Cortrosyn)	0.25 mg IM, IV to diagnose adrenal insufficiency—plasma cortisol measured, urine and/or blood	ACTH stimulation test; hypersensitivity reactions range from fever to anaphylaxis, various methods of testing may be used
adrenocorticotropic hormone	50 U—same as above	
ammonium chloride	0.1 g/kg PO to diagnose renal disease; timed hourly urine specimens are collected and measured for acidity pH	A loading test considered positive when the urine does not become more acid after the drug has been administered
arginine	0.5 g injected IV to diagnose diabetes, liver or kidney disease, pituitary tumors	Timed blood samples are collected before and after the dose and measured for either glucagon or prolactin. Exaggerated glucagon response indicates diabetes, liver, or renal response. A decrease in prolactin level indicates possible pituitary tumor.
betazole hydrochloride (Histalog)	1.5 mg/kg injected SC, IM for gastric analysis. Timed specimens of gastric secretions are collected from a nasogastric tube that is inserted before the test	Gastric analysis may be done to diagnose duodenal or gastric ulcers, gastric cancer, pernicious anemia; drug may cause allergic reactions including anaphylaxis
bethanecol chloride (Urecholine)	10–50 mg PO or 2.5 mg SC to measure enzyme function; serum amylase is measured after dose	Plasma amylase should rise after drug
calcium gluconate	15 mg/kg IV infusion administered over 4 h. Timed urine and blood samples are collected before and after drug is administered and measured for calcitonin, calcium, creatinine, phosphorus, parathyroid hormone.	Various tests may be done to diagnose thyroid cancer, parathyroid disease, osteomalacia, kidney disease, vitamin D intoxication
chlorpromazine (Thorazine)	25 mg IM administered to diagnose tumors of hypothalmus; timed blood samples collected before and after dose and measured for prolactin	A positive test occurs when prolactin levels do not rise as expected after dose
clomiphene citrate (Clomid)	100 mg PO every 24 h × seven doses; blood samples are collected before and after dose and measured for follicle-stimulating and lutenizing hormones	Test done to diagnose abnormalities of gonadotropin associate with pituitary disorders; may produce cystic ovarian changes, multiple pregnancies
cortisone	200 mg PO or predisone 40 mg PO to diagnose parathyroid disease, sarcoidosis, breast and other cancers, Addison's disease. Serum calcium is measured before and during each day of dosage	
deferoxamine mesylate (Desferal Mesylate)	10 mg/kg IM, IV to diagnose abnormalities of iron metabolism and iron poisoning; urine specimens are collected and measured for iron	Also used in the treatment of iron poisoning; may produce allergic reactions (anaphylaxis, pruritus, rash), diarrhea, dysuria, abdominal and leg cramps, tachycardia
deoxycorticosterone acetate	10 mg IM every 12 hours for 3 days to diagnose aldosteronism; timed plasma renin and 24-h urine for sodium, potassium, creatine collected before and after dose	Suppression test; positive test occurs when levels do not fall in urine and plasma
dexamethasone (Decadron and others)	0.5 mg or 2 mg PO every 6 h × eight doses to diagnose Cushing's syndrome and other abnormalities of adrenal hypersecretion; plasma cortisol and 24-h urines for ketosteroids collected before and after the dose	Suppression test; test results and interpretation vary according to dose used
D-xylose	5 or 25 g PO in 250 ml of water to diagnose intestinal malabsorption; timed blood and urine specimens collected for D-xylose excretion	Absorption test; a positive test occurs when urine levels of D-xylose decrease instead of increase

TABLE 28–2 (*cont.*)

Drug	Diagnostic Use	Comments/Precautions
edrophonium hydrochloride (Tensilon)	2 mg IV; 8 mg IV in 8 s if necessary to diagnose myasthenia gravis	A positive test occurs when the patient has a short temporary improvement of strength without tongue twitching that is typical in persons without myasthenia gravis; may produce respiratory paralysis that can be reversed with atropine sulfate; also used to determine optimum dose for patients after diagnosis
fludrocortisone (Florinef)	0.2 mg PO every 8 h × nine doses to diagnose primary aldosteronism; timed plasma renin and urine specimens for aldosterone are collected before and after dose	Suppression test that is positive when plasma renin falls while urine aldosterone either is unchanged or rises
fluorescein (Alefluor and others)	1 drop of 1% ophthalmic solution or moistened strip applied to cornea	Dye that enables physician to examine cornea for trauma; may produce burning, erythema, stinging
	5 ml (500 mg) of 10% solution or 3 ml (750 mg) of 25% solution IV	Dose to measure circulation time or visualize eye circulation; may produce headache, paresthesia, nausea, vomiting, metallic taste, anaphylaxis
folic acid (Folate)	15 mg—300 μg PO, IM to diagnose folate deficiency or malabsorption; blood, urine and/or bone marrow samples may be collected before and after dose	Dose varies according to test; smaller doses administered for absorption test; larger doses for therapeutic response test (for deficiency states)
fructose	30–50 g in 200 ml of water to diagnose absorption; timed blood and urine specimens collected before and after dose	Plasma and urine levels rise abnormally when malabsorption or liver disease present
furosemide (Lasix)	8 mg PO to diagnose primary aldosteronism as a cause for hypertension; plasma renin collected before and after dose	A screening test that is positive when plasma levels fall after the dose; patient must remain upright for 4 h after dose
galactose	40 g in 250 ml water or 1 mg/kg IV of 50% solution over 4–5 min to diagnose liver disease; timed blood and urine specimens collected before and after dose	A tolerance test that is positive in patients with cirrhosis, hepatitis, and metastatic liver cancer
glucagon	Glucagon may be injected IM or IV to diagnose adrenal or pancreatic tumors, diabetes; timed blood and urine specimens are collected before and after dose	Stimulation, suppression and tolerance tests may be done; dose varies according to specific test; anticipate and prepare for possible hypoglycemic reactions
glucose	Glucose may be administered orally or IV to diagnose diabetes mellitus; timed blood and urine specimens are collected before and after dose	Several tests may be done. Abnormal rises and falls in plasma and urine glucose indicate diabetes
histamine phosphate	May be administered parenterally or by inhalation for gastric analysis or to test bronchial reaction, respectively; may also be used to diagnose adrenal tumor	Rarely used because of potentially fatal adverse responses; see betazole hydrochloride
human chorionic gonadotropin hormone (HCG) (Android HCG, Follutein, and others)	2,000–3,000 IU IM every 24 h × four doses to diagnose hypogonadism; plasma testosterone measured before and after the dose	Stimulation test
hydrochlorothiazide (Esidrex, Oretic, others)	50 mg PO twice daily for 7–10 days to diagnose hyperparathyroidism, juvenile osteoporosis, vitamin D intoxication	Timed serum and urine specimens for calcium are collected before and after dose; anticipate diuresis; observe for hypokalemia
hydrocortisone	40 mg PO every 8 h × 10 days; serum calcium specimen collected before and during dose	Suppression test to diagnose a variety of diseases including Addison's disease, sarcoidosis, breast and other cancers
insulin	Various doses SC, IV to diagnose hypoglycemia, endocrine disease, glomerular filtration rates, insulin antibodies, or types of diabetes; timed blood specimens collected before and after dose	Antibodies, clearance, suppression, or tolerance tests may be done. Dose administered and substances measured vary with specific test; watch for hypoglycemia

TABLE 28–2 *(cont.)*

Drug	Diagnostic Use	Comments/Precautions
lactose, maltose, or sucrose	1–2 g/kg PO in water to diagnose malabsorption syndromes, timed blood specimens are collected before and after dose	Absorption test that is positive for malabsorption when serum glucose remains normally low after dose
levodopa (Dopar, Larodopa)	500 mg PO to diagnose pituitary disease; timed serum specimens collected before and after dose	Stimulation and suppression tests may be done; substances measured include growth hormone or prolactin depending upon specific test
methacoline	10–30 mg SC to diagnose atropine or belladonna poisoning	A positive test for poisoning occurs when the patient does not develop a typical facial flush, sweating, tearing, runny nose, increased salivation and peristalsis
metyrapone (Metopirone)	750 mg PO every 4 h × six doses to diagnose adrenal or pituitary disease; serum cortisol and 24-h urine ketosteroids are collected before and after dose	A stimulation test
pentagastrin (Peptavlon)	6 μg/kg SC to measure gastric secretion, pepsin and intrinsic factor in stomach; timed specimens are collected before and after dose through a nasogastric tube	May produce borborygmi, dizziness, faintness, flushing, nausea, tachycardia, urge to defecate
phentolamine mesylate (Regitine)	Less than 5 mg IM, IV is injected to diagnose pheochromocytoma (adrenal tumor) as a cause of hypertension	Blood pressure readings are taken serially before, during and after dose; may produce abdominal or anginal pain, cardiac arrhythmia, nausea, vomiting, or diarrhea
propranolol (Inderal)	40 mg PO with 1 mg glucagon M to diagnose pituitary disorders; timed blood specimens are collected before and after doses and growth hormone levles are measured	A stimulation test; arginine, insulin, or levodopa may also be used
secretin	5 μg/kg IV infusion for 1 h to diagnose Zollinger–Ellison syndrome. Timed blood gastrin specimens are collected before and after dose.	
thyroid hormones	Various thyroid hormones may be given to diagnose thyroid diseases. Timed blood specimens are collected before and after dose and measured for circulating hormone level.	Suppression and stimulation tests may be done. Thyroid-stimulating hormone, thyroid-releasing hormone, thyroxine may be administered depending upon specific test
tolbutamide (Orinase)	25–40 mg/kg–1 g po to diagnose pancreatic tumors or hypoglycemia; timed blood glucose and insulin specimens are collected before and after the dose	Watch for hypoglycemia
tubocurarine chloride	0.1–0.5 mg injected to diagnose myasthenia gravis; may also be used to diagnose pain caused by compression of nerve root	A positive test for myasthenia gravis occurs when the patient experiences muscle weakness or other symptoms after the dose
vitamins	Vitamins may be administered to diagnose deficiency states or intoxication; blood or urine samples may be collected before and after data	Vitamin A, vitamin B_{12}, vitamin C may be used in saturation absoption, tolerance tests

TABLE 28–3 Contrast Agents

Contrast Agent	Diagnostic Use	Comments and Precautions
barium sulfate (Barosperse, Esophotrast, others)	Swallowed or instilled rectally for x-ray examinations of GI system including barium enema, upper GI series	May produce allergic reactions, nausea, vomiting, diarrhea may occur; fecal impaction may occur; follow hospital procedures for enemas, laxatives, fluids after x-ray examination

TABLE 28–3 (*cont.*)

Contrast Agent	Diagnostic Use	Comments and Precautions
diatrizoate meglumine (Hypaque, Hypaque Cysto, others)	Various concentrations and preparations may be injected or instilled for angiocardiograms, aortograms, arthrograms, cerebral angiograms, cholangiograms, discograms, peripheral arteriograms and venograms, cystourethrograms, excretion urethrograms, splenoportograms, CT scan of head	May produce serious or fatal reaction, especially in patients with iodine allergy; review hospital procedures for patient preparation
diatrizoate meglumine and diatrizoate sodium (Hypaque-M and others)	Various preparations and concentrations may be swallowed, injected, or instilled for angiocardiograms, aortograms, coronary arteriograms, urograms, venograms, hysterosalpingograms	May produce serious or fatal allergic reactions, especially in patients with iodine allergy; review hospital procedures for patient preparation
diatrizoate meglumine and iodipamide meglumine (Sinografin)	Instilled into uterus for hysterosalpingogram	Same as above
diatrizole sodium (Hypaque and others)	Various concentrations and preparations may be swallowed, injected or instilled for x-ray examination of GI tract, retrograde pyelograms, urethrograms, CT scan of the head, cerebral and peripheral angiograms, aortograms, venograms, cholangiograms, hysterosalpingograms, splenoportograms	Same as above
ethiodized oil (Ethodiol)	Injected into lymph system for lymphograms or instilled into uterus for hysterosalpingograms	May produce pulmonary embolism during lymphogram
iocetamic acid (Cholebrine)	Swallowed for oral cholecystogram	May produce nausea, vomiting, heartburn; allergic reactions may occur, especially in persons with iodine allergy
iodamine meglumine (Renovue)	Various concentrations may be injected IV or instilled for urograms, CT scan of the brain	May cause allergic reactions, especially in patients with iodine allergy
iodipamide meglumine (Cholografin)	Various concentrations are injected IV for cholecystograms or cholangiograms	May cause allgeric reactions, especially in patients with iodine allergy
iopanoic acid (Telapaque)	Tablets are swallowed one at a time 2–5 min the night before cholecystogram	May produce nausea, vomiting, diarrhea; allergic reactions may occur, especially in patients with iodine allergy
iophendylate (Pantopaque)		May interfere with thyroid function tests using iodine for several years; may produce headache, nausea, mild temperature elevations, backache
iothalamate meglumine (Conray)	Various concentrations may be injected into arteries, veins, or ducts; or instilled into bladder, uterus, kidney, pelvis for urograms, venograms, cholangiograms, endoscopic retrograde cholangiopancreatography	May cause allergic reactions, especially in patients with iodine allergy
iothalamate meglumine and iothalamate sodium (Vasconray)	May be injected into arteries, veins, chambers of the heart for CT scan of the brain, aortograms, angiocardiograms, selected coronary arteriorgrams, selected renal arteriograms, excretion urethrograms	Same as above
iothalamate sodium (Angio-Conray; Conray-325, 400)	Various concentrations and preparations may be injected into arteries, veins, heart chambers for CT scan of the brain, aortograms, angiocardiograms, excretion urethrograms	Same as above
ipodate calcium (Oragrafin) *or* iopodate sodium (Bilivist)	Swallowed the night before oral cholecystogram	May cause nausea, vomiting, diarrhea, dysuria, headache, abdominal pain; may cause allergic reactions, especially in patients with iodine allergy
metrizamide (Amipaque)	May be injected for arteriograms or injected into subarachnoid space of spinal canal for myelogram or CT of the brain or spinal cord	May cause allergic reaction, including anaphylaxis; nausea and vomiting, mild temperature elevations; dizziness, hearing or visual disturbances; seizures

TABLE 28–3   (cont.)

Contrast Agent	Diagnostic Use	Comments and Precautions
propyliodine oil suspension (Dionosil Oil)	Instilled into the trachea or bronchial tree for bronchograms	May cause allergic reactions, especially in patients with iodine allergy; transient fever, malaise, and aching joints may occur
radioactive isotopes	Various radioactive isotopes may be swallowed or injected for scans of the brain, heart, lungs, liver, kidneys, spleen, pancreas, bones	
tyropanoate sodium (Bilopaque Sodium)	Swallowed for oral cholecystogram	Contains iodine; may cause allergic reactions, especially in patients with iodine allergy; not recommended for patients with severe liver or kidney disease

Abbreviations: CT, computed tomography; GI, gastrointestinal.

EXERCISE

The list below contains examples of nursing implications for patients receiving diagnostic drugs or contrast agents. In the space to the right of each statement, provide the reasons you think the nursing implication is important. One example is given.

Nursing Implication	Reason
1. Record allergies prominently on the chart, on the requisition for the test, and on the patient's identification band.	
2. Describe, in advance and using nontechnical language, what sensations the patient can expect after a diagnostic drug or contrast agent is administered.	
3. Know where the emergency drugs, supplies, and equipment are located before administering a diagnostic drug in the hospital, clinic, or doctor's office.	Many diagnostic drugs and contrast agents can cause anaphylaxis. The nurse needs to know where emergency materials are located in order to respond immediately in case this life-threatening event occurs.
4. Observe for local reactions such as erythema, warmth, tenderness, swelling after a diagnostic or contrast agent is administered IV.	
5. Label all specimens of body fluids immeidately when assisting in a diagnostic study.	
6. Administer enemas, laxatives, fluids according to instructions when assisting with x-ray examinations and other diagnostic studies.	

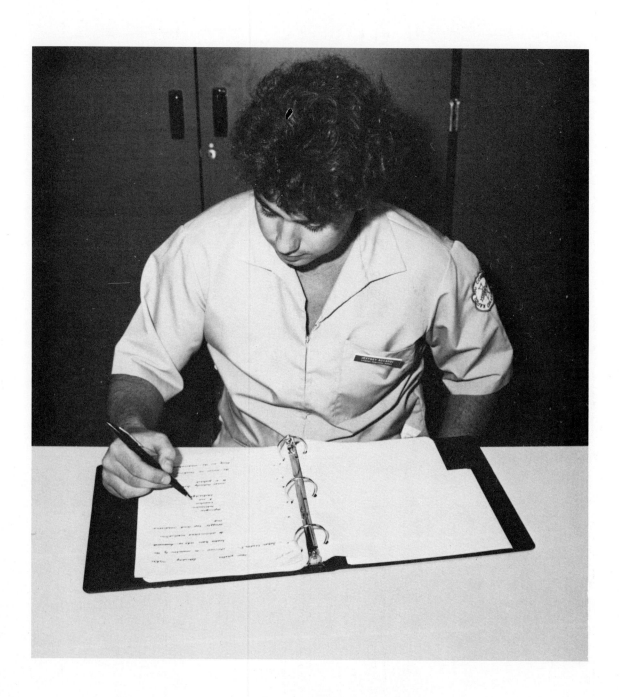

Section VIII

ARITHMETIC REVIEW

Chapter 29 | ROMAN AND ARABIC NUMERALS

EXPECTED BEHAVIORAL OUTCOMES

After completing Chapters 29 through 33, you should return to the expected behavioral outcomes and evaluate your ability to:

1. Use numbers in both the Arabic and Roman systems and convert numbers from one system to the other.
2. Add, subtract, multiply and divide fractions, decimals, and percents.
3. Change fractions, decimals, or percents into each of the other systems.
4. Construct and interpret a ratio.
5. Complete the arithmetic review quiz at the end of the section with a high degree of accuracy as determined by your instructor.

In order to read and interpret prescriptions and orders written by the doctor, the nurse uses two systems of numbers or numerals. Both Arabic and Roman systems are used in expressing dosages of drugs, and therefore are reviewed below.

NUMBERS OR NUMERALS

Arabic System.

This system uses ten arithmetic symbols 0, 1, 2, 3, 4, 5, 6, 7, 8, 9. All other numbers are composed of two or more of these symbols. These same symbols are used to express fractions (¼) or decimals (0.5).

Roman System.

This system uses the letters I, V, X, L, C, D, and M as symbols and combines them in definite ways to express whole numbers. The letters express amounts as follows:

I = 1	C = 100
V = 5	D = 500
X = 10	M = 1,000
L = 50	

In expressing numbers by the Roman system, certain rules must be followed:
    1. Some letters may be repeated in sequence, but never more than three times. (The letters V, L,

and D, of course, are never repeated, because their values when doubled are expressed by X, C, and M, repectively.) Examples of letters repeated in sequence:

$$III = 3$$
$$XXX = 30$$

2. When letters representing numbers of lesser value follow letters representing larger numbers, the lesser values are added to the larger number.

EXAMPLE: VIII = 5, 1, 1, 1, or 8

3. When letters representing numbers of lesser value precede letters representing larger numbers, the lesser value is subtracted from the larger number.

EXAMPLE: IX = 10 − 1, or 9

4. When letters representing numbers of lesser value are placed between numbers of higher value, the lesser value is subtracted from the larger amount it precedes.

EXAMPLE: XXIV = 10 + 10 + 5 − 1 = 24

1. Write as Roman numerals:
   a. 8_____.
   b. 13_____.
   c. 26_____.
   d. 29_____.
   e. 61_____.

   f. 72_____.
   g. 81_____.
   h. 105_____.
   i. 250_____.
   j. 510_____.

2. Write as Arabic numerals:
   a.   VI_____.
   b.   XIV_____.
   c. XXXIX_____.
   d.   XC_____.
   e. LXXV_____.

   f.   XLV_____.
   g.   LXV_____.
   h. LXXXVI_____.
   i.   MD_____.
   j.   MCD_____.

Chapter 30 | FRACTIONS

The physician often orders only part of a dose already on hand. When the nurse calculates the dose, fractions must be used. A fraction is part of a whole amount. When a whole amount is divided into two or more equal parts, a fraction may be used to identify the parts and their relationship to the whole. It is expressed as two numbers separated by a line.

EXAMPLES: ⅓, ⅔, ⅝, ¾, ⅘

PARTS OF A FRACTION

The parts of a fraction are the numerator or upper number, and the denominator or lower number.

EXAMPLE: $\dfrac{1 \text{ (numerator)}}{3 \text{ (denominator)}}$

KINDS OF FRACTIONS

Proper Fraction

A *proper fraction* has a numerator or upper number that is smaller than the denominator or lower number.

EXAMPLE: $\dfrac{1 \text{ (numerator is smaller than the denominator)}}{3 \text{ (denominator is larger than the numerator)}}$

Improper Fraction

An *improper fraction* has a numerator or upper number that is larger than the denominator or lower number.

EXAMPLE: $\dfrac{4 \text{ (numerator is larger than the denominator)}}{3 \text{ (denominator is smaller than the numerator)}}$

Complex Fraction

A *complex fraction* is one in which the numerator or upper number and the denominator or lower number or both are fractions.

EXAMPLES: $\dfrac{\frac{1}{2} \text{ (numerator is a fraction)}}{7 \text{ (denominator is a whole number)}}$

$\dfrac{3 \text{ (numerator is a whole number)}}{\frac{1}{2} \text{ (denominator is a fraction)}}$

$\dfrac{\frac{1}{2} \text{ (numerator is a fraction)}}{\frac{1}{4} \text{ (denominator is a fraction)}}$

Mixed Number

A *mixed number* is made up of a whole number and a fraction.

EXAMPLE: $3\frac{1}{3}$, $5\frac{1}{8}$, $2\frac{1}{2}$, $2\frac{1}{8}$, $9\frac{1}{6}$

Identify the following:

	a	b	c
1.	8 _____.	$^{10}/_9$ _____.	$7\frac{1}{5}$ _____.
2.	$\dfrac{\frac{1}{3}}{\frac{1}{8}}$ _____.	$\dfrac{\frac{1}{3}}{6}$ _____.	$\frac{1}{3}$ _____.
3.	$\frac{1}{120}$ _____.	$\dfrac{1\frac{1}{8}}{4\frac{1}{2}}$ _____.	$10\frac{1}{2}$ _____.
4.	$1\frac{4}{5}$ _____.	$^{16}/_{15}$ _____.	145 _____.
5.	$^{40}/_{50}$ _____.	$^{30}/_{10}$ _____.	$^{100}/_{150}$ _____.

CHANGING FRACTIONS TO LOWER TERMS

Some fractions can be changed to lower terms. This is done by dividing both the numerator and the denominator by the same number. This number should be the largest possible number that will go into the numerator and the denominator. Another term that describes this procedure is reducing fractions.

EXAMPLE: $\frac{4}{8}$ divided by $\frac{4}{4}$ equals $\frac{1}{2}$

Change the following fractions to their lowest terms:

	a	b	c
1.	$^{100}/_{150} =$	$^2/_8 =$	$^{16}/_{20} =$
2.	$^5/_{15} =$	$^{25}/_{75} =$	$^2/_4 =$
3.	$^5/_{10} =$	$^2/_6 =$	$^{50}/_{100} =$
4.	$^{32}/_{64} =$	$^8/_{16} =$	$^8/_{32} =$
5.	$^6/_{18} =$	$^{10}/_{15} =$	$^{10}/_{25} =$

CHANGING IMPROPER FRACTIONS TO MIXED NUMBERS OR WHOLE NUMBERS

Improper fractions are changed to mixed or whole numbers by dividing the numerator or upper number by the denominator or lower number.

EXAMPLES: $8/4 = 8$ divided by $4 = 2$ (a whole number)
$6/5 = 6$ divided by $5 = 1\frac{1}{5}$ (a mixed number)

$$\begin{array}{r} 1\frac{1}{5} \\ 5\overline{)6} \\ \underline{5} \\ 1 \end{array}$$

Change the following improper fractions to mixed or whole numbers:

	a	b	c
1.	$4/2 =$	$9/7 =$	$15/10 =$
2.	$30/5 =$	$150/100 =$	$120/120 =$
3.	$90/75 =$	$12/6 =$	$9/6 =$
4.	$80/45 =$	$3/2 =$	$16/15 =$
5.	$21/19 =$	$200/100 =$	$14/12 =$

Changing Mixed Numbers to Improper Fractions

Mixed numbers may be changed to improper fractions by:

1. Multiplying the whole number by the denominator or lower number of the fraction.
2. To this answer adding the numerator or upper number of the fraction.
3. Placing the sum or answer arrived at over the denominator of the fraction.

EXAMPLE: To change $4\frac{2}{3}$ (mixed number) to an improper fraction
4 (whole number) is multiplied by 3 (denominator) $= 12$
2 (numerator) is added to sum $= 12 + 2 = 14$
14 or sum is placed over denominator $3 = 14/3$

Thus: $4\frac{2}{3} = \dfrac{(4 \times 3) + 2}{3} = 14/3$

Change the following mixed numbers to improper fractions:

	a	b	c
1.	$15\frac{1}{2} =$	$3\frac{1}{2} =$	$2\frac{3}{8} =$
2.	$8\frac{1}{6} =$	$10\frac{2}{3} =$	$1\frac{1}{2} =$
3.	$9\frac{2}{7} =$	$6\frac{1}{3} =$	$10\frac{1}{2} =$
4.	$50\frac{1}{2} =$	$14\frac{1}{7} =$	$4\frac{1}{2} =$
5.	$2\frac{3}{4} =$	$5\frac{1}{5} =$	$7\frac{2}{5} =$

MULTIPLYING WHOLE NUMBERS AND FRACTIONS

Whole numbers may be multiplied by fractions by:

1. Multiplying the whole number by the numerator of the fraction.
2. Placing the sum or answer over the denominator. (The result will be an improper fraction.)
3. Changing the improper fraction to a mixed number.

EXAMPLE: To multiply 4 by $\frac{2}{5}$:

$$4 \text{ (whole number)} \times 2 \text{ (numerator)} = 8$$

$$\frac{8 \text{ (sum)}}{5 \text{ (denominator)}}\text{(improper fraction)}$$

$$\frac{8}{5} = 8 \div 5 = 5\overline{)8}\begin{smallmatrix}1\\ \frac{5}{3}\end{smallmatrix} = 1\frac{3}{5} \text{ (mixed number)}$$

Multiply the following whole numbers and fractions:

a	**b**	**c**
1. $7 \times \frac{1}{2} =$	$15 \times \frac{2}{3} =$	$4 \times \frac{1}{2} =$
2. $8 \times \frac{2}{3} =$	$9 \times \frac{2}{3} =$	$15 \times \frac{2}{5} =$
3. $8 \times \frac{3}{8} =$	$24 \times \frac{5}{8} =$	$4 \times \frac{3}{8} =$
4. $5 \times \frac{2}{5} =$	$10 \times \frac{1}{2} =$	$11 \times \frac{1}{4} =$
5. $9 \times \frac{1}{4} =$	$21 \times \frac{1}{3} =$	$18 \times \frac{1}{6} =$

Multiplying Two Fractions

Two fractions may be multiplied by:

1. Multiplying the numerators or upper numbers.
2. Multiplying the denominators or lower numbers.
3. Reducing the new fraction to its lowest term.

EXAMPLE: To multiply $\frac{3}{4} \times \frac{2}{5} = \dfrac{3 \times 2}{4 \times 5} = \frac{6}{20} = \frac{3}{10}$ (reduced to lowest term)

Multiply the following fractions:

a	**b**	**c**
1. $\frac{5}{6} \times \frac{1}{3} =$	$\frac{3}{5} \times \frac{2}{3} =$	$\frac{7}{8} \times \frac{2}{5} =$
2. $\frac{3}{4} \times \frac{2}{3} =$	$\frac{6}{7} \times \frac{7}{8} =$	$\frac{5}{8} \times \frac{3}{4} =$
3. $\frac{4}{5} \times \frac{3}{5} =$	$\frac{5}{8} \times \frac{1}{2} =$	$\frac{2}{3} \times \frac{1}{6} =$
4. $\frac{3}{8} \times \frac{4}{5} =$	$\frac{7}{9} \times \frac{5}{6} =$	$\frac{1}{3} \times \frac{3}{8} =$
5. $\frac{10}{11} \times \frac{1}{3} =$	$\frac{11}{12} \times \frac{4}{5} =$	$\frac{9}{10} \times \frac{3}{4} =$

MULTIPLYING MIXED NUMBERS

Mixed numbers may be multiplied by:

1. Changing the mixed numbers to improper fractions.
2. Multiplying the numerators.
3. Multiplying the denominators.
4. Reducing the new fraction to its lowest term.

EXAMPLE: To multiply $2\frac{1}{2} \times 4\frac{1}{3} = \frac{5}{2} \times \frac{13}{3}$ (changed to improper fractions):

$$\frac{5 \times 13}{2 \times 3} = \frac{65 \text{ (numerators multiplied)}}{6 \text{ (denominators multiplied)}}$$

$$\frac{65}{6} = 65 \div 6 = 6\overline{)65}\begin{smallmatrix}10\frac{5}{6} \text{ (lowest term)}\\ \frac{6}{5}\end{smallmatrix}$$

EXAMPLE: To multiply 4 (whole number) × 4⅔ (mixed number):

$$^4/_1 \times {}^{14}/_3 \text{ (changed to improper fractions)}$$

$$\frac{4 \times 14}{1 \times 3} = \frac{56}{3} \text{ (numerators multiplied)} \atop \text{ (denominators multiplied)}$$

$$^{56}/_3 = 56 \div 3 = 3\overline{)56} \quad \begin{array}{r} 18^2/_3 \text{ (lowest term)} \\ \hline \end{array}$$

$$\begin{array}{r} 3 \\ \hline 26 \\ 24 \\ \hline 2 \end{array}$$

Multiply the following mixed numbers:

a	b	c
1. 4⅔ × 4⅛ =	3⅗ × 2½ =	3 × 3⅜ =
2. 6⅛ × 7⅓ =	5⅗ × 2¼ =	5 × 2⅗ =
3. 6 × 6⅓ =	2⅔ × 3⅗ =	7⅛ × 4¼ =
4. 8⅔ × 5¼ =	9 × 9½ =	9⅓ × 5¼ =
5. 5 × 4¼ =	2 × 1½ =	10½ × 3¼ =

DIVIDING FRACTIONS

Fractions may be divided by:

1. Inverting the divisor (divisor is the number by which another number is divided). Inverting is done by reversing the numerator and the denominator of the fraction.
2. After inverting the divisor, multiply.

EXAMPLE: To divide ¾ by ⅔ (⅔ is the divisor):

¾ ÷ 3/2 (divisor has been inverted)
¾ × 3/2 (division sign has been changed to multiplication)

$$\frac{3 \times 3}{4 \times 2} = \frac{9}{8} = 8\overline{)9} \quad \begin{array}{r} 1\tfrac{1}{8} \text{ (reduced to lowest term)} \\ \hline 8 \\ \hline 1 \end{array}$$

3. Mixed numbers may be divided in the same manner. The mixed numbers must be changed to improper fractions before dividing is done.

EXAMPLE: A mixed number divided by a fraction. To divide 3¾ by ⅔:

3¾ ÷ ⅔ = ¹⁵/₄ × 3/2 (mixed number has been changed to improper fraction, and divisor has been inverted)

$$\frac{15 \times 3}{4 \times 2} = \frac{45}{8} = 8\overline{)45} \quad \begin{array}{r} 5\tfrac{5}{8} \text{ (lowest term)} \\ \hline 40 \\ \hline 5 \end{array}$$

EXAMPLE: A mixed number divided by a mixed number.

To divide 2⅔ by 4⅖ = ⁸/₃ ÷ ²²/₅ (mixed numbers have been changed to improper fractions)

$^8/_3 \times {}^5/_{22}$ (divisor has been inverted, and division sign has been changed to multiplication sign)

$$\frac{8 \times 5}{3 \times 22} = {}^{40}/_{66} = {}^{20}/_{33} \text{ (reduced to lowest term)}$$

Divide the following fractions and mixed numbers:

a	**b**	**c**
1. $1^1/_3 \div {}^1/_2 =$	$6 \div {}^1/_3 =$	$6^1/_2 \div 2 =$
2. $^7/_9 \div {}^4/_5 =$	$5 \div {}^1/_5 =$	$5^1/_5 \div 5^2/_5 =$
3. $^3/_4 \div {}^1/_2 =$	$7^1/_2 \div 5^1/_5 =$	$8 \div {}^1/_4 =$
4. $4^1/_2 \div 2^1/_4 =$	$^2/_3 \div {}^1/_6 =$	$^4/_5 \div {}^3/_5 =$
5. $10 \div 1^1/_2 =$	$3 \div {}^1/_3 =$	$^2/_3 \div {}^3/_4 =$

Chapter 31 | DECIMAL FRACTIONS

A *decimal fraction* is a way of expressing a fraction whose denominator is ten or a multiple of ten. The decimal point is a dot. All numbers to the *left* of the decimal point are *whole numbers.* All the numbers written to the *right* of the decimal point are *decimal fractions* that have a denominator of ten or a multiple of ten. The first place to the right of the decimal point is for tenths; the second place is for hundredths; and the third place is for thousandths, and so on. Throughout this text a decimal fraction will be referred to as a "decimal."

EXAMPLES:
0.1	one-tenth
0.01	one-hundredth
0.001	one-thousandth
1.	one
10.	ten
100.	one hundred
1.1	one and one-tenth
10.01	ten and one-hundredth

Explain the following:

1. 0.5 _____.
2. 5.5 _____.
3. 10.01_____.
4. 2.5 _____.
5. 1.5 _____.

6. 5.2 _____.
7. 1.3 _____.
8. 1.05 _____.
9. 0.005_____.
10. 25.05 _____.

DIVIDING DECIMALS AND WHOLE NUMBERS BY DECIMALS AND WHOLE NUMBERS

A decimal may be divided by a whole number by:

1. Dividing in the usual manner and placing the decimal point in the quotient (answer) directly above the decimal point in the dividend (the number to be divided).

EXAMPLE: To divide 5.5 by 5:

$$
\begin{array}{r}
1.1 \\
5\overline{)5.5} \\
\underline{5} \\
5 \\
\underline{5}
\end{array}
$$

A decimal has been divided by a whole number. The decimal point in the quotient has been placed directly above the decimal point in the dividend.

A whole number may be divided by a decimal by:

1. Moving the decimal point in the divisor to the right as many places as necessary to make the divisor a whole number.

2. Placing a decimal point after the whole number and then moving that decimal point in the dividend the same number of places to the right as the decimal point in the divisor was moved. Zeros are added to the whole number as necessary in order to move the decimal point.

3. Dividing in the usual manner.

EXAMPLE: To divide 55 by 0.2:

$$
0.2\overline{)55} = 0.2\overline{)55.0} = 02\overline{)550}
\begin{array}{r}
275 \\
\underline{4} \\
15 \\
\underline{14} \\
10 \\
\underline{10}
\end{array}
$$

A whole number has been divided by a decimal. The decimal point in the divisor was moved one place to the right to make the divisor a whole number. A decimal point was placed in the dividend and moved the same number of places as the decimal point in the divisor.

A decimal may be divided by a decimal by:

1. Making the divisor a whole number by moving the decimal point to the right.
2. Moving the decimal point in the dividend the same number of places to the right as the decimal point in the divisor was moved.
3. Dividing in the usual manner.
4. Placing the decimal point in the quotient directly above the decimal point in the dividend.

EXAMPLE: To divide 5.25 by 2.5:

$$
2.5\overline{)5.25} \quad = \quad
\begin{array}{r}
2.1 \\
25\overline{)52.5} \\
\underline{50} \\
25 \\
\underline{25}
\end{array}
$$

A decimal has been divided by a decimal. The decimal point in the divisor was moved one place to the right to make the divisor a whole number. The decimal point in the dividend was moved one place (the same number of places the decimal point in the divisor was moved). The decimal point in the quotient was placed directly above the decimal point in the dividend.

Divide the following decimals:

a	b	c
1. $52.5 \div 5.2 =$	$40.5 \div 5.5 =$	$8.5 \div 2.5 =$
2. $100.25 \div 50.5 =$	$30.3 \div 3.3 =$	$25.5 \div 2.5 =$
3. $25.25 \div 2.25 =$	$14.5 \div 2.5 =$	$12.2 \div 2.1 =$
4. $3.25 \div 3.2 =$	$4.45 \div 1.125 =$	$50.5 \div 25.5 =$
5. $10.5 \div 5.5 =$	$5.125 \div 2.5 =$	$82.5 \div 0.02 =$

MULTIPLYING DECIMALS BY WHOLE NUMBERS AND BY DECIMALS

Decimals can be multiplied by whole numbers and decimals by:

1. Multiplying in the usual way.
2. Pointing off the total number of decimal places moving from right to left.

EXAMPLE: To multiply 5.25×5:

$$
\begin{array}{r}
5.25 \\
\times\ 5 \\
\hline
26.25
\end{array}
$$

A decimal has been multiplied by a whole number. Two decimal places have been pointed off in the answer, because there are two decimal places in 5.25, the number that was multiplied.

EXAMPLE: To multiply 5.25×5.5:

$$
\begin{array}{r}
5.25 \\
\times\ 5.5 \\
\hline
2625 \\
2625 \\
\hline
28.875
\end{array}
$$

A decimal has been multiplied by a decimal. Three decimal places have been pointed off in the answer, because there were two decimal places in 5.25, the number multiplied, and one decimal place in 5.5, the multiplier.

Multiply the following decimals and whole numbers:

a	b	c
1. $40.1 \times 4.01 =$	$2.55 \times 20.5 =$	$3.33 \times 2.02 =$
2. $4.25 \times 2.5 =$	$3.03 \times 6.3 =$	$7.125 \times 0.25 =$
3. $5.25 \times 3.5 =$	$140 \times 2.5 =$	$4.25 \times 50 =$
4. $50.5 \times 25.5 =$	$35.25 \times 8.5 =$	$100.5 \times 20 =$
5. $23.5 \times 8.3 =$	$85.05 \times 3.05 =$	$7.05 \times 7.5 =$

CHANGING DECIMALS TO FRACTIONS

Decimals can be changed to fractions by:

1. Identifying the correct number of places to the right of the decimal point in order to select the denominator of the fraction.
2. Removing the decimal point.
3. Placing the appropriate denominator under the number.
4. Reducing the fraction to lowest terms.

EXAMPLE: To change 0.05 to a fraction:

05 (decimal point has been removed)

$$\frac{05}{100}$$ (proper denominator has been placed under number)

$5 \mid \dfrac{\cancel{05}}{\cancel{100}} = \dfrac{1}{20}$ (reduced to lowest term)

Change the following decimals to fractions:

a	b	c
1. 0.35 =	0.3 =	0.04 =
2. 0.5 =	0.2 =	0.002 =
3. 0.1 =	0.55 =	0.75 =
4. 0.4 =	0.005 =	0.001 =
5. 0.01 =	0.8 =	0.07 =

CHANGING COMMON FRACTIONS TO DECIMALS

Common fractions can be changed to decimals by dividing the numerator of the fraction by the denominator of the fraction. When dividing any number, remember that:

1. The number being divided is the *dividend*.
2. The number by which dividend is divided is the *divisor*.
3. The answer is called the *quotient*.

EXAMPLE: To change ½ to a decimal:
1 is the numerator (the number to be divided or the dividend)
2 is the denominator (the number by which the dividend is to be divided)

$$
\begin{array}{r}
0.5 \text{ (a decimal)} \\
\tfrac{1}{2} = 2\overline{)1.0} \\
\underline{1\ 0}
\end{array}
$$

Note: 2 will not go into 1; therefore, a decimal point is placed immediately after the 1 in the dividend, and a zero is added. When a decimal point is placed in the dividend, a decimal point also must be placed directly above in the quotient or answer. In this case the quotient becomes a decimal.

ROUNDING OFF

When common fractions are changed to decimal fractions, the division does not always come out even. For example, when the fractions ⁵⁄₆, ³⁄₈, and ³⁄₇ are changed to decimals, the division comes out as follows:

EXAMPLES:

a	b	c
0.8333 *or* 0.83	0.375 *or* 0.38	0.428 *or* 0.43
⁵⁄₆ = 6)5.000	³⁄₈ = 8)3.000	³⁄₇ = 7)3.000
4 8	2 4	2 8
20	60	20
18	56	14
20	40	60
18	40	56
2		4

In such instances, the decimal fraction usually is rounded off to the nearest hundredth. The following procedure may be used:

1. If the last number of the fraction is less than 5, it is dropped; for example, in example a, above, the answer would be 0.83.
2. If the last number of the fraction is 5, it is dropped and the preceding number is raised 1. (See example b, above.)
3. If the last number of the fraction is more than 5, it is dropped and the preceding number is raised by 1. (See example c, above.)

Note: It is not usually necessary to carry a decimal fraction out more than two places before rounding off.

Change the following fractions to decimals:

a	b	c
1. $1/8 =$	$1/4 =$	$1/6 =$
2. $4/5 =$	$2/3 =$	$3/5 =$
3. $7/8 =$	$5/6 =$	$3/4 =$
4. $1/3 =$	$3/8 =$	$5/8 =$
5. $1/5 =$	$5/7 =$	$2/5 =$

Chapter 32 | PERCENTAGES

Percentage means parts per 100. The term *percent* is usually indicated by the symbol %.

> EXAMPLE: 5% is actually 5 parts per 100.
> Expressed as fraction: $5/100$.
> Expressed as a decimal: 0.05

CHANGING PERCENTS TO FRACTIONS

When a percent is a whole number, mixed number, or fraction, it can be changed to a fraction by:

1. Omitting the percent sign.
2. Writing the whole number, mixed number, or fraction as the numerator.
3. Writing 100 as the denominator.
4. Reducing the resulting fraction to lowest term.

> EXAMPLE: To change 5% (whole number) to a fraction:
>
> $$5\% = 5/100 = 1/20 \text{ (fraction reduced to lowest term)}$$
>
> To change $1/2$% (fraction) to a fraction:
>
> $$1/2\% = \frac{1/2}{100} = 1/2 \div 100/1 = 1/2 \times 1/100 = 1/200 \text{ (fraction reduced to lowest term)}$$
>
> To change $5 1/2$% (mixed number) to a fraction:
>
> $$5 1/2\% = \frac{5 1/2}{100} = 11/2 \div 100/1 = 11/2 \times 1/100 = 11/200 \text{ (fraction reduced to lowest term)}$$

Change the following percents to fractions:

	a	b	c
1.	$50\% =$	$25\frac{1}{5}\% =$	$\frac{1}{5}\% =$
2.	$\frac{1}{3}\% =$	$4\frac{1}{2}\% =$	$2\frac{1}{4}\% =$
3.	$6\% =$	$\frac{1}{8}\% =$	$3\frac{1}{2}\% =$
4.	$12\% =$	$15\% =$	$15\frac{1}{2}\% =$
5.	$\frac{4}{5}\% =$	$12\frac{1}{2}\% =$	$30\% =$

CHANGING FRACTIONS TO PERCENTS

Fractions can be changed to percents by:

1. Multiplying by 100.
2. Reducing to lowest terms and writing as a mixed number.
3. Adding the percent symbol.

EXAMPLE: To change $\frac{1}{2}$ to a percent:

$$\tfrac{1}{2} \times {}^{100}/_1 = {}^{100}/_2 = 50\%$$

Change the following fractions to percents:

	a	b	c
1.	$\frac{1}{6} =$	$\frac{1}{20} =$	$\frac{1}{10} =$
2.	$\frac{1}{5} =$	$\frac{1}{80} =$	$\frac{1}{15} =$
3.	$\frac{3}{5} =$	$\frac{1}{8} =$	$\frac{1}{4} =$
4.	$\frac{3}{4} =$	$\frac{4}{5} =$	$\frac{2}{5} =$
5.	$\frac{1}{100} =$	$\frac{1}{50} =$	$\frac{1}{25} =$

CHANGING PERCENTS TO DECIMALS

Percent can be changed to a decimal by removing the percent sign, and then:

1. If the percent is a whole number, dividing by 100. This is done by moving the decimal point two places to the left.

EXAMPLE: To change 10% to a decimal: $10\% = 10. = 0.1$ (decimal)

2. If the percent is written as a fraction or mixed number, change to a decimal and then move decimal point two places to the left.

EXAMPLE: To change $\frac{1}{5}\%$ to a decimal:

$$\frac{1}{5}\% = \frac{1}{5} = 5\overline{)1.0} \quad \begin{array}{r} 0.2 = 0.002 \text{ (decimal)} \\ \underline{1\ 0} \\ 0 \end{array}$$

EXAMPLE: To change $3\frac{1}{2}\%$ to a decimal:

$$3\frac{1}{2}\% = 3\frac{1}{2} = \frac{7}{2} = 2\overline{)7.0} \quad \begin{array}{r} 3.5 = 0.035 \text{ (decimal)} \\ \underline{6} \\ 1\ 0 \\ \underline{1\ 0} \end{array}$$

Change the following percents to decimals:

	a	b	c
1.	$5\% =$	$2\% =$	$\frac{1}{4}\% =$
2.	$\frac{1}{8}\% =$	$75\% =$	$7\frac{1}{2}\% =$
3.	$\frac{3}{4}\% =$	$50\% =$	$40\% =$
4.	$4\frac{1}{4}\% =$	$5\frac{1}{2}\% =$	$\frac{3}{5}\% =$
5.	$2\frac{1}{2}\% =$	$6\% =$	$6\frac{1}{5}\% =$

CHANGING DECIMALS TO PERCENTS

A decimal may be changed to a percent by:

1. Multiplying by 100; to do this, move the decimal point two places to the right.
2. Adding the percentage sign.

EXAMPLE: To change 0.5 to a percent:

$$0.5 = 50. = 50\%$$

Change the following decimals to percents:

a	b	c
1. $0.1 =$	$0.01 =$	$0.05 =$
2. $0.8 =$	$5.5 =$	$2.5 =$
3. $0.25 =$	$0.125 =$	$3.5 =$
4. $4.5 =$	$5.25 =$	$0.7 =$
5. $7.5 =$	$0.75 =$	$0.4 =$

Chapter 33 | RATIOS

A *ratio* is a way of expressing a fractional part of a whole. In a ratio, the numerator of the fraction is written in front of the denominator instead of over it.

> EXAMPLE: In a ratio, the fraction ¹/₂ would be written 1:2 or 1-2.
> The symbol : or – is placed between the numbers of the ratio.

When using a ratio with drugs, always consider the first number as the amount of drug in the solution and the second number the total amount of solution.

> EXAMPLE: In a 1:2 solution there is one part drug, two parts of solution.

Many drugs are prepared in solution; for this reason the bedside nurse should be able to interpret a ratio.

Write the following fractions as ratios:

	a	b	c
1.	¹/₈_____	²/₅_____	³/₅_____
2.	¹/₁₂_____	¹/₁,₅₀₀_____	¹/₂,₀₀₀_____
3.	¹/₄_____	¹/₁₀₀_____	¹/₁,₀₀₀_____
4.	¹/₅₀₀_____	¹/₃_____	¹/₈₀_____
5.	¹/₁₀_____	¹/₅₀_____	¹/₇₅_____

CHANGING A RATIO TO A PERCENT OR DECIMAL

A ratio is changed to a percent or decimal in the same way that a fraction is changed to a percent or decimal.

EXAMPLE: To change the ratio 1:50 to a percent:

$$1:50 \text{ (ratio)} = \frac{1}{50} \text{ (fraction)} = \frac{1}{50} \times \frac{100}{1} = 2\%$$

EXAMPLE: To change the ratio 1:50 to a decimal:

$$1:50 \text{ (ratio)} = \frac{1}{50} \text{ (fraction)} = 50\overline{)1.00} \quad \frac{0.02 \text{ (decimal)}}{\underline{1\ 00}}$$

Change the following ratios to percents and to decimals:

Ratio	a Percent	b Decimal
1. 1:3 =		
2. 1:100 =		
3. 1:1,000 =		
4. 1:500 =		
5. 1:150 =		
6. 1:200 =		
7. 1:4 =		
8. 1:8 =		
9. 1:2,000 =		
10. 1:4,000 =		

CHANGING A PERCENT TO A RATIO

This is the same as changing a percent to a fraction (see p. 364).

EXAMPLE: To change 50% to a ratio:

$$50\% \text{ (per cent)} = 50 = \frac{50}{100} \text{ (fraction)} = \frac{1}{2} \text{ (reduced to lowest term)} =$$
$$\frac{1}{2} = 1:2 \text{ (ratio)}$$

Change the following percents to ratios:

a	b	c
1. 10% =	80% =	40% =
2. 70% =	30% =	5% =
3. ½% =	¼% =	1% =
4. 20% =	75% =	15% =
5. 2% =	60% =	25% =

CHANGING A DECIMAL TO A RATIO

This is the same as changing a decimal to a fraction (see pp. 361–362).

EXAMPLE: To change 0.5 to a ratio:

$$0.5 \text{ (decimal)} = \frac{5}{10} \text{ (fraction)} = \frac{1}{2} \text{ (reduced to lowest term)} =$$
$$\frac{1}{2} = 1:2 \text{ (ratio)}$$

Change the following decimals to ratios:

a	b	c
1. 0.2 =	0.05 =	0.001 =
2. 0.002 =	0.005 =	0.25 =
3. 0.025 =	0.075 =	0.1 =
4. 0.01 =	0.75 =	0.8 =
5. 0.4 =	0.6 =	0.0001 =

ARITHMETIC POSTTEST

Directions: Solve the following problems. Circle the answer you believe to be correct. If you believe the correct answer is not given circle NG (not given).

---

1. Change $1/75$ to a percent.

   a. 75%   **b.** $1\frac{3}{4}$%   **c.** $\frac{3}{4}$%   **d.** $1\frac{1}{3}$%   **e.** NG

---

2. Change 1:1,000 to a fraction.

   a. $\frac{1}{2}$ **b.** $\frac{1}{100}$ **c.** $\frac{1}{10}$ **d.** $\frac{1}{50}$ **e.** NG

---

3. Change 2.5 to a percent.

   a. 2%   **b.** 250%   **c.** 25%   **d.** 2.5%   **e.** NG

---

4. Change $\frac{1}{2}$% to a decimal.

   a. 0.02   **b.** 0.002   **c.** 0.5   **d.** 0.005   **e.** NG

---

5. Change 4% to a fraction.

   a. $\frac{1}{4}$ **b.** $\frac{1}{20}$ **c.** $\frac{1}{25}$ **d.** $\frac{1}{50}$ **e.** NG

---

6. Change $30/18$ to a mixed or whole number.

   a. $1\frac{1}{4}$ **b.** $1\frac{1}{2}$ **c.** 3   **d.** $1\frac{2}{3}$ **e.** NG

---

7. Divide $25.5 \div 5$.

   a. 51   **b.** 1.5   **c.** 5.1   **d.** 15   **e.** NG

---

8. Multiply 50.5×1.5.

   a. 7.5   **b.** 75   **c.** 4.5   **d.** 5   **e.** NG

---

9. Change 0.2 to a ratio.

   a. 1:500   **b.** 2:5   **c.** 1:50   **d.** 1:5   **e.** NG

---

10. Reduce $18/21$ to lowest term.

    a. $\frac{3}{14}$ **b.** $\frac{1}{7}$ **c.** $\frac{6}{7}$ **d.** $\frac{3}{7}$ **e.** NG

---

11. Change $\frac{1}{2}$% to a fraction.

    a. $\frac{1}{200}$ **b.** $\frac{1}{2}$ **c.** $\frac{1}{20}$ **d.** $\frac{1}{50}$ **e.** NG

---

12. Change $\frac{1}{5}$% to a decimal.

    a. 0.5   **b.** 0.002   **c.** 0.005   **d.** 0.02   **e.** NG

---

13. Change 5% to a ratio.

    a. 1:20   **b.** 1:200   **c.** 1:2   **d.** 1:5   **e.** NG

---

14. Change $\frac{1}{3}$ to a percent.

    a. 30%   **b.** 3%   **c.** $33\frac{1}{3}$%   **d.** $66\frac{2}{3}$%   **e.** NG

---

15. Multiply 20.05×3.1.

    a. 62.155   **b.** 6215.5   **c.** 5261.5   **d.** 612.55   **e.** NG

---

16. Change 10% to a decimal.

    a. 0.01   **b.** 0.1   **c.** 0.5   **d.** 0.005   **e.** NG

---

17. Change $\frac{2}{3}$ to a percent.

    a. $66\frac{2}{3}$%   **b.** 33%   **c.** 75%   **d.** 60%   **e.** NG

---

18. Change 8% to a fraction.

    a. $\frac{4}{5}$ **b.** $\frac{2}{5}$ **c.** $\frac{2}{25}$ **d.** $\frac{5}{8}$ **e.** NG

19. Divide $12.2 \div 0.2$.

    a. 6.1 **b.** 2.6 **c.** 6.2 **d.** 62 **e.** NG

20. Multiply 32.25×4.6.

    a. 1,438.50 **b.** 148.350 **c.** 185.430 **d.** 158.340 **e.** NG

21. Divide $30.6 \div 6$.

    a. 5.1 **b.** 50.1 **c.** 0.51 **d.** 5 **e.** NG

22. Multiply $0.25 \times 1,000$.

    a. 0.025 **b.** 250 **c.** 25 **d.** 52 **e.** NG

23. Reduce $^{75}/_{750}$ to lowest term.

    a. $^{1}/_{2}$ **b.** $^{1}/_{4}$ **c.** $^{1}/_{100}$ **d.** $^{1}/_{10}$ **e.** NG

24. Multiply $3^{1}/_{2} \times 3^{1}/_{4}$.

    a. $12^{1}/_{4}$ **b.** $12^{1}/_{2}$ **c.** $13^{1}/_{2}$ **d.** 13 **e.** NG

25. Divide $^{2}/_{3} \div ^{1}/_{3}$.

    a. 3 **b.** 2 **c.** $^{1}/_{6}$ **d.** $^{1}/_{2}$ **e.** NG

26. Divide $6^{1}/_{2} \div 1^{1}/_{3}$.

    a. $4^{7}/_{8}$ **b.** $3^{1}/_{2}$ **c.** $4^{1}/_{4}$ **d.** $4^{1}/_{3}$ **e.** NG

27. Change $81^{1}/_{8}$ to an improper fraction.

    a. $^{648}/_{8}$ **b.** $^{649}/_{8}$ **c.** $^{469}/_{8}$ **d.** $^{469}/_{9}$ **e.** NG

28. Change 40% to a ratio.

    a. 1:2 **b.** 1:5 **c.** 2:5 **d.** 3:5 **e.** NG

29. Divide $75 \div 0.5$.

    a. 0.325 **b.** 150 **c.** 3.250 **d.** 1.50 **e.** NG

30. Change 0.75 to a percent.

    a. $^{3}/_{4}\%$ **b.** 25% **c.** 0.25% **d.** 75% **e.** NG

31. Change 1:3 to a decimal.

    a. 13.3 **b.** 0.3 **c.** 0.67 **d.** 0.003 **e.** NG

32. Change 5.25 to a percent.

    a. 0.25% **b.** 525% **c.** 5.5% **d.** 5% **e.** NG

33. Change 50% to a ratio.

    a. 1:50 **b.** 1:20 **c.** 1:5 **d.** 1:2 **e.** NG

34. Divide $^{7}/_{8} \div ^{1}/_{4}$.

    a. $3^{1}/_{4}$ **b.** $^{1}/_{4}$ **c.** $^{3}/_{8}$ **d.** $^{1}/_{2}$ **e.** NG

35. Reduce $^{1,500}/_{6,000}$ to lowest term.

    a. 4 **b.** $^{1}/_{4}$ **c.** 6 **d.** $^{1}/_{6}$ **e.** NG

36. Multiply $14^{1}/_{2} \times$ by $2^{1}/_{8}$.

    a. $28^{1}/_{8}$ **b.** $30^{13}/_{16}$ **c.** $29^{3}/_{4}$ **d.** $36^{1}/_{2}$ **e.** NG

37. Reduce $^{100}/_{150}$ to lowest term.

    a. $^{2}/_{3}$ **b.** $^{1}/_{5}$ **c.** $^{1}/_{3}$ **d.** $^{1}/_{15}$ **e.** NG

38. Multiply $8^{1}/_{5} \times 2^{1}/_{2}$.

    a. $16^{4}/_{5}$ **b.** $18^{1}/_{2}$ **c.** $18^{1}/_{10}$ **d.** $19^{1}/_{10}$ **e.** NG

39. Divide $45 \div \frac{3}{5}$.

      a. 75 **b.** $22\frac{1}{2}$ **c.** $23\frac{1}{5}$ **d.** 90 **e.** NG

40. Change $\frac{4,000}{200}$ to a mixed or whole number.

      a. 200 **b.** 40 **c.** 20 **d.** $2\frac{1}{4}$ **e.** NG

41. Multiply $\frac{1}{4} \times \frac{1}{4}$.

      a. $\frac{1}{8}$ **b.** $\frac{1}{6}$ **c.** $\frac{2}{3}$ **d.** 2 **e.** NG

42. Reduce $\frac{30}{450}$ to lowest term.

      a. $\frac{1}{5}$ **b.** $\frac{1}{3}$ **c.** $\frac{1}{10}$ **d.** $\frac{3}{5}$ **e.** NG

43. Multiply $1\frac{3}{4} \times \frac{4}{7}$.

      a. 1 **b.** $\frac{1}{7}$ **c.** 4 **d** $\frac{2}{7}$ **e.** NG

44. Multiply $\frac{2}{3} \times \frac{1}{4}$.

      a. $\frac{1}{2}$ **b.** $\frac{1}{7}$ **c.** $\frac{1}{6}$ **d.** $1\frac{1}{7}$ **e.** NG

45. Change $16\frac{1}{2}$ to an improper fraction.

      a. $\frac{23}{2}$ **b.** $\frac{32}{2}$ **c.** $\frac{33}{2}$ **d.** $\frac{18}{2}$ **e.** NG

46. Multiply $2.5 \times 1,000$.

      a. 250 **b.** 25,000 **c.** 25 **d.** 0.25 **e.** NG

47. Divide $500 \div 1,000$.

      a. 25 **b.** 0.5 **c.** 500 **d.** 0.05 **e.** NG

48. Divide $50 \div 0.25$.

      a. 0.02 **b.** 0.2 **c.** 20 **d.** 200 **e.** NG

49. Divide $100 \div 0.5$.

      a. 20 **b.** 50 **c.** 200 **d.** 2 **e.** NG

50. Divide $5 \div 1,000$.

      a. 200 **b.** 20 **c.** 0.5 **d.** 0.05 **e.** NG

APPENDIXES

| GLOSSARY

absorption. The taking up of a substance into or across body tissue.

acetylcholine. A substance released at the parasympathetic and skeletal nerve endings, which acts as a chemical transmitter and may be necessary for the rhythmical activities of the heart.

acidifying agent. A drug given to render the body fluids more acid.

acidosis. The depletion of the alkaline reserve in the body.

addiction. A pattern of drug use that involves preoccupation with getting and using drugs and a tendency to relapse after withdrawal.

adhesive. The property of sticking together.

adrenalectomy. Surgical excision of the adrenal gland.

adrenergic. A drug that stimulates body parts that are innervated by the sympathetic nervous system.

adrenolytic. A drug that prevents the action of circulating epinephrine on effector cells; an adrenergic blocking agent.

adsorption. The taking up of a substance by attracting other particles or materials to a surface.

adverse response. A reaction to a drug that is unfavorable, unintended, and does not benefit the patient.

aerohalor. An instrument consisting of a discharge chamber and interchangeable mouth- and nosepieces, used to administer solid aerosols to the upper and lower respiratory tracts.

aerosol. The suspension of a drug to be administered as a fine spray or mist.

agitation. An abnormal restlessness.

agranulocytosis. An acute disease characterized by a sudden drop in the production of leukocytes. Frequently caused by the administration of certain drugs.

aldosterone. A hormone secreted by the adrenal cortex to regulate the metabolism of sodium, chloride, and potassium.

alkalinizing agents. A drug given to render the body fluids more alkaline.

alkaloids. Basic organic compounds containing carbon, hydrogen, nitrogen, and oxygen found in the seeds, roots, and leaves of plants. Many are prepared synthetically.

alkalosis. Opposite of acidosis. A pathologic condition in which the alkaline content of the blood increases beyond the norm or there is an abnormal decrease in the acid content.

allergen. Any substance that causes an allergic reaction, such as pollens, food, drugs, and so forth.

allergy. An abnormal reaction to a substance that under the same conditions is harmless to the average person.

alleviate. To lessen or relieve.

amphetamines. A group of synthesized compounds, with chemical and pharmacologic properties similar to those of ephedrine, that stimulate the sensory cortex and produce alertness.

ampule. A small sealed glass container, the contents of which are sterile.

analgesic. A drug given for the relief of pain.

anaphylaxis. An immediate exaggerated allergic reaction that is life threatening.

androgens. Hormones that are responsible for the normal development and maintenance of spermatogenesis and male sexual characteristics.

anesthesia. A state induced by a drug or other agent that causes a loss of sensation and may or may not cause loss of consciousness.

anethesiologist. A physician who specializes in prescribing and administering anesthetic agents.

anesthetic. An agent that produces insensibility to pain or touch.

angiocardiogram. Film of the heart and great vessels taken after the introduction of an opaque material into a blood vessel or heart chamber.

angioedema. A sudden appearance of swelling of the skin or mucous membranes; may result from allergy and produce obstruction of breathing.

angiogram. Film of the blood vessels after the injection of a suitable opaque substance.

anorexia. Loss of appetite.

antacid. A drug that neutralizes acidity of the gastric juices or other secretions.

anthelmintic. A drug given to kill or expel intestinal worms.

antiadrenergic. A drug that depresses the sympathetic nervous system.

antiamebic. A drug that cures or prevent infection from amebae.

antianxiety. A drug given to lessen anxiety states by blocking stimuli to the central nervous system.

antiarrhythmic agent. A drug that relieves or prevents disturbances in heart rate, regularity, conduction pathway, or origin of heartbeat.

antibiotic. A medication produced by a living organism and effective against bacteria.

antibodies. Protein substances produced by the body in response to the presence in the bloodstream of a foreign agent or antigen.

anticoagulant. A drug that delays the clotting time of the blood.

anticonvulsant. A drug that relieves or prevents convulsions.

antidepressant. A drug given to elevate moods of depression.

antidiarrheal. A drug that checks excessive bowel movements.

antidiuretic. A drug given to lessen the flow of urine.

antidote. Any substance that neutralizes the effects of a poison.

antiemetic. A drug that prevents or relieves vomiting.

antigens. Substances, usually protein in nature, that when introduced into the body will stimulate the production of antibodies.

antihistamine. A drug that antagonizes the effects of histamine and is used to prevent or relieve allergic reactions.

antihypertensive. A drug that is used to reduce blood pressure.

antilipemic. A drug that lowers serum cholesterol.

antimalarial. A drug that prevents or relieves malaria.

antimetabolite. A substance tht retards the growth of malignant cells, by interfering with the cells' growth and metabolism.

antimuscarinic. A lessening of the peristaltic movement of the stomach and intestines and a decrease of gastric secretions.

antipruritic. A substance used to control iching.

antipyretic. A drug that tends to reduce a fever.

antiseptic. A substance that prevents the growth of disease-producing germs.

antispasmodic. A drug that will prevent or relieve muscular spasms.

antitoxin. An immunizing agent composed of antibodies that neutralize certain toxins produced by disease-causing microorganisms; administered to provide passive immunity.

antitussive. A drug that is used to suppress coughing.

aortogram. Film of aorta after introduction of an opaque material.

apathy. A lack of feeling or emotions.

apical. Pertaining to the apex or climax. In the case of the apical pulse, it is the point at which the maximum impulse of the heart can be detected. This point is at the fifth level intercostal space of the chest.

approximate. Nearly or about accurate.

aqua. Water.

aqueous. Watery.

aromatic. Having an agreeable and spicy odor.

arteriogram. 1. Films of an artery or system of arteries after the injection of a suitable opaque substance. 2. Tracing of the arterial pulse.

astringent. A substance that constricts the skin and mucous membranes.

ataractic. A drug that promotes calmness and composure; useful in the treatment of some mental and emotional disorders.

ataxia. Uncoordinated muscle activity, especially during ambulation; may occur as an adverse response to drug therapy.

atomizer. An instrument for throwing a fine spray.

azotemia. The presence of nitrogen-containing substances in the blood. Uremia.

bactericidal. Being destructive to bacteria.

bactericide. A chemical agent that destroys bacteria or other pathogenic microorganisms.

bacteriostatic. A chemical agent that prevents the growth of bacteria or other pathogenic microorganisms.

bacterium. Microorganisms that are nonmotile and non-spore-forming.

benign. Not progressive, recurring, or malignant.

borborygmus. A rumbling noise that occurs as gas is propelled through the intestines; may occur as an adverse response to drug therapy.

calibrated. Marked in graduation.

cancer. A malignant growth. A growth of disorganization in which body functions are interrupted causing the body cells to lose their proper nutrition.

capsule. A small soluble container for drugs.

carcinoma. A malignant tumor composed of epithelial tissue.

cardiotonic. A drug that strengthens cardiac contractions.

carminative. A drug or substance given to relieve gas and distention of the intestinal tract.

cathartic. A drug that increases and hastens the evacuation of the bowel.

caustic. A substance capable of burning, corroding, or destroying tissue.

chemotherapy. The treatment of disease by chemical substances that have specific, toxic effects on microorganisms but are not harmful to a patient.

chloasma. The discoloration of circumscribed areas of the skin.

cholangiogram. Films of the gallbladder and bile ducts after the introduction of a contrast agent.

cholecystogram. Films of the gallbladder after the introduction of an opaque dye.

cholinergic. A drug that stimulates the parasympathetic nervous system.

cholinergic blocker. A drug given to block the action of the parasympathetic nervous system.

choriocarcinoma. A malignant growth formed from the epithelium of the chorionic villi (the fingerlike processes that form from the outer fetal membranes).

coagulant. A drug that hastens the clotting of blood.

coefficient. Any numeral placed before a symbol as a multiplier.

compounding. The preparing of a medicine from two or more ingredients.

contraceptive. An agent that prevents pregnancy; an oral contraceptive is a drug that prevents pregnancy by inhibiting or suppressing ovulation.

contraindicated. A situation that indicates the inappropriateness of a treatment that otherwise would be advisable.

contrast agent. A drug administered to highlight various body parts so that they can be visualized by x-ray examination or a scanner.

convulsant. A drug given to cause convulsions in cases of depression.

corrosive. A chemical used to produce necrosis; may be employed to cauterize ulcers and remove warts.

counterirritant. A drug that irritates the unbroken skin, thereby causing stimulation of the sensory nerve endings and bringing relief from pain that originates in the viscera.

cryptorchism. The failure of one or both testes to descend from the abdominal cavity into the scrotum.

crystals. A natural solid that has definite form.

cumulative. The act of becoming larger by successive additions. Drugs are said to have a cumulative action if, when taken into the body in small doses, they are not eliminated, but accumulate in the system causing toxic symptoms.

cutaneous. Relating to the skin.

cycloplegic. A drug that produces paralysis of the ciliary structure of the eyes.

cystitis. Inflammation of the urinary bladder.

cystogram. Film of the urinary bladder after the introduction of opaque material.

decimal. Numbered by tens.

demulcent. A soothing agent, usually used to protect the mucous membrane.

denominator. The part of a fraction below the line.

depressant. A drug that tends to decrease the activities of the body parts.

detergent. A cleaning agent.

deteriorate. To decline gradually.

diagnostic. Pertaining to the act of recognizing an illness from the symptoms.

digestant. A substance that promotes the digestion of food in the gastrointestinal tract.

dilate. To distend or enlarge in size.

dilute. To reduce in strength or make thinner.

disinfectant. A substance that destroys disease-producing organisms.

dissociative anesthesia. One that causes an individual to become unaware of the environment.

distilled. Purified by the process of condensation.

diuretic. A substance given to increase the flow of urine.

dividend. The number or quantity to be divided.

divisor. The number or quantity by which another number or quantity is divided.

dose. A measured quantity of drug to be given at a stated time.

drug. A substance that acts on living protein in the body.

drug history. A part of the assessment phase of the nursing process during which the nurse collects and appraises information about the patient's past and present use of prescribed and non-prescribed drugs.

drug interaction. An adverse response produced when two or more drugs are administered at the same time. Drug–food interaction may occur as an adverse response of certain drug and food combination.

drug tolerance. An adverse response that occurs when a patient does not receive the same benefits from a drug or a dose that has previously been helpful; cross-tolerance is the same response to a similar drug.

dyscrasia. A condition in which there is an imbalance in the normal constituents.
   blood d. A condition in which there is an abnormal distribution of the blood elements.

dyskinesia. A difficulty in moving.

dystonia. An impairment of muscle tone.

ectoparacide. A drug that kills head and/or body lice.

electrolyte. Any compound that separates into charged ions, capable of conducting an electric current, when it is dissolved in water. The most common are sodium, potassium, chloride, and magnesium.

elixir. A drug preparation that is made palatable by the addition of alcohol, sugar, and an aromatic substance.

emetic. A drug that produces vomiting.

emollient. A substance that softens and soothes the skin.

emulsion. A solution in which fine particles of one solution are suspended in another solution.

enteric. Pertaining to the intestinal tract.

enteric coated. Coating on a pill or other medicine that prevents it from dissolving before it reaches the small intestine.

equation. An expression of two values that are equal.

equivalent. Being of equal or the same value.

erythrokinetics. The quantitative study of the in vivo (within the living organism, human body) production and destruction of red blood cells.

escharotic. A drug given to increase eschar development, i.e., one that causes sloughing.

estrogen. The female hormone secreted by the graafian follicle or the ovary.

euphoria. A marked feeling of well-being.

expectorant. A drug that aids in the elimination of mucus or other secretions from the trachea or lungs.

expiration. The act of coming to an end.

extract. A preparation that contains all the original qualities in concentrated form.

extravasation. The escape of a fluid from its conductor (such as a needle) into the body tissues.

fasciculation. The spontaneous contractions of several muscle fibers that are supplied by a single motor nerve fiber.

fibrinogen. A substance necessary for blood clotting. It is a protein found in the blood that by its thrombin action is converted into fibrin. Clotting factor 1.

flatulence. An excessive formation of gas in the gastrointestinal tract.

formula. (1) A recipe. (2) A symbolic expression of the composition of a substance.

fungicide. A substance that inhibits or prevents the growth of fungi.

germicide. A preparation or drug that kills germs.

glaucoma. A disease of the eyes characterized by increased intraocular pressure.

glycosides—cardiac. A group of drugs derived from plants (e.g., digitalis from foxglove) that upon hydrolysis yield sugar and other substances that strengthen cardiac contractions.

hallucinogen. A drug that causes symptoms similar to those present in mental disorders.

hemostatic. A drug that checks the flow of blood.

hepatotoxic. A drug that causes damage to the liver.

hiatus. An opening.
   h. hernia. The protrusion of the stomach or

other abdominal organ through the esophageal opening into the diaphragm.

hirsutism. An abnormal growth of hair.

hormone. The secretion of a ductless gland.

hydrolysis. The act of splitting a substance into simpler forms by the additon or removal of water.

hyperglycemia. The excessive amount of sugar in the blood.

hyperreflexia. An exaggeration of the reflexes.

hypnotic. A drug or medication that produces sleep.

hypochloremia. A diminishing of the chlorides in the blood.

hypodermic. Given or introduced beneath the skin.

hypoglycemia. The abnormal low level of sugar in the blood.

hypoglycemic. A drug used in the treatment of diabetes mellitus.

hyponatremia. A deficiency of sodium in the blood.

hypothermia. A lowered temperature. It may be the result of a physical disorder or induced therapeutically.

idiosyncrasy. An unusual susceptibility to a drug or other substance.

immune serum. An immunizing agent that contains human antibodies collected from human donors; administered to provide temporary passive immunity.

immunosuppressive. A drug that inhibits the patient's immune system.

infection. A state produced by the invasion and multiplication of microorganisms in the body.

Infusion. The introduction of fluids into a vein by gravity.

inhalation. The drawing of gases or vapor into the lungs.

insoluble. Cannot be dissolved.

instillation. The procedure of introducing a liquid into a cavity.

intra-. A prefix that signifies into or within.

intradermal. Within the tissues of the skin.

intramuscular. Within the muscle.

intraocular. Within the eye.

intraspinal. Within the spine.

intravenous. Within the vein.

inunction. The act of rubbing a medication into the skin.

irritant. A drug that stimulates or hastens healing by causing a mild irritation when applied to an abraded or inflamed area of the skin or mucous membrane.

keratitis. Inflammation of the cornea of the eye.

keratolytic. A drug used to soften and loosen keratinized (horny) epithelium.

keratosis. The formation of a horny growth.

laxative. A mild cathartic that produces one or two bowel movements without discomfort.

legal. Lawful.

lethal. Deadly or fatal.

lichenification. A thickening or hardening of the skin.

liniment. A preparation thinner than an ointment applied to the skin by rubbing, such as a counterirritant or anodyne.

lipoma. A fatty tumor.

lymphoblastic. Producing lymphocytes.

lymphoblastoma. A malignant lymphoma in which cells resembling lymphoblasts predominate.

lymphocytoma. A malignant lymphoma in which mature lymphocytes predominate.

lymphoma. A primary tumor of lymphoid tissue.

lymphosarcoma. A malignancy of the lymphoid tissue.

malignant. A tendency to become progressively worse.

masculinization. The production of masculine characteristics in women.

maximum. The largest amount possible.

medication. The use of healing agents.

medication administration record (MAR). A written list of all medications the patient is receiving.

medicinal. Having healing qualities.

medicine. A drug or remedy.

melanizing agent. A drug that adds or removes pigment from the skin.

melanoma. A dark-pigmented growth.
   malignant m. A growth consisting of a dark mass of cells that has a high potential to metastasize.

minimum. Smallest or least amount possible.

miotic. A drug that causes the pupil of the eye to contract.

miscible. Capable of being mixed.

monoamine oxidase inhibitors. A group of drugs administered as antidepressants; associated with many serious food and drug interactions.

myalgia. Muscular pain.

mydriatic. A drug that causes the pupil of the eye to dilate.

narcotic. A drug that relieves pain and causes stupor or sleep.

narcotic antagonist. A drug that offsets the effects of narcotic analgesia.

negligence. The failure to exercise the care needed under the circumstances.

neoplasm. An abnormal growth of new tissue. Tumor.

nephrotic syndrome. A condition involving massive edema, proteinuria, and kidney disease.

nephrotoxic. A drug that damages the kidneys.

neuroleptic. A drug, particularly an anesthetic agent, that reduces the number of stimuli reaching the central nervous system and creates euphoria.
n. analgesics. Drugs that cause a state of psychic indifference without producing sleep.

numerator. The top or upper number of a fraction.

nursing assessment. The first phase of the nursing process during which the nurse gathers information about the patient and determines its significance.

nursing care plan. A written map that describes the assistance to be provided by the nurse to the patient.

nursing diagnosis. A written description of a potential or actual deficit in self-care that can be helped by choosing and using specific nursing actions.

nursing goals and objectives. Written statements that describe what will be acheived by nursing actions.

nursing implications. The relationship of information about drug therapy to specific actions to be taken by the nurse.

nursing orders. Written statements that describe specific nursing actions to be taken to achieve goals and objectives.

nursing process. A systematic method of assisting the patient with self-care; composed of several interrelated steps or phases: assessment, diagnosis, goal setting, implementation, evaluation, and revision.

nystagmus. An involuntary rhythmic movement of the eyeballs either with horizontal, rotary, or vertical movements.

occult. Hidden, obscure; not easily recognized or seen.

ocular. Pertaining to the eyes or vision.

ointment. A soft, fatty substance having soothing or healing action.

oophorectomy. Surgical removal of the ovaries.

ophthalmo-. A combining form that means the eyes.

orthostatic. Pertaining to the upright position.

orthostatic hypotension. A drop in blood pressure that occurs when a person assumes a sitting or standing position; an adverse response to many drugs.

ototoxic. A drug that damages hearing and/or vestibular function.

palatable. Pleasing to the taste.

palliative. A process of relieving symptoms without curing the disease.

parasympathetic drug. Cholinergic blocking drug that destroys or inhibits impulses from the parasympathetic nervous system.

parasympathomimetic drug. Cholinergic drug that produces effects resulting in the stimulation of the parasympathetic.

parenteral. By a route other than the gastrointestinal tract.

paresthesia. An abnormal sensation resulting from a disorder of the sensory nervous system.

paroxysmal. Sudden, periodic attacks of a symptom, such as a cough.

peripheral. Away from the center—such as the outer parts of the body.

pharmacist. An individual qualified to prepare and dispense drugs.

pharmacodynamics. The study of the action of drugs on the living organism.

pharmacology. The study of drugs and their effects on the body.

pharmacopoeia. A book describing drugs, usually an official authority or standard.

pharmacotherapeutics. The study of the action of drugs in the presence of disease.

photosensitivity. The sensitivity to light.

physical dependence. An adverse response in which the patient experiences symptoms of withdrawal after a drug is discontinued.

pill. A medication in the form of a hard ball intended to be taken whole.

placebo. An inactive substance substituted for medicine to satisfy a patient's desire for a drug.

polydipsia. Excessive thirst.

powder. A collection of small particles of a solid.

prescription. A written order for dispensing drugs, signed by a doctor.

progesterone. The female hormone secreted by the corpus luteum of the ovary.

proteinuria. Protein in the urine.

prothrombin. That which is converted into thrombin by extrinsic thromboplastin during the second stage of blood clotting.

pruritus. An itching. It may accompany many skin disorders, and some systemic disorders, such as diabetes mellitus.

psoriasis. A chronic skin condition characterized by bright red patches covered with silvery scales.

psychedelic. A drug that is capable of inducing altered states of perception, thought, feeling, including visual and auditory hallucinations.

psychic energizer. A drug that is stimulating and energy producing.

psychostimulant. A drug that is both stimulating and energy producing.

psychotropic. A drug that modifies mental activities.

purgative. A drug that causes watery stools and some griping.

pyelogram. Film of the kidney and ureters after the introduction of a suitable contrasting substance.

quotient. The quantity resulting when one number has been divided by another.

radiomimetic. An agent that is nucleotoxic and locally vesicant, used in the treatment of certain neoplastic diseases.

radiopaque drug. A substance impenetrable to x-rays; used as a diagnostic tool.

radium. A highly radioactive chemical element found in uranium. Symbol Ra.

radon. A colorless, gaseous radioactive element produced by disintegration of radium.

ratio. A way of expressing the fractional part of a whole.

resistance. A condition in which pathogens are no longer killed or inhibited by an agent that has previously been effective.

rhabdosarcoma. A sarcoma containing striated muscle fibers.

rhinorrhea. A profuse mucous discharge from the nose.

rubefacient. 1. A reddening of the skin. 2. A substance that causes reddening of the skin.

saccharin. An artificial sweetener that is much sweeter than sugar; may be used in cases of diabetes mellitus or obesity, or when the use of sugar is contraindicated.

sarcoma. A malignant growth of connective tissue, bones, cartilige, and tendons.
  reticulum cell s. A malignant lymphoma in which the cells are derived from the reticuloendothelium, or tissue having both reticular and endothelial properties.

schizophrenia. A chronic state of mental deterioration to the point that it is impossible to distinguish reality from fantasy. May be accompanied by hallucinations and delusions.

sedative. A drug that quiets or allays excitement.

seminoma. A tumor of the testes.

shock. A sudden vital depression of the entire body—may be caused by emotion or injury.

solute. A substance dissolved in a liquid.

solution. A liquid that contains a dissolved substance.

solvent. A liquid in which other substances have been dissolved.

specific. A drug that cures a specific disease or condition.

spirits. An alcoholic solution that contains a volatile substance.

sprue. A chronic debilitating disease involving the gastrointestinal system in which foods, particularly fats, are imperfectly absorbed from the small intestines.

sterile. Free from living material that might cause disease.

stimulant. Anything that will temporarily increase functional activity.

stomatitis. An inflammation of the mouth mucosa.

subcutaneous. Beneath the skin.

sublingual. Beneath the tongue.

superinfection. A new infection that develops when normal bacterial flora are destroyed by an antibiotic administered for a primary infection.

suppository. A semisolid medicated substance shaped like a cone and inserted into the rectum, vagina, or urethra.

susceptible. Capable of being affected.

sympatholytic drug. Adrenergic blocking drug that destroys or inhibits impulses from the sympathetic nervous system.

sympathomimetic drug. Adrenergic drug that produces effects similar to those caused by stimulation of the sympathetic nervous system.

syndrome. The constant grouping of a set of symptoms to the point that it constitutes an identifiable pattern.

synergize. To harmonize, such as two drugs that produce an effect that neither alone could produce.

synthetic. Prepared or produced artificially.

syrup. A concentrated, aqueous solution of sugar usually containing a medicine.

tablet. A small disk of compressed medicated powder.

therapy. Treatment of disease.

thiazide diuretics. Synthetic compounds that tend to increase the excretion of sodium and chloride. Benzothiadiazides.

tic douloureux. Trigeminal neuralgia. A painful disorder of the fifth cranial nerve.

tincture. A diluted alcoholic solution of a drug. The standard concentration of powerful drugs is 10%.

tolerance. Power of resistance. Ability to take a drug without any harm; *see also* drug tolerance.

tonic. A medicine given to increase the strength of the patient generally.

topical. Local or regional.

toxic. Poisonous.

toxicology. The study of the poisonous or toxic effects produced by overdosage.

toxoid. An immunizing agent composed of toxins of specific microorganisms that have been altered to make them harmless; administered to provide active acquired immunity.

tranquilizer. A drug that acts to reduce mental tension or anxiety.

troche. A small, dry medicated disk, usually intended to be dissolved in the mouth; also referred to as a lozenge.

tumor. An abnormal growth of cells. May be benign or malignant.

urogram. Films of any part of the urinary tract.

urticaria. An allergic reaction manifested by the sudden appearance of smooth, slightly elevated whitish patches on the skin.

vaccine. An immunizing agent composed of weakened or dead bacteria, rickettsiae, or viruses; administered to provide active acquired immunity.

vasoconstrictor. A drug that causes the blood vessels to constrict.

vasodilator. A drug that causes the blood vessels to dilate.

venogram or *phlebogram.* 1. Films of a vein after the injection of a suitable opaque substance. 2. A tracing of the venous pulse.

vitamin. One of a group of organic substances necessary for normal nutrition.

volatile. Evaporates or vaporizes easily.

wheal. A localized area of edema on the skin surface, often causing severe itching. May be artificially produced or a manifestation of urticaria.

Wilms' tumor. A tumor (sarcoma) of the kidneys usually occurring in infants or small children.

SUGGESTED READINGS

BOOKS

ABRAMS, ANNE C.: *Clinical Drug Therapy: Rationale for Nursing Practice.* Lippincott, Philadelphia, 1983.

AMERICAN HOSPITAL FORMULARY SERVICE, McEvoy, G. (ed.): *Drug Information* 85. American Society of Hospital Pharmacists, Bethesda, MD, 1985.

ATKINSON, L. D., and MURRAY, M. E.: *Fundamentals of Nursing: A Nursing Process Approach.* Macmillan, New York, 1985.

DORLAND'S ILLUSTRATED MEDICAL DICTIONARY. Saunders, Philadelphia, 1981.

EISENHAUER, L. A., AND GERALD, M. C.: *The Nurse's 1984-85 Guide to Drug Therapy: Drug Profiles for Patient Care.* Prentice-Hall, Englewood Cliffs, NJ, 1984.

GILMAN, A. G., AND GOODMAN, L. S.: *Goodman and Gilman's The Pharmacological Basis of Therapeutics* (7th ed). Macmillan, New York, 1985.

GOVONI, L. E., and HAYES, J. E.: *Drugs and Nursing Implications* (5th ed.). Appleton-Century-Crofts, East Norwalk, CT, 1985.

LUCKMAN, J. and SORENSON, K. C.: *Medical-Surgical Nursing: A Pathophysiologic Approach.* Saunders, Philadelphia, 1980.

MASON, M. A., and BATES, G. F.: *Basic Medical-Surgical Nursing.* Macmillan, New York, 1984.

MASON, M. A., BATES, G. F., and SMOLA, B. K.: *Workbook in Basic Medical-Surgical Nursing* (3rd ed.). Macmillan, New York, 1984.

MILLER, M. A., and LEAVELL, L.: *Kimber-Gray-Stackpole's Anatomy and Physiology* (17th ed.). Macmillan, New York, 1977.

ROBINSON, C. H.: *Basic Nutrition and Diet Therapy* (4th ed.). Macmillan, New York, 1980.

TIETZ, N. W.: *Clinical Guide to Laboratory Tests.* Saunders, Philadelphia, 1983.

PERIODICALS

American Journal of Nursing. American Journal of Nursing Co., New York.

Journal of Practical Nursing. National Association for Practical Nurse Education and Service, St. Louis, MO.

Nurses' Drug Alert. Michael J. Powers Co., Millburn, NJ. (Also appears as a regular feature in *American Journal of Nursing.*)

Nursing Clinics of North America. Saunders, Philadelphia.

Nursing 86. Springhouse Corp., Springhouse, PA.

Nursing 86 Drug Handbook. Springhouse Corp., Springhouse, PA.

Nursing Photobook Series. Giving Medications. Intermed Communications, Springhouse, PA.

Nursing Photobook Series. Managing IV Therapy. Intermed Communications, Springhouse, PA.

ANSWERS TO ODD-NUMBERED CASE STUDIES, EXERCISES, AND PROBLEMS

CHAPTER 1

Case Study 1

1. Drugs prescribed for Mrs. Jones include: ampicillin (IV), guaifenesin (Robitussin) (PO), and normal saline by inhalation.
2. Ampicillin is prescribed to treat disease by killing microorganisms that are causing it. Guaifenesin (Robitussin) is prescribed to relieve the symptom of cough by promoting the expectoration of mucus. Normal saline is also prescribed to promote the expectoration of mucus and thus relieve cough and congestion.
3. Roles of the nurse related to drug therapy for Mrs. Jone include:
   a. Patient's assistant; administers drug therapy because of education that has built the knowledge and skill to do so, education that the patient does not possess; offers frequent fluids to Mrs. Jones because she is probably too weak to do this alone.
   b. Health team member: collects, labels, and sends a sputum specimen prior to beginning drug therapy; administers drug therapy prescribed by the physician; observes, records, reports the patient's response to drug therapy by taking vital signs, recording characteristics of the patient's sputum, observing and recording patient's appearance.
   c. Activity coordinator: coordinates patient's trip to x-ray examination so that it does not interfere with medication and intermittent positive-pressure breathing (IPPB) therapy; coordinates collecting the patient's sputum before beginning drug therapy.
   d. Patient teacher: teaches the patient and or family what to report in the way of potential side effects of drug therapy.
4. Major laws afecting drug therapy for Mrs. Jones include licensure laws that permit the physician to prescribe drug therapy, the pharmacist to prepare and dispense the prescribed drugs, and the nurse to administer drug therapy. In addition, food and drug acts are federal laws that provide standards for purity and effectiveness for each of the drugs prescribed for Mrs. Jones.
5. Health team members that participate in drug therapy for Mrs. Jones include:

    a. Dietitian: provides the fluids according to the physician's order. Additional fluids help the body to eliminate end products of microorganisms killed by the antibiotic (ampicillin). Additional fluids also help to liquefy respiratory secretions and thus help expectorants (guaifenesin and normal saline) to be more effective.

    b. Laboratory technologist: examines the sputum culture to identify organisms. Prepares a report that identifies specific organisms present in the sputum and specific drug known to be effective for each organism identified. Drug therapy may be adjusted on the basis of this report.

    c. Licensed practical/vocational nurse: collects the sputum before starting drug therapy; prepares the equipment needed to begin intravenous administration; explains drug therapy to the patient; administers drugs according to the physician's order and hospital policy; records the administration of drug therapy; observes, records, reports the patient's response to drug therapy; teaches the patient to report side effects.

    d. Pharmacist: prepares and dispenses drug therapy prescribed by the physician; maintains a drug profile according to local custom; reports the potential for drug interactions and similar problems to the physician and/or nurse; acts as a resource person for other members of the health team.

    e. Physician: prescribes drug therapy according to Mrs. Jones's condition; evaluates Mrs. Jones's medical response to therapy.

    f. Respiratory therapist: administers and records normal saline by inhalation (IPPB) according to the physician's prescription. Evaluates the patient's response to therapy.

  6. Trends in drug therapy that affect nursing practices for Mrs. Jones may include some or all of the following:

- The nurse may have to look up one or more of the drugs prescribed in order to maintain a current base of knowledge and skill.
- The nurse needs to be especially alert to the potential for drug interaction since Mrs. Jones is receiving combination therapy.
- The nurse should know what foods and fluids should be included or avoided in order for Mrs. Jones to obtain maximum benefit from drug therapy.
- Mrs. Jones's drug therapy is likely to be dispensed in a unit dose system. Although dosage calculation may not be needed, the nurse will still need to pay close attention to reading labels, identifying the patient correctly, and recording accurately and completely.
- The nurse will need to monitor Mrs. Jones's IV administration site carefully and calculate the IV flow rate accurately.
- A drug profile may be kept for Mrs. Jones. Changes in the profile may be reported by the pharmacist to the nurse.
- Mrs. Jones's hospital stay is likely to be short. She may need to continue drug therapy at home. The nurse needs to consider early patient teaching, written instructions, and possible referral if necessary.
- In collecting a drug history, the nurse needs to obtain information about other drugs the patient may be taking including nonprescribed drugs purchased over-the-counter, substances that may be used for recreation (to get high), and prescribed drugs taken prior to hospitalization.

CHAPTER 3

Case Study 3

1. Using a head-to-toe method and the guide provided in the case study, the nursing observations in the case study include:

    a. Neck and chest: Lungs sounded congested. Respiratory rate was 32 beats/min and shallow. Apical rate was 110.

    b. Extremities: Both feet were edematous.

    c. Skin: The color was grayish. The skin was moist and cool.

2. Digoxin works directly on the heart muscle to help it contract more strongly and effectively.

3. a. Wash the hands before preparing the dose.

    b. Pour the drug from its container to the patient's cup without touching it with your fingers.

    c. Assist the patient to swallow the dose by tipping the cup into the mouth. Do not touch the medication with your hands.

    d. Wash the hands after the dose has been administered.

4. Read all directions of the package before opening it. Ask for a demonstration of the supplies from the charge nurse, in-service instructor, or your clinical instructor. Determine how to make a correct charge for the supplies.

5. These drugs should be stored in a locked container according to hospital policy (either alphabetically, in individual patient compartments or in a similar orderly manner). These drugs should be stored apart from external drugs since they are taken internally.

CHAPTER 4

Answers to Arithmetic Pretest

1. b	**11.** a	**21.** e	**31.** c	**41.** a
3. e	**13.** a	**23.** a	**33.** b	**43.** c
5. a	**15.** d	**25.** a	**35.** c	**45.** d
7. c	**17.** d	**27.** e	**37.** e	**47.** d
9. d	**19.** d	**29.** e	**39.** a	**49.** a

CHAPTER 5

Exercises

1. 104°F.
3. 98.6°F.
5. 96.8°F.
7. 36.6°C.
9. 37.8°C.

CHAPTER 6

Metric Quiz

1. 0.5 L = 500 ml
3. 5,000 m = 5 km
5. 0.25 L = 250 ml
7. 100 mg = 0.1 g
9. 250 mg = 0.25 g
11. 2 mg = 0.002 g
13. 500 mg = 0.5 g
15. 2.5 L = 2,500 ml
17. 125 ml = 0.125 L
19. 1.5 g = 1,500 mg
21. 1,000 mm = 1 m
23. 0.0025 g = 2.5 mg
25. 2,500 g = 2.5 kg
27. 2,000 ml = 2 L
29. 3.5 g = 0.0035kg

CHAPTER 7

Apothecaries' System Quiz

1. 4 ft = 48 in.
3. ʒ $\overline{ss}$ = ʒ iv
5. ʒ vi = ʒ XLVIII
7. gr XLV = ʒ ¾
9. gr CXX = ʒ ii
11. 72 in. = 2 yd
13. ʒ xxxii = 2 pt
15. 3 yd = 9 ft
17. ʒ iv = ʒ xxxii
19. gr. CLXXX = ʒ iii

21. 0.25 mi = 1,320 ft
23. ʒ iii = 180 m
25. ʒ s̄s̄ = gr. CCXL
27. 18 in. = ¹/₂ yd
29. ʒ viii = ʒ i

CHAPTER 8

Converting from One System to Another

1. gr xxx = 2 g
3. 80 lb = 36.5 kg
5. gr i = 60 mg
7. 2,000 mg = gr xxx
9. 60 cm = 24 in.
11. 60 m = 4 ml
13. gr viis̄s̄ = 0.5 g
15. gr i = 0.06 g
17. 10 ml = ʒ iis̄s̄
19. 500 mg = gr viis̄s̄
21. 150 lb = 68.2 kg
23. 15 ml = ʒ s̄s̄
25. gr XLV = 3,000 mg
27. 25 in. = 62.5 cm
29. 176 lb = 80 kg

CHAPTER 9

Conversion Exercises

Converting Household Measures

1. 2 glassfuls = 16 oz
3. 8 tsp = 4 dessertspoonfuls
5. 6 tbsp = 3 oz

Converting to Household Equivalents

1. 30 ml = 2 tbsp
3. 120 ml = 8 tbsp
5. 15 ml = 1 tbsp

CHAPTER 9

Measurements Quiz

1. a	**11.** a	**21.** c	**31.** b	**41.** a
3. d	**13.** b	**23.** e (300 mg)	**33.** d	**43.** b
5. b	**15.** b	**25.** c	**35.** e (64 ml)	**45.** a
7. d	**17.** e (36.7°C)	**27.** d	**37.** a	**47.** c
9. c	**19.** e (gr is̄s̄)	**29.** c	**39.** e (104°F)	**49.** a

CHAPTER 10

Dosage Calculation Problems

1. $\dfrac{0.125 \text{ mg}}{0.25 \text{ mg}} \times 1 = x$

$x = $ ¹/₂ tablet

3. $\dfrac{2.5 \text{ mg}}{5 \text{ mg}} \times 1 = x$

$\qquad x = 0.5$ tablet ($\frac{1}{2}$ tablet)

5. $\dfrac{0.1 \text{ mg}}{0.05 \text{ mg}} \times 1 = x$

$\qquad x = 2$ tablets

Dosage Calculation Quiz

1. $\dfrac{20,000 \text{ U}}{100,000 \text{ U}} \times 5 = x$

$\qquad x = 1$ ml

3. $\dfrac{50,000 \text{ U}}{150,000 \text{ U}} \times 1 = x$

$\qquad x = 0.3$ ml

5. $\dfrac{10 \ \mu g}{30 \ \mu g} \times 1 = x$

$\qquad x = 0.3$ ml

7. $\dfrac{25 \text{ mg}}{100 \text{ mg}} \times 1 = x$

$\qquad x = 0.25$ ml

9. $\dfrac{15 \text{ mg}}{10 \text{ mg}} \times 1 = x$

$\qquad x = 1.5$ ml

11. $\text{gr } x = \dfrac{650 \text{ mg}}{325 \text{ mg}} \times 1 = x$

$\qquad x = 2$ tablets

13. $\dfrac{20 \text{ mEq}}{5 \text{ mEq}} \times 1 = x$

$\qquad x = 4$ ml

15. through 24. Answers to these questions will vary according to the amount of diluent the student elects to add. The key factor in calculating the correct dose is the concentration of the resulting solution after the diluent has been added. The concentration or strength becomes the dose on hand in the dosage calculation formula.

CHAPTER 11

Exercises

	U100		U40	
Milliliters	**Minims***		**Milliliters**	**Minims***
1. 0.5	7.5, 8			
3. 0.6	9, 9.6			
5. 0.55	8.25, 8.8			
7. 0.75	11.3, 12			
9. 0.3	4.5, 4.8		0.75	11.3, 12

*Two answers in minims are provided. The first answer is correct if the student uses 15 m as the conversion. The second answer is correct if the student uses 16 m as the conversion. Where possible, the student should select the conversion factor that provides a whole number.

CHAPTER 12

Exercises

1. Young's rule; 0.2 g.
3. Fried's rule; 4 mg.
5. Clark's rule; gr iii.

CHAPTER 15

Drug Administration Quiz

1. a
3. **a.** The right patient.
   b. The right drug.
   c. The right dose.
   d. The right route.
   e. The right time.
5. **a.** Call the physician if the written order is unclear.
   b. Call the pharmacy for further information about a drug.
   c. Consult a reference book for additional information about a drug.
7. **a.** Compare the medicine card or profile to the name on the patient's identification bracelet.
   b. Ask the patient to give his or her name.
9. c
11. a, d
13. b
15. c
17. b
19. d
21. a, b, c, d
23. a, b
25. a, b, c
27. **a.** Children or adults in the sitting, standing, or lying position.
   b. Place two fingers just below the acromion process and the other hand around the upper arm at the point of the axillary fold.
   c. Injection sites lies in a small rectangle of the lateral surface between the landmarks.
   d. 90°.
   e. Cannot be used for repeated injections or amounts greater than 1 ml.
29. **a.** Adults who are not malnourished and children over the age of 3 years should be placed in the prone position with the toes pointed inward and the entire buttock exposed.
   b. An imaginary line is drawn horizontally across the exposed buttock at the top of the gluteal fold. Another imaginary line is drawn vertically from the top of the iliac crest to the bottom of the buttock. An alternate method is to draw an imaginary diagonal line from the greater trochanter of the femur up to the posterior superior iliac spine of the hip.
   c. The injection sites lie in the upper outer quadrant or above and outside the diagonal line.
   d. 90°.
   e. Not recommended for children under 3 years and malnourished adults. Gluteal arteries and sciatic nerves in the area, therefore site selection must be done carefully. The site must be fully exposed to identify landmarks.
31. **a.** Children and adults may be in the sitting, standing, or lying position.
   b. The fleshy portion of the arm, abdomen, thighs, or buttocks.
   c. Injections sites lie in the SC tissue that you pick up between your thumb and index finger.
   d. 45°.
   e. Do not massage or aspirate when injecting heparin sodium or insulin into the sc tissue.
33. **a.** Adults and children should be placed in the prone position with the toes pointed inward.
   b. The entire buttock is exposed and the dorsogluteal (gluteus medius) site is located in the same manner as answer 29 above.

   c. See answer 29 above.

   d. See answer 29 above.

   e. Change the needle after drawing medication into the syringe. Add 2 to 3 minims of air to the syringe. Retract the skin of the dorsogluteal area laterally and tautly with the heel of your free hand before locating the injection site and hold it in this way during the entire injection. Wait 10 s after injecting before removing the needle. Do not massage the injection site. Use alternate buttocks for subsequent injections.

35. a. Report the error as soon as it is discovered to the charge nurse.

   b. Notify the physician if it has not already been done.

   c. Observe the patient carefully for an adverse drug reaction. Consult the pharmacist or reference books if necessary to get additional information about a possible reaction.

   d. Carry out any precautionary measures ordered by the physician.

   e. Chart the error and what was done.

   f. Fill out an incident report as required by the hospital.

CHAPTER 16

Case Study 5

 1. Meperidine should be underlined twice.

 2. Narcotic analgesia depresses the central nervous system by binding to special receptors on all membranes of neurons in the brain.

 3. Mr. Najita is experiencing acute pain.

 4. The student's list of nursing actions should include:

   a. Assess Mr. Najita for duration and location of pain, respiratory rate, elapsed time since last dosage, and extent of relief.

   b. Use safety measures that prevent accidents and injury (raise siderails, place call bell and other needed items close at hand, remove smoking materials, caution the patient not to get up without assistance).

   c. Check the drug history to see if there is a possibility for drug interactions.

   d. Check with Mr. Najita about allergy.

   e. Monitor blood pressure and respiratory rate; report hypotension and respiratory rate below 12 breaths/min before administering narcotic analgesia.

   f. Monitor IV flow rate carefully to prevent dehydration and retained secretions in the tracheobronchial tree.

 5. The student's list of nursing actions should include:

   a. Use a combination of pain relieving methods.

   b. Medicate Mr. Najita early before the pain becomes severe.

   c. Convey a confident, caring attitude when administering the injection.

   d. Rotate injection sites to encourage complete absorption.

   e. Check back in 30 to 40 min to see if pain relief has been effective for Mr. Najita.

 6. The nurse's response should begin with another assessment of Mr. Najita's pain. A second feature of the response is to check with the registered nurse, surgeon, or anesthesiologist for possible adjustment of the preanesthetic medication. The patient may develop respiratory depression and/or hypotension if medicated at 6 PM for pain and medication again at 7 PM with the preanesthetic. A third feature of the nurse's response is to check to see if the operative consent has been signed, before administering the next dose of narcotic analgesia. If the operative consent has not been signed, the nurse should check with the registered nurse, head nurse, or surgeon according to hospital policy.

 7. The nurse should check to see that an operative consent has been signed before administering narcotic analgesia. In some hospitals, the patient may not provide legal consent when influenced by narcotic analgesia.

 8. a. 75 mg: x ml = 50 mg: 1 ml

   $50\,x = 75$

   $x = 1.5$ ml

   b. 0.4 mg: x ml = 0.5 mg:1 ml

   $0.5\,x = 0.4$

   $x = 0.8$ ml

   c. 50 mg: x ml = 50 mg: 1 ml

   $50x = 50$

   $x = 1$ ml

   Total volume   1.5 ml Meperidine hydrochloride

                + 0.8 ml Atropine sulfate

                <u> 1.0 ml Hydroxyzine hydrochloride</u>

                3.3 ml

9. Factors selected by the student should contain the following essential features:
   a. The total volume to be injected exceeds the maximum amount of 3 ml. Thus two injections at different sites will be needed.
   b. The narcotic analgesia is administered in one intramuscular site.
   c. Atropine and hydroxyzine hydrochloride may be mixed in the same syringe using the following calculations:
      (1) Calculate the volume of atropine sulfate to be administered: 0.8 ml.
      (2) Calculate the volume of hydroxyzine hydrochloride to be administered: 1 ml.
      (3) Add the results from steps 1 and 2 together to calculate the total volume to be injected: 1.8 ml.
      (4) After cleansing both containers, withdraw 0.8 ml of atropine sulfate.
      (5) Withdraw 1 ml of hydroxyzine hydrochloride. The total volume in the syringe should now be 1.8 ml.
   d. The medication should be injected using the Z-tract method because hydroxyzine hydrochloride is one of the ingredients.
10. Essential nursing implications to be considered during and after the general anesthesia include:
    a. Provide preoperative instruction for Mr. Najita about measures that will be used to assist recovery from anesthesia.
    b. Administer the preanesthetic medication on time.
    c. Speak slowly in low tones; call the patient by name.
    d. Follow safety rules in the operating room.
    e. Check the patient frequently during surgery for pressure areas of impaired circulation to extremities.
    f. Prevent chilling during surgery by covering body parts not in the operative field.
    g. Provide extra blankets to reduce shivering when the patient is recovering from anesthesia.
    h. Develop a postoperative plan that includes a regular sequence of postoperative coughing, turning, deep breathing, leg exercises, ambulation.
    i. Check the anesthesia record postoperatively to note the duration, type of agents used, and the patient's response.
    j. Record a urine output that falls below 30 ml/h.
    k. Monitor vital signs and record tachycardia, pulse irregularities, slowing respirations.
    l. Listen to Mr. Najita's bowel sounds; observe for abdominal distention.

CHAPTER 16

Exercise 1

Drug	Patient's Condition	Intended Effects	Adverse Responses	Nursing Implications
diazepam (Valium)	Preoperative Anxious Seizures	Relaxation Relief of anxiety Anticonvulsant	CNS: headache, vertigo, light-headedness* CVS: increased heart rate, hypotension Respiratory system: decreased respiratory rate GI system: weight gain, nausea GU system: irregularities, sexual dysfunction, withdrawal symptoms, nightmares	1. Observe and document behavior. 2. Administer larger doses at bedtime if permitted 3. Use safety measures 4. Patient must avoid stimulants, alcohol, nonprescribed drugs 5. Patient to consult MD as part of family planning 6. Use nondrug measures that convey caring 7. Encourage patient to carry drug identification
amitryptyline hydrochloride	Depressed	Relief of depression by tricyclic antidepressant	CNS: fatigue, visual disturbances CVS: arrythmias, hypotension, MI, CHF GU: urinary retention, sexual dysfunction GI system: dry mouth, constipation, weight gain	1. Observe and document patient behavior. 2. Report behavior that indicates possible suicide. 3. Develop a warm and caring relationship. 4. Check the patient's mouth to be certain oral medication has been swallowed.

Exercise 1 (*Cont.*)

Drug	Patient's Condition	Intended Effects	Adverse Responses	Nursing Implications
			skin: rash *musculoskeletal* system: joint pains, tremors *drug interactions*: many	5. Use nondrug measures. 6. Patient must avoid abrupt withdrawal, alcohol, nonprescribed drugs. 7. Check specifically for adverse responses. 8. Check specifically for drug interactions. 9. Encourage patient to carry drug identification. 10. Patient to consult MD as part of family planning. 11. Encourage a regular program of exercise and rest.

*Abbreviations: CHF, congestive heart failure; CNS, central nervous system; CVS, cardiovascular system; GI, gastrointestinal; GU, genitourinary; MI, myocardial infarction.

CHAPTER 17

Case Study 7

1. Drugs that should be underlined include: atropine, Xylocaine viscous, spinal anesthesia, bethanecol chloride (Urecholine).
2. Atropine: anticholinergic; Xylocaine viscous: topical anesthetic; spinal anesthesia: local anesthetic; bethanecol chloride (Urecholine): cholinergic.
3. Topical anesthesia to the mucous membranes of the mouth, pharynx, esophagus is produced by swallowing Xylocaine viscous. Nursing implications include:
    a. Check for allergies and obtain blood pressure and pulse before administering initial dose.
    b. If NPO order is changed, do not offer food or fluids for 45 to 60 min after administering.
    c. Observe for adverse responses such as dizziness, drowsiness, hypotension, bradycardia, increased effects if administered with meperidine for pain.
    d. Locate emergency drugs, supplies, and equipment on your nursing unit before administering a local anesthetic.
4. Spinal anesthesia may have been selected for one or more of the following reasons:
    • Does not produce nausea or vomiting if the patient has eaten before surgery
    • Does not cause hypotension and respiratory depression.
    • Recovery period is usually shorter.
    • May be safer if the patient also has cardiovascular or respiratory disease.
5. Local anesthetics used for spinal anesthesia include: dibucaine hydrochloride (Nesacaine), lidocaine hydrochloride (Xylocaine), mepivacaine hydrochloride (Carbocaine), prilocaine hydrochloride (Citanest), procaine hydrochloride (Novocain), tetracaine hydrochloride (Pontocaine). A record of the specific agent used for Mr. Jones may be located on the anesthesia record and in the postoperative note.
6. Mr. Jones has been placed on bedrest in a flat position to prevent post–spinal anesthesia headache.
7. Nursing implications associated with spinal anesthesia for Mr. Jones include:
    • Monitor vital signs frequently during recovery period.
    • Maintain IV fluid intake as ordered to prevent dehydration. Record output also.
    • Observe for return of movement and sensation from the waist down.
    • Palpate the bladder frequently to detect urinary retention.
    • Protect anesthetized parts from injury.
8. The physician has ordered bethanecol chloride (Urecholine) to relax the urinary sphincter and promote voiding.

9. Nursing actions before bethanechol chloride (Urecholine) is administered should include:
   - Maintain IV fluid intake as ordered.
   - Palpate Mr. Jones's bladder frequently to detect urinary retention.
   - Administer analgesic as needed so that pain does not interfere with voiding.
   - Provide privacy for Mr. Jones.
   - Assist Mr. Jones in standing up to void.
   - Run water to encourage voiding.
10. Place a measured amount of warm water in the urinal and encourage Mr. Jones to urinate in the warm water.

Matching Exercise

1. A
2. D
3. E
4. F
5. I
6. B
7. H
8. J
9. G
10. C

CHAPTER 18

Case Study 9

1. Thrombophlebitis means you have clot in the vein of your leg and it is causing inflammation along that vein.
2. Initial observations of the affected leg might include: swelling, warmth, tenderness, positive Homan's sign (pain in the back of the knee on the affected leg when the foot is dorsiflexed). Mrs. Cronin may also have fever and tachycardia.
3. The intended effect of heparin is to prevent the thrombus from enlarging and extending.
4. Observations that would indicate an adverse response to heparin include hypersensitive responses such as chills, fever; urticaria; hemorrhage or bleeding, especially from the gastrointestinal tract, vagina (Mrs. Cronin is postpartum), or urinary system; thrombocytopenia (a reduction in circulating thrombocytes).
5. The partial thromboplastin time (PPT) will be measured to monitor the patient's response to heparin. A therapeutic range lies between 15 and 120 s.
6. The prothrombin time (PT) will be measured to monitor the patient's responses to warfarin sodium. A therapeutic range lies between 15 and 30 s.
7. The following guidelines should be used to administer heparin by the subcutaneous route:
   a. Select a tuberculin syringe (1 ml) and a very small-gauge short needle (e.g., no. 26, ½ in.).
   b. After the correct dose has been measured, aspirate 0.1 ml air into the syringe and position it at the plunger end.
   c. Select an injection site on the abdomen or in the iliac area away from muscle and other deeper tissue. Rotate sites.
   d. Grasp 2.5 to 5 cm (1 to 2 in.) of subcutaneous tissue between the thumb and fingers of one hand.
   e. Inject the needle at a 90° angle (perpendicular) to the skin.
   f. After the heparin dose has been injected, clear the needle with the 0.1 ml of air in the syringe.
   g. Apply firm pressure over the injection site for 1 to 2 min.
   h. Drugs may be injected directly into segments of varicose veins. The drugs, called *sclerosing agents*, produce imflammation, scarring, and occlusion of diseased veins. This, in turn, moves venous blood into deeper veins.
   i. Protamine sulfate.
   j. Phytonadione (vitamin K).

Case Study 11

1. Digoxin is intended to improve myocardial contraction for Mr. Scarlotti.
2. *Digitalis toxicity* is a potentially fatal adverse response that results from accumulation of too much drug.

Toxicity may produce fatal cardiac arrhythmias. Statements in the case study that should indicate increased risk for digitalis toxicity include: age 82 (the very young and very old are more likely to develop toxicity), serum Na, K stat (low serum potassium is associated with toxicity).

3. Questions for Mr. Scarlotti should contain the following essential elements:
   a. Have you had any nausea or vomiting since you started taking this medication?
   b. Have there been changes in your appetite?
   c. Have you noticed any of these symptoms: drowsiness and fatigue, headache, muscle weakness, pain numbness or tingling on your face, blurred vision, borders or halos around objects, any other vision changes?

4. The dose should be held while the registered nurse and/or physician is notified. In some cases, the physician may order the dose to be administered. In other cases, the dose may be omitted.

5. Digitalizing dose.

6. Maintenance dose.

7. An effective dose would result in increased urine output, decreased weight, improvement of dyspnea, better skin color, decreased pulse rate, reduction of edema if present.

Exercises

1. The student's list should contain the following essential instructions:
   a. These are nitroglycerin tablets. Your doctor has prescribed them to relieve your chest pain. They work very fast to temporarily widen the blood vessels in your heart.
   b. At the first sign of chest pain, you should stop all activity and place 1 nitroglycerin tablet under your tongue.
   c. If the first tablet does not relieve the pain, you may take another one in 5 minutes.
   d. Please call me if the second tablet does not relieve your pain in 3 to 5 minutes.
   e. Sometimes these tablets cause headache, dizziness, light-headedness. Please let me know if that happens to you. I'll want to check your blood pressure at that time.
   f. Whenever you take a tablet, please mark the time down. I'm leaving 10 tablets in this bottle. If they run low, let me know.
   g. Keep the tablets away from light and out of reach of visitors and others.

3. The effects of antiarrhythmic drugs on the four characteristics of the heart are summarized in the table below.

Name of Drug	Contractility	Automaticity	Rhythmicity	Conductivity
atropine	No effect	Increases	No effect	Increases
bretylium tosylate	Increases	Decreases	Increases	Decreases
disopyramide phosphate	No effect	Decreases	No effect	Decreases
lidocaine hydrochloride	No effect	Decreases	No effect	No effect
phenytoin	No effect	Decreases	No effect	Increases
procainamide	No effect	Decreases	No effect	Decreases
propranolol	No effect	Decreases	No effect	Decreases
quinidine sulfate	No effect	Decreases	No effect	Decreases
verapamil	No effect	Decreases	No effect	Decreases

CHAPTER 19

Exercise 1

1. Ammonium chloride acts on the urine causing it to become more acid.
2. Thiazide diuretics act on the kidney tubules to increase the excretion of sodium, chloride, and water. This effect causes diuresis.
3. Clomiphene citrate acts on the ovaries to stimulate ovulation and promote fertility and conception.
4. Clotrimazole acts in the vagina to kill or inhibit the growth of yeasts causing vaginitis.
5. Nitrofuradantin acts in the bladder to inhibit the growth of bacteria causing cystitis.
6. Ovulen acts on the ovaries to inhibit ovulation and prevent pregnancy.
7. Oxytocin injections act on the uterus to stimulate uterine contractions.
8. Testosterone is a male hormone that acts on male and female reproductive organs, skin, hair, oil glands, and muscles to regulate the development of sexual characteristics.

Case Study 13

1. Additional information from Mrs. Lopez that the student will need includes: usual voiding practices, usual types and amounts of daily fluid intake, drug allergies, previous infections of the urinary tract and vagina.
2. The physician will probably order a clean catch urine for culture and sensitivities to identify the specific organisms causing the urinary tract infection. In addition, the physician will probably do a pelvic examination and vaginal smear to identify organisms causing vaginitis.
3. Specific teaching associated with methanamine mandelate includes:
   * Take 2 tablets of this medication four times each day at the same time every day until the entire supply is used up. The best way to do it is to take two tablets with each meal and two more at bedtime. This will add up to four times per day.
   * Drink 3 to 4 qt of fluids each day while you are taking this drug. When the urine is acid, the drug works better so drink about 1 qt of cranberry juice per day as part of your total fluid intake. Coffee, tea, and colas irritate the bladder so avoid these or drink decaffeinated beverages.
   * Urinate when you first notice the sensation; do not delay voiding after you feel the urge.
   * Dry the perineal area from front to back after urinating, defecating, and bathing.
   * Be sure to return for another urine culture as the doctor has instructed. The only way to know for certain that the infection is gone is to examine the urine to make sure there are no more bacteria in it.
4. Additional patient teaching that Mrs. Lopez will need includes:
   * Insert the tablet high into the vagina with the applicator every night.
   * Continue using the vaginal tablets for the entire 7 days even if the drainage stops or your menses begins.
   * Call the doctor if symptoms worsen or you develop blistering, burning, stinging, or swelling.
   * Wear a light pad to protect your clothing from staining by the medication.
   * Avoid nonprescribed vaginal douches and sprays, constricting clothing and nylon underwear, wet bathing suits; get plenty of rest and a balanced diet.
   * Ask your sexual partner to wear a condom for sexual intercourse during drug therapy.
5. Nursing implications associated with the use of oral contraceptives include:
   * Check Mrs. Lopez's blood pressure because oral contraceptives are linked to an increased incidence of hypertension.
   * Observe Mrs. Lopez's skin for rashes, chloasma.
   * Ask Mrs. Lopez if she has experienced nausea, vomiting, weight gain, breast tenderness, visual disturbances, vaginal bleeding; report positive findings to the registered nurse or physician.
   * Ask Mrs. Lopez if she smokes and encourage her to stop if necessary because the risk of cardiovascular disease is greatly increased in women who smoke and use oral contraceptives.
   * Teach Mrs. Lopez how to look for thrombosis or thrombophlebitis (pain, tenderness, swelling, erythema, especially in the calf or inner aspect of the thigh) and to report symptoms immediately because the incidence of this condition is greatly increased in women who use oral contraceptives.
6. The student's response should contain the following features:
   * That is a good question to ask.
   * Did she tell the physician about the oral contraceptives?
   * An offer to check with the physician or registered nurse to get the question answered.
7. The student's explanation should contain the following features:
   * Certain diseases that a person in the hospital might have may make him or her more susceptible to urinary tract infections.
   * Pregnancy makes a person more susceptible to urinary tract infection.
   * Catheters may be inserted into the bladder during surgery or certain tests done on the urinary tract may make a person more susceptible to urinary tract infection.

CHAPTER 20

Exercise: Multiple-Choice Questions

1. c
3. b
5. c
7. d
9. d

CHAPTER 21

Case Study 15

1. Cimetidine suppresses the secretion of gastric acid by blocking the effects of histamine. Oral suspension antacids neutralize gastric acids that have already been secreted.
2. Adverse responses that may devlop in Mr. Grayner include: headache, confusion, slurred speech, constipation or diarrhea, gynecomastia, diminished sexual interest and performance, malaise, myalgia, skin rash, fever, drug interactions. The patient taking an oral suspension antacid may develop constipation (aluminum hydroxide) or diarrhea (magnesium hydroxide), kidney stones, rising levels of aluminum, calcium, or magnesium depending upon the specific preparation. Patients taking either kind of antacid may experience interference with other drug absorption, rebound hypersecretion.
3. Nursing implications associated with Mr. Grayner's drug therapy include:
   • Assist in the nursing assessment; report sodium restriction, liver or kidney disease that may affect Mr. Grayner's response to drug therapy.
   • Prevent drug interactions by administering cimetidine at least 1 h before or 2 h after other drugs.
   • Assess, report, and record characteristics of Mr. Grayner's pain, if present, and bowel movements.
   • Instruct Mr. Grayner to report changes in sexual interest and performance to the physician.
   • Instruct Mr. Grayner not to stop taking the drug abruptly.
   • Instruct Mr. Grayner to avoid substances that increase gastric irritation: coffee, tea, cola, alcohol, cigarettes.

CHAPTER 21

Exercise 1

1. The two major categories are antidiarrheals and laxatives.
2. Patient symptoms for each category include:
   a. Antidiarrheals: increased number of stools; loose, semiliquid, or watery stools; abdominal cramps; nausea, vomiting, or weakness; increased frequency.
   b. Laxatives: a reduction in the number of stools, a reduction in the frequency of bowel movements, increased hardness of stools.
3. Two sample patient conditions for each category:
   a. Antidiarrheals: ulcerative colitis, infection, systemic disease.
   b. Laxatives: hemorrhoids, lack of exercise, insufficient dietary fiber and/or fluid intake; a habit of ignoring the urge to defecate.
4. Major adverse responses for each category:
   a. Antidiarrheals.
      (1) Adsorbents and protectives may interfere with absorption of other drugs.
      (2) Opiate derivatives have potential for abuse.
      (3) Preparations with atropine may cause dry mouth, rash, dizziness, and urinary retention.
      (4) Opiate derivatives produce many drug interactions.
   b. Laxatives.
      (1) Allergic reactions.
      (2) Interference with absorption of other drugs.
      (3) Laxative abuse syndrome.
      (4) Fluid and electrolyte imbalance.
      (5) Nausea, cramping, diarrhea, abdominal distress.
5. Five major nursing implications for each category of drugs:
   a. Antidiarrheals.
      (1) Measure and record characteristics of every stool.
      (2) Record and report related symptoms such as nausea, vomiting, abdominal pain, weakness, sudden onset of abdominal distention.
      (3) Anticipate the patient's need for rapid and easy access to the bathroom or bedpan; provide additional toilet paper.
      (4) Use safety measures to prevent slips and falls from hurried trips to the bathroom.
      (5) Cleanse and dry the skin thoroughly and gently after each bowel movement.
      (6) Monitor daily weight, fluid and food intake.

b. Laxatives.
   (1) Gather and record information during the nursing assessment about the patient's usual pattern of elimination.
   (2) Seek additional information before administering a laxative to a patient with abdominal pain, colic, nausea, or vomiting.
   (3) Use safety measures to prevent slips and falls from hurried trips to the bathroom.
   (4) Encourage an increase of dietary fiber, fluids, exercise.
   (5) Teach the patient to establish and maintain a regular time for bowel movements.

CHAPTER 22

Exercise 1

	Thyroid drugs	Antithyroid drugs
Patient's condition	Hypothyroidism	Hyperthyroidism
Actions and uses	To restore normal blood levels of circulating thyroid hormones	To decrease thyroid function by inhibiting manufacture of thyroid hormones, damaging the gland, or suppressing pituitary hormones that stimulate thyroid gland
Adverse responses	Angina, tachycardia, arrythmias, palpitations, symptoms of hyperthyroidism	Skin rashes and purpura; anemias, joint pain and stiffness, paresthesias, headache, nausea, drug fever, hepatitis, nephritis, iodine anaphylaxis, allergy or intoxication
Nursing implications	Assist with nursing history; administer oral preparations on an empty stomach; monitor laboratory studies; report pulse of more than 100 beats/min, changes in rhythm or regularity; instruct the patient not to change drugs	Assist with nursing history; administer oral preparations with or after meals; monitor laboratory studies; report adverse responses

CHAPTER 23

Exercise 1: Examples of Answers and Organization of Information About Antihistamines and Immunosuppressives

Descriptive Categories	Antihistamines	Immunosuppressives
Effects on allergy/ immune response	Antagonizes the effects of histamine that occur during an hypersensitive response	Suppress the natural immune response
Patient's condition	Allergic conjunctivitis, allergic rhinitis, hay fever, dermatitis, drug allergy	Preoperative or postoperative organ transplantation, autoimmune disease, neoplastic disease
Actions and uses	Prevent or relieve allergic symptoms	Prevent or relieve organ transplant rejection; kill cancer cells

Descriptive Categories	Antihistamines	Immunosuppressives
Adverse responses	Sedation, lassitude, anorexia, nausea, vomiting, dryness of mouth, throat, urinary retention, drug interactions	Increased susceptibility to infection and tumor formation, genetic damage, destruction of normal cells
Nursing implications	Report and record information about allergies; administer oral drugs with meals to prevent gastrointestinal symptoms; know where emergency drugs are located; use safety measures that prevent accidents from sedative effects	Report fever and other signs of infection; observe for bleeding in gums, skin, urine, stools, vagina; report and record jaundice and crystals in the urine.

CHAPTER 24

Case Study 17

1. Information that should be underlined and associated rationale includes:
   - Benign prostatic hypertrophy: produces urinary retention and stasis that is associated with a high potential for urinary tract infection.
   - Transurethral resection of the prostate: involves the introduction of surgical instruments into the urinary tract to remove the prostate gland and provides a route for pathogens to enter the body.
   - General anesthesia: temporarily paralyzes normal respiratory defenses against pathogens in the respiratory tract and increases the potential for respiratory infection.
   - Temperature, pulse respiration (TPR): the temperature elevation, tachycardia are signs of possible infection.
   - Foley catheter: provides a route of entry for pathogens; increases the potential for urinary tract infection.
   - Malaise, myalgia: these are common symptoms of infection.
2. Additional information is needed about Mr. Mason's respiratory status: Are the lung sounds clear? Is there a cough?
3. The following diagnostic tests can be anticipated: chest x-ray film, urine culture and sensitivities, sputum culture (if the lung sounds are not clear or Mr. Mason has a cough).
4. Sample explanations for Mr. Mason include:
   - Chest x-ray examination: an x-ray film of your lungs to try to locate the cause of your fever and other discomfort.
   - Urine culture and sensitivities: a laboratory test that tells whether or not the urine is infected and what specific germs are causing the infection; if germs are present, part of the test involves identifying which drugs are best able to kill them.
   - Sputum culture and sensitivities: same as urine but the test is done on mucus that you cough up from the deepest part of your lungs.
5. Actions and uses of gentamicin include: an aminoglycoside that kills or inhibits the growth of gram-negative aerobic bacteria such a Pseudomonas, Proteus, *Staphylococcus aureus*; used primarily for the patient with urinary tract infection, respiratory infection, infected burns, peritonitis, meningitis.
6. A sample explanation of blood tests ordered for Mr. Mason is: the doctor has ordered blood tests every 3 days while you are on this drug in order to keep track of its effects on your kidneys.

7. **Major Adverse Responses**	**Sample Nursing Actions for Detection or Prevention***
Ototoxicity	Ask the patient about tinnitus, disturbances of hearing or equilibrium before each dose; report positive findings before administering a dose
Nephrotoxicity	Monitor available laboratory reports to anticipate clinical responses; encourage fluid intake of 3–4 L/day if permitted by the physician
Acute muscular paralysis and apnea	Administer intravenous doses over 30–60 min as prevention; know where emergency drugs and equipment are located; conduct more frequent observations in patients at risk
Resistance	Maintain the dose schedule exactly as ordered; rotate injection sites to encourage complete absorption; do not mix with other drugs in the same syringe

Major Adverse Responses	Sample Nursing Actions for Detection or Prevention*
	Use nondrug measures that prevent the spread of infection, enhance the patient's recovery from infection, and prevent nosocomial infection in hospitalized patients*

*Encourage students to specify what nursing actions prevent the spread of infection, enhance the patient's recovery from infection, and prevent nosocomial infections in hospitalized patients.

8. Amikacin, kanamycin, netilmicin, streptomycin, tobramycin

Exercise 1: Sentence Completion Exercise

1. Antimicrobial agents are drugs that kill or inhibit the growth of bacteria, fungi, and viruses.
2. The physician usually orders a culture and sensitivity test before the first dose of antibiotic because the selection of a specific drug depends on its ability to kill or inhibit the growth of the specific pathogen causing infection.
3. Three nursing actions related to the collection of specimens for culture and sensitivities include:
   a. Collect the specimen before starting the first dose of an antimicrobial agent.
   b. Avoid contaminating the specimen with other organisms during the collection procedure.
   c. Label the specimen correctly and send it to the microbiology laboratory immediately.
4. Three specific nursing implications related to the administration of cephalosporins for infection include:
   a. Report penicillin allergy before administering the first dose, and anticipate a possible change of drug.
   b. Administer oral preparations with full glass of water on an empty stomach to encourage complete absorption.
   c. Caution the patient not to drink alcohol while taking a cephalosporin to prevent a drug–alcohol interaction.
5. Three nursing implications that enhance the effects of tetracyclines in a patient with infection include:
   a. Administer oral preparations on an empty stomach if possible to encourage complete absorption.
   b. Do not administer with milk, cheese, iron supplements, antacids that may interfere with complete absorption.
   c. Adminster IV preparations slowly according to the manufacturer's directions; do not adminster with other drugs at the same time.

CHAPTER 25

Case Study 19

1. Antineoplastic agents that should be underlined in the case study include mechlorethamine, vincristine, and procarbazine.
2. The hormone that should be circled is prednisone.
3.

Drug	Effect on Malignant Cells	Effect on Normal Cells
mechlorethamine	Kills malignant cells by preventing cell reproduction and growth	Has same effect on normal cells, especially those of bone marrow, hair, skin, and mucous membranes, nervous system, urinary system
vincristine (Oncovin)	Kills malignant cells by preventing cell reproduction and growth at a different stage of cell life than above	Has same effect on normal especially those of the bone marrow, nervous system, gastrointestinal system, skin, hair, and mucous membranes
prednisone	Suppresses inflammatory response and reduces symptoms both of disease and those produced during chemotherapy	May cause toxic effects in every body system
procarbazine	Kills malignant cells by preventing cell reproduction and growth; is also linked to the development of new malignant cells	Same as drugs above

4. Major Adverse Response	Nursing Action for Detection or Prevention
Infection	Inspect the mouth daily for oral lesions.
	Wash hands carefully before and after caring for Miss Toma.
Nausea, vomiting, other gastrointestinal symptoms	Administer prescribed antiemetics before chemotherapy is administered
	Monitor intake and output
Bleeding	Inspect body openings, body discharges, mucous membranes and skin daily for signs of bleeding
	Use safety measures to prevent accidents and injuries

5. Five nursing actions to increase Miss Toma's comfort and well-being could include:
   a. Encourage Miss Toma to eat a balanced diet and drink sufficient fluids. Request help from the dietitian if necessary.
   b. Assist the patient with scrupulous oral and personal hygiene.
   c. Suggest wearing scarves, wigs, or hats to Miss Toma for alopecia.
   d. Provide emotional support for Miss Toma through active listening, identifying and praising strengths.
   e. Offer backrubs and similar comforting measures regularly.
   f. Report Miss Toma's questions and concerns to the registered nurse or physician.

CHAPTER 27

Problems

1. Drugs may be applied to the skin or mucous membranes of the eyes, ears, mouth, vagina, rectum.
3. Elase is a topical enzyme that may be used for debridement of wounds, burns, and ulcers because it digests protein.
5. Adverse responses to methoxsalen for the patient with vitiligo include: burns, blisters, pruritus, nausea, vomiting, higher rates of skin cancer.
7. Before inserting an enema tip into the patient's rectum you would lubricate it with petrolatum.
9. Lindane is a drug used for the person with head and body lice.
11. Pilocarpine is a miotic drug that may be used to constrict pupils and reduce intraocular pressure in patients with glaucoma.
13. Povidone-iodide is an antiseptic commonly used as a preoperative scrub. (Other answers may be acceptable depending on local custom.)
15. Haloprogin may be applied as a spray by the person with a fungal infection of the skin.
17. Homatropine is a mydriatic drug that may be used to dilate the pupils during examination of the eye.
19. Vitiligo is a progressive loss of skin pigment that causes patchy areas of pink or white skin.

CHAPTER 28

Exercise 1

1. D
2. S
3. S
4. D, S
5. D, S
6. D
7. D
8. D
9. D
10. D

CHAPTER 29

Roman Numerals (pp. 351–352)

1. a. $8 = VIII$
   c. $26 = XXVI$
   e. $61 = LXI$
   g. $81 = LXXXI$
   i. $250 = CCL$

Arabic Numerals (p. 351)

2. a. $VI = 6$
   c. $XXXIX = 39$
   e. $LXXV = 75$
   g. $LXV = 65$
   i. $MD = 1,500$

CHAPTER 30

Identification of Fractions and Mixed Numbers (pp. 353–354)

	a	b	c
1.	Whole number	Improper fraction	Mixed number
3.	Simple fraction	Complex fraction	Mixed number
5.	Simple fraction	Improper fraction	Simple fraction

Changing Fractions to Lower Terms (p. 354)

	a	b	c
1.	$100/150 = 2/3$	$2/8 = 1/4$	$16/20 = 4/5$
3.	$5/10 = 1/2$	$2/6 = 1/3$	$50/100 = 1/2$
5.	$6/18 = 1/3$	$10/15 = 2/3$	$10/25 = 2/3$

Changing Improper Fractions to Mixed or Whole Numbers (p. 355)

	a	b	c
1.	$4/2 = 2$	$9/7 = 1\,2/7$	$15/10 = 1\,1/2$
3.	$90/75 = 1\,1/5$	$12/6 = 2$	$9/6 = 1\,1/2$
5.	$21/19 = 1\,2/19$	$200/100 = 2$	$14/12 = 1\,1/6$

Changing Mixed Numbers to Improper Fractions (p. 355)

	a	b	c
1.	$15\,1/2 = 31/2$	$3\,1/2 = 7/2$	$2\,3/8 = 19/8$
3.	$9\,2/7 = 65/7$	$6\,1/3 = 19/3$	$10\,1/2 = 21/2$
5.	$2\,3/4 = 11/4$	$5\,1/5 = 26/5$	$7\,2/5 = 37/5$

Multiplying Whole Numbers and Fractions (pp. 355–356)

	a	b	c
1.	$7 \times 1/2 = 3\,1/2$	$15 \times 2/3 = 10$	$4 \times 1/2 = 2$
3.	$8 \times 3/8 = 3$	$24 \times 5/8 = 15$	$4 \times 3/8 = 1\,1/2$
5.	$9 \times 1/4 = 2\,1/4$	$21 \times 1/3 = 7$	$18 \times 1/6 = 3$

Multiplying Two Fractions (p. 356)

	a	b	c
1.	$5/6 \times 1/3 = 5/18$	$3/5 \times 2/3 = 2/5$	$7/8 \times 2/5 = 7/20$
3.	$4/5 \times 3/5 = 12/25$	$5/8 \times 1/2 = 5/16$	$2/3 \times 1/6 = 1/9$
5.	$10/11 \times 1/3 = 10/33$	$11/12 \times 4/5 = 11/15$	$9/10 \times 3/4 = 27/40$

Multiplying Mixed Numbers (pp. 356–357)

	a	b	c
1.	$4 2/3 \times 4 1/8 = 19 1/4$	$3 3/5 \times 2 1/2 = 9$	$3 \times 3 3/8 = 10 1/8$
3.	$6 \times 6 1/3 = 38$	$2 2/3 \times 3 3/5 = 9 3/5$	$7 1/8 \times 4 1/4 = 30 9/32$
5.	$5 \times 4 1/4 = 21 1/4$	$2 \times 1 1/2 = 3$	$10 1/2 \times 3 1/4 = 34 1/8$

Dividing Fractions and Mixed Numbers (pp. 357–358)

	a	b	c
1.	$1 1/3 \div 1/2 = 2 2/3$	$6 \div 1/3 = 18$	$6 1/2 \div 2 = 3 1/4$
3.	$3/4 \div 1/2 = 1 1/2$	$7 1/2 \div 5 1/5 = 1 23/52$	$8 \div 1/4 = 32$
5.	$10 \div 1 1/2 = 6 2/3$	$3 \div 1/3 = 9$	$2/3 \div 3/4 = 8/9$

CHAPTER 31

Explanation of Decimals (p. 359)

1. $0.5 =$ five-tenths
3. $10.01 =$ ten and one-hundredth
5. $1.5 =$ one and five-tenths
7. $1.3 =$ one and three-tenths
9. $0.005 =$ five-thousandths

Dividing Decimals (p. 360)

	a	b	c
1.	$52.5 \div 5.2 = 10.10$	$40.5 \div 5.5 = 7.36$	$8.5 \div 2.5 = 3.4$
3.	$25.25 \div 2.25 = 11.22$	$14.5 \div 2.5 = 5.8$	$12.2 \div 2.1 = 5.81$
5.	$10.5 \div 5.5 = 1.91$	$5.125 \div 2.5 = 2.05$	$82.5 \div 0.02 = 4.125$

Multiplying Decimals and Whole Numbers (p. 361)

	a	b	c
1.	$40.1 \times 4.01 = 160.801$	$2.55 \times 20.5 = 52.275$	$3.33 \times 2.02 = 6.7266$
3.	$5.25 \times 3.5 = 18.375$	$140 \times 2.5 = 350.0$	$4.25 \times 50 = 212.50$
5.	$23.5 \times 8.3 = 195.05$	$85.05 \times 3.05 = 259.4025$	$7.05 \times 7.5 = 52.875$

Changing Decimals to Fractions (pp. 361–362)

	a	b	c
1.	$0.35 = 7/20$	$0.3 = 3/10$	$0.04 = 1/25$
3.	$0.1 = 1/10$	$0.55 = 11/20$	$0.75 = 3/4$
5.	$0.01 = 1/100$	$0.8 = 4/5$	$0.07 = 7/100$

Changing Fractions to Decimals (p. 362)

a	b	c
1. $1/8 = 0.125$	$1/4 = 0.25$	$1/6 = 0.17$
3. $7/8 = 0.875$	$5/6 = 0.83$	$3/4 = 0.75$
5. $1/5 = 0.2$	$5/7 = 0.71$	$2/5 = 0.4$

CHAPTER 32

Changing Percents to Fractions (p. 364)

a	b	c
1. $50\% = 1/2$	$25 1/5 \% = 63/250$	$1/5 \% = 1/500$
3. $6\% = 3/50$	$1/8 \% = 1/800$	$3 1/2 \% = 7/200$
5. $4/5 \% = 1/125$	$12 1/2 \% = 1/8$	$30\% = 3/10$

Changing Fractions to Percents (p. 365)

a	b	c
1. $1/6 = 16.67\%$	$1/20 = 5\%$	$1/10 = 10\%$
3. $3/5 = 60\%$	$1/8 = 12 1/2 \%$	$1/4 = 25\%$
5. $1/100 = 1\%$	$1/50 = 2\%$	$1/25 = 4\%$

Changing Percents to Decimals (p. 365)

a	b	c
1. $5\% = 0.05$	$2\% = 0.02$	$1/4 \% = 0.0025$
3. $3/4 \% = 0.0075$	$50\% = 0.5$	$40\% = 0.4$
5. $2 1/2 \% = 0.025$	$6\% = 0.06$	$6 1/5 \% = 0.062$

Changing Decimals to Percents (p. 366)

a	b	c
1. $0.1 = 10\%$	$0.01 = 1\%$	$0.05 = 5\%$
3. $0.25 = 25\%$	$0.125 = 12.5\%$ *or* $12 1/2 \%$	$3.5 = 350\%$
5. $7.5 = 750\%$	$0.75 = 75\%$	$0.4 = 40\%$

CHAPTER 33

Fractions Written as Ratios (pp. 367–368)

a	b	c
1. $1/8 = 1:8$	$2/3 = 2:5$	$3/5 = 3:5$
3. $1/4 = 1:4$	$1/100 = 1:100$	$1/1,000 = 1:1,000$
5. $1/10 = 1:10$	$1/50 = 1:50$	$1/75 = 1:75$

Changing Ratios to Percents and to Decimals (pp. 367–368)

	a	b
Ratio	Percent	Decimal
1. 1:3	$33 1/3 \%$	0.33
3. 1:1,000	$1/10 \%$	0.001
5. 1:150	$2/3 \%$	0.0067
7. 1:4	25%	0.25
9. 1:2,000	$1/20 \%$	0.0005

Changing Percents to Ratios (p. 368)

a	b	c
1. $10\% = 1:10$	$80\% = 4:5$	$40\% = 2:5$
3. $\frac{1}{2}\% = 1:200$	$\frac{1}{4}\% = 1:400$	$1\% = 1:100$
5. $2\% = 1:50$	$60\% = 3:5$	$25\% = 1:4$

Changing Decimals to Ratios (p. 368)

a	b	c
1. $0.2 = 1:5$	$0.05 = 1:20$	$0.001 = 1:1,000$
3. $0.025 = 1:40$	$0.075 = 3:40$	$0.1 = 1:10$
5. $0.4 = 2:5$	$0.6 = 3:5$	$0.0001 = 1:10,000$

ARITHMETIC POSTTEST (ODD-NUMBERED PROBLEMS)

1. d	**11.** a	**21.** a	**31.** b	**41.** e ($\frac{1}{16}$)
3. b	**13.** a	**23.** d	**33.** d	**43.** l
5. c	**15.** a	**25.** b	**35.** b	**45.** c
7. c	**17.** a	**27.** b	**37.** a	**47.** b
9. d	**19.** e (61)	**29.** b	**39.** a	**49.** c

Index

5th Ed.

BATES - FITCH - LARSON - MOONEY
BASIC DRUG THERAPY &
Arithmetic Review